THE
ROYAL INFIRMARY
OF EDINBURGH

❦ · ❦ · ❦

1929—1979

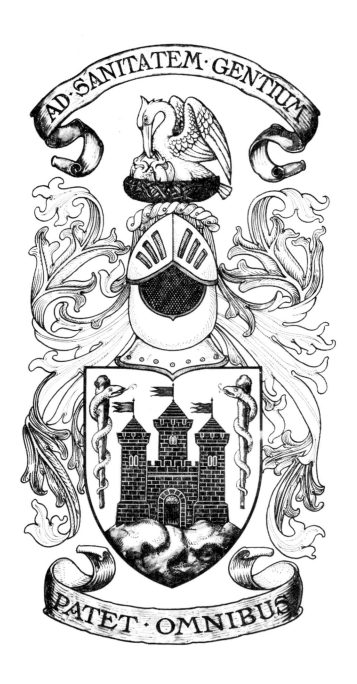

Coat of Arms granted to the Managers of the Royal
Infirmary of Edinburgh in 1914

THE
ROYAL INFIRMARY
OF EDINBURGH

❦ · ❦ · ❦

1929—1979

E. F. CATFORD

1984

SCOTTISH ACADEMIC PRESS
EDINBURGH

Published by
Scottish Academic Press Ltd,
33 Montgomery Street
Edinburgh EH7 5JX

SBN 7073 0279 x

Design, typography, lay-outs by T. L. Jenkins, Edinburgh

Printed and bound in Edinburgh, Scotland
by Clark Constable   Edinburgh   London   Melbourne

Contents

❧ · ❧ · ❧

Illustrations

Foreword

BY THE HON. LORD ROSS

It may seem surprising to some that a judge should write the Foreword to this book, but lawyers have had a long association with the Infirmary. In 1727, before the first hospital was built, a Voluntary Bond was entered into by certain subscribers, who were respectively three advocates and two writers to the signet. Moreover, the Managers in 1730 included one of the Senators of the College of Justice, one of the Faculty of Advocates, and one of the Society of Writers to the Signet: and four of the six representatives of the contributors were respectively the Lord President of the Court of Session, the Lord Justice Clerk, the Lord Advocate and the Solicitor-General. As the author has pointed out in Chapter I, the effect of the arrangements made for the Board of Managers in 1870 was that there should always be at least four lawyers and four medical men on the Board. Even after the introduction of the National Health Service, and before the reorganisation of 1974, there was usually at least one member of the legal profession on the Board of Management, and I had the honour to be the last representative of that profession on the Board when it was dissolved in 1974. These then are my credentials for writing this Foreword.

Dr. Logan Turner's book, covering the first two hundred years, is, of course, a classic, and those wishing to study the history of the Royal Infirmary of Edinburgh, must turn to that work first. But much has happened since the Bicentenary in 1929, and all who are interested in the Royal Infirmary must be grateful to Mr. Catford for bringing the history of this great institution up to date.

In this work, Mr. Catford has described the Royal Infirmary during the half century ending in 1979. He has dealt with the administration and fund-raising so necessary in the days when the Infirmary was a voluntary hospital. By citing from the contemporary records, he has succeeded in capturing some of the flavour of the period about which he is writing. Although all this is in the past, the dedication and faith of the men who administered the voluntary hospital is worth recording along with the similar devotion and loyalty of the medical staff who in these days gave their services without payment. It is of interest too to read of how the Infirmary fared in the upheaval of the years of the Second World War.

At a time like the present, when there is widespread discussion about the National Health Service and about its future, it is enlightening to read the author's account of the introduction of the National Health Service, and of the changes which ensued after the new administration took over. All this is not merely part of the history of the Infirmary, it is part of the social history of our country.

In the fourth chapter, Mr. Catford gives an account of the planning towards the new Infirmary. In this he has been kinder to all concerned than others might have been in view of the twenty years which elapsed between the meeting in June 1955 to consider the plan for rebuilding and the placing of the main contract for the building of Phase I in 1975. One cannot help remarking that if decisions had been taken sooner, a new hospital might by now have been in existence, and the history of the Royal Infirmary would have been somewhat different. However, this is no fault of the historian!

In subsequent chapters, the author traces in considerable detail the various developments in the Infirmary during the Sixties and Seventies. He deals with the new buildings, with the different departments and with the leading personnel involved. He also has something to say about the reorganisation of 1974, as to the merits of which I content myself with saying that opinions may well differ!

The seventh chapter faithfully records various changes in Medicine during the fifty years being reviewed, and these have, of course, been numerous and far reaching. The point is rightly made that throughout its history the Infirmary has not merely treated patients but has also trained doctors. For the Royal Infirmary is a teaching hospital, and many doctors throughout the world must have had their first introduction to clinical medicine at the Royal Infirmary. Many nurses too have received their early or subsequent training in the Infirmary. In the final chapter, after referring to the work of the archivists, the author describes the celebrations which attended the anniversaries of 1979.

The book also contains two Appendices compiled by Mr. Donald McIntosh, who has played an important part in the preparation of this book. Mr. Catford, I am sure, would have found the writing of this book much more difficult without the help of someone like Donald McIntosh whose knowledge of and affection for the Royal Infirmary are well-known. Appendix II with the names of medical and surgical officers is of special interest, and will be very useful for reference purposes.

But a great hospital is more than just an institution about which facts can be assembled and statistics quoted. A hospital at once inspires both apprehension and affection in the hearts of its patients, it has an atmosphere and an ethos of its own which is quickly communicated to all who resort there, and no one who has ever entered the doors of the Royal Infirmary can have left without being aware of the general spirit of kindness and caring which pervades the hospital at all levels.

Within Edinburgh and the surrounding country, there cannot be many families who have not had occasion to be grateful to the Royal Infirmary at some time throughout the past five decades. The Royal Infirmary is very much "Edinburgh's Hospital", and the citizens of Edinburgh and the inhabitants of its environs have every reason to take pride in their hospital. But they also have a great respect for the Infirmary. In some other cities and towns with Royal Infirmaries, the hospital has become known by its initials. Thus in Dundee, the Dundee Royal Infirmary was usually referred to as the "D.R.I.". In Edinburgh, on the other hand, the Infirmary is invariably referred to as "The Royal".

But most of all, it is appropriate that the author has recorded, sometimes by name and sometimes not, the men and women who have devoted their lives to the maintenance of the hospital over these five decades. To the surgeons and physicians, the nursing staff, the paramedical staff, the administrators, the domestic staff, the maintenance staff, the porters and to all who have worked there, society owes a debt of gratitude. All such persons have contributed to the Infirmary, and have helped to make it the great institution which it is, and **Mr.** Catford has done them and all of us a great service in writing this history. The Infirmary itself, in whichever form it continues, is a monument to all who have served there, but this book too will serve as their well merited memorial. This literary work deserves to be read by all who are interested in the Royal Infirmary, and I wish the book and its author well.

November 1983   DONALD M. ROSS

Acknowledgements

I would like first to express my gratitude to The Hon. Lord Ross who, in the midst of his busy life and great responsibilities as a Senator of the College of Justice, has yet found time to contribute the Foreword to this book.

When I was invited to write a 'sequel' to Dr. A. Logan Turner's *Story of a Great Hospital* which had brought the history of the Royal Infirmary of Edinburgh up to 1929 I felt some trepidation for the task was clearly going to be a formidable one. It has proved also to be a fascinating one, thanks largely to the help I received from many sources.

I am grateful to the Lothian Health Board who gave me access to minutes and reports of the authorities successively responsible for the administration of the Royal Infirmary since 1929. At the outset I had the privilege of meeting a number of physicians, surgeons and others who, having retired after long and distinguished careers in the Infirmary, kindly recounted recollections of life there in the 1930s, bringing that period vividly alive. More than a score of Heads of Departments provided memoranda summarising more recent events in their own fields, often supplemented by interviews; and I gained much by talking with members of staff at many levels. I began to list all those who had helped in these and other ways but when the list, still incomplete, had reached 100 names it became clear that they could not be thanked individually. I hope, therefore, that all will understand that omission does not indicate lack of appreciation.

There are two, however, whose help cannot be allowed to go unrecorded. First, the late Mrs Patricia Eaves-Walton, Archivist to the Infirmary and the Lothian Health Board. She gave cheerfully of her time and professional knowledge to guide me through the labyrinth of documents under her charge. Her death in 1981 meant a severe loss to everyone concerned with research into Edinburgh's medical history.

Next must come Mr. Donald McIntosh, F.R.C.S.E. who was Senior Consultant Surgeon to the Royal Infirmary until his retiral in 1976. From his lifetime experience as surgeon, as Board of Management member and as Chairman of the South Lothian District Surgical Division and the Lothian Health Board's Area Medical Committee he distilled a wealth of advice for my benefit. He kindly read the manuscript at several stages, guiding me safely past many pitfalls and rescuing me from others. He provided the tabular statement in Appendix I and compiled the lists of senior staff which form Appendix II.

For all that co-operation I am indeed grateful. Mistakes that remain are my own, as also are opinions not otherwise attributed.

Among those not directly connected with the Infirmary who also helped were Librarians whose readiness to do so was, as always, invaluable: Miss J. P. S. Ferguson at the Royal College of Physicians of Edinburgh, Miss Dorothy Wardle at the Royal College of Surgeons of Edinburgh and the staffs of the University of Edinburgh Main and Medical Libraries, the Central City Library and the Library of the Scottish Health Services Centre, Edinburgh. My thanks, too, are due to my wife who typed the first draft of the manuscript and provided helpful comments and criticisms.

I would also like to thank: Professor J. P. Duguid C.B.E., of the Bacteriology Department, Dundee University, who provided information about the early use of penicillin in Edinburgh; Mr. James A. Ross, M.B.E. for allowing me to use excerpts from his book *The Edinburgh School of Surgery after Lister*; the Royal College of Physicians of Edinburgh for permitting me to quote from a 1957 Report on Scottish Teaching Hospitals; and the Editors of *The Scotsman* and *The Edinburgh Evening News* for giving permission to quote from those papers and from the former *Edinburgh Evening Dispatch*.

Finally, I am grateful to those who provided photographs, or permitted the use of copyright photographs, as shown in the following list.

E. F. C.

	Plate Nos.
Editors of:—	
Edinburgh Evening News	7, 35, 36
Nursing Mirror	15
Scotsman	3, 4, 19, 20, 22, 32
Scottish Daily Record	18
Scottish Field	13, 31
Professor Emeritus Ronald H. Girdwood, P.R.C.P.E.	10
Picker International Ltd., London	5
Dr. A. E. Ritchie, C.B.E., F.R.S.E.	9
Robb and Campbell Harper, Ltd., Edinburgh	25
Royal Infirmary of Edinburgh Archives	1, 11, 12, 14, 16, 17, 21, 23, 26, 27, 34
University of Edinburgh-Medical Illustration Department	6, 8, 24, 28, 30, 33 and frontispiece
University of Edinburgh Obstetrics Department	29

(Plate No. 2 is from a photograph by the Author.)

Introduction

The Bicentenary of the Royal Infirmary of Edinburgh was celebrated in 1929. A few years later Dr. A. Logan Turner's book *Story of a Great Hospital* appeared in commemoration of that event. His book tells of the growth of the Infirmary from its earliest days as the 'little house' at the head of Robertson's Close into a world famous teaching hospital with 1,000 beds, the largest voluntary hospital in the country. His book ends with the words:

> What of the future! It would be idle, perhaps unprofitable in 1929, the bicentenary year, to predict what the future may have in store for the Royal Infirmary of Edinburgh. Recent legislation has made it competent for County and Town Councils to submit schemes for the reorganisation of hospital facilities and to provide treatment for sick persons within their area; and to take reasonable steps to secure full co-operation with every voluntary hospital, university or medical school within or serving the area of the Council. It is possible that a new system of hospital administration may profoundly affect the status of the Royal Infirmary in the years to come. Perchance the cross roads have been reached and, in the misty haze of uncertainty, it is difficult to discern along which route, indicated by the signposts, the voluntary hospital will travel in order to fulfil its destiny.

Clearly, the coming of the municipal hospitals in the wake of the Local Government (Scotland) Act of 1929 and the discussions which were then taking place in many quarters about the growing need for co-ordination of hospital services had made it clear to Dr. Logan Turner, as to many others, that changes lay ahead. But it is unlikely that he foresaw the Royal Infirmary moving from its position as a voluntary hospital administered by an independent Board of Managers in virtual isolation from other hospitals, to become a state-owned hospital, holding a key place in a network of hospitals in south-east Scotland with a total of some 13,000 beds. Nor could he have foreseen the immense advances in medical knowledge and in medical and associated techniques that would so greatly affect the story of the Infirmary in the years ahead.

Much, indeed, has changed in the half-century since 1929. It is the aim of this book to chronicle the changes and to show how the Infirmary, under varying forms of management, has sought to keep pace with complex developments in medical knowledge and practice. If, for the moment, we leave out of account the all-important contributions of Sir James Y. Simpson in the 1840s and those of Lord Lister in the 1870s it can reasonably be accepted that in the medical and hospital fields, there have been more and greater advances during the last fifty years than in the whole of the previous two hundred. In the achievement of many of these, the Infirmary has played its part.

At the bi-centenary service in Edinburgh's High Kirk of St. Giles in November

1929, The Very Reverend Charles L. Warr, Dean of the Thistle and Chapel Royal, prophesied great changes when he said: 'A greater future lies before the Infirmary; the enterprise of wider expansion is at hand which, in due time, will be brought to full fruition by the proud and generous impulse of the citizens.' No doubt he had in mind the proposals for expansion then being formed for which a special appeal for voluntary contributions was shortly to be launched and which, ten years later, culminated in the opening of the Simpson Memorial Maternity Pavilion and the Florence Nightingale Nurses Home. But his words might also be applied to the coming, after nearly twenty years, of the National Health Service and the great advances in the Infirmary and in other hospitals which that made possible.

Though much has changed in the Royal Infirmary scene, much has remained the same. For one thing, David Bryce's Scottish baronial buildings, reminiscent of Holyrood Palace, still stand overlooking Lauriston Place and the Meadows as they have stood since 1879, though with the open spaces between their many wings now almost wholly built upon. Despite dreams and much sustained effort in planning, during the 1960s, when it was confidently believed that within a decade the old buildings would be replaced upon their own site by a fully equipped modern hospital, its lay-out and design directed to the needs of the 1980s and beyond, the old familiar buildings are still there. All, or almost all are now likely to remain for a good many years housing, as effectively as adaptation and ingenious improvisation can achieve, the latest scientific devices and equipment to support the skills of the hospital physicians, surgeons, nurses and other staff. The replacement of those old buildings has become a slower process than was then thought.

There is another sense in which things have not changed. Nowadays 'the Royal' is an integral part of a broad complex of hospitals. Nevertheless, to many of those who live in Edinburgh and a wide surrounding area, it continues to be in a special sense *their* hospital to which they still feel a special attachment. This is not surprising. For generations, in times of sickness and accident, they and their families have found help in its wards and clinics, full of faith in the skill of the Infirmary's physicians and surgeons to cure them, in the efficiency of its nurses and in the desire of the whole hospital community to contribute to their comfort while in hospital and to their speedy return to the world outside.

Among the changes that have taken place has been the growth in numbers of that hospital community—physicians, surgeons, nurses, members of the paramedical professions, technicians, caterers, porters, cleaners and others. In 1929 the medical and surgical staff, including clinical tutors and residents was rather more than 100. The corresponding figure for 1979 was nearly 500 and, if all groups of staff are counted, the totals are—for 1929, about 1,100 and for 1979 just over 4,000.

For this growth in numbers there are many reasons. First, although the number of beds in the general hospital has not increased (in 1929 it was 1,100; in 1979, excluding the Simpson Memorial Maternity Pavilion, it was about 1,000) their use has greatly intensified because patients spend less time in hospital. In 1929 the average stay in hospital was 25 days in medical wards and 14 in surgical wards. In 1979 the overall average stay in hospital was 10 days. So, while 19,600 in-patients were dealt with in 1929, there were 30,300 in 1979, involving an obvious increase in the amount of care and attention required, not only because of the larger number of patients, but also because of the more intensive and elaborate treatments many of them now receive.

The number of out-patients has also much increased. In 1929 there were 65,000 new out-patients and their attendances during the year totalled about 195,000; in 1979 the figures were 128,500 and 516,300 respectively. For all, in-patients and out-patients alike, the scientific tests and procedures now used far exceed in number and complexity those undertaken fifty years ago and they require the services of a great variety of professional and technical staff highly skilled in disciplines and processes of which many were then unknown. To add to all this there was, throughout these fifty years, a gradual and necessary reduction in weekly hours of work. Consider, as just one example of this, the nurse's lot. In 1929 her working week was one of 56 hours or possibly more; by 1979 a nurse's tours of duty were based on a working week of 40 hours (since reduced to $37\frac{1}{2}$) and while in training the nurse is given time to attend lectures to which, formerly, she was required to go in her off-duty periods.

Taking all these factors together, the growth in hospital staff is no more than the logical accompaniment of progress. Likewise, the growth in cost to the community of the vital services provided by a great hospital such as the Royal Infirmary of Edinburgh should be seen as the necessary price to be paid if we are to have available at all times to all who need them, not just the medical, surgical and nursing skills and sympathetic care that the Infirmary has always provided, but also the most modern scientific aids to diagnosis, treatment and cure, enabling full benefit to be gained from those skills and that care.

I

The Nineteen-thirties

Voluntary Hospital Days

Today, after thirty-five years of hospital provision by the National Health Service, it is easy to forget that the Royal Infirmary previously carried on its essential work and built up its world-wide reputation as a centre of healing and medical teaching while dependent entirely on two sources of voluntary support. On the one hand, the services of its physicians and surgeons were given without payment, other than limited honoraria in respect of clinical teaching. For livelihood they relied on private practice in their own consulting rooms and in nursing homes—practices which might build up only slowly over several years—and on payment by colleges or university if they also held appointments as lecturers or professors. For many of those recently qualified and holding junior posts, their service was possible only if they had some private means or a family able to tide them over. The fact that their hospital work brought a wide range of experience, enhanced expertise and a professional reputation which assisted the growth of their private practice does not diminish the value of their contribution. Without their services so freely given, the voluntary hospital system could neither have survived so long nor achieved the standard at which it eventually handed on its task, and its personnel, to the new system.

On the other hand, there was the direct financial help given by the public to the hospital. Voluntary hospitals such as the Infirmary were dependent almost entirely on legacies, donations and subscriptions, with no guarantee from one year to the next that necessary funds would be forthcoming. The Infirmary, because of its reputation, was more fortunate than some hospitals for it had been well endowed over the years though by no means always with the amount necessary to make desired extensions and improvements.

The organisation and administration of any large hospital is bound to be a complex matter involving many skills. It was, in one respect, even more complex when in addition to the organising of its services there was a constant need to seek funds so that much time and effort were taken up by the mechanics of fund-raising. In a striking if rather superficial way, this can be demonstrated simply by thumbing through the pages of any of the annual reports of the voluntary Board of Managers. For example, in the report for 1929-30 only 37 pages are devoted to describing the work of the hospital during the year while 98 pages contain closely-printed lists of the legacies, donations and subscriptions received.

As the Board of Managers of necessity placed much emphasis on the fund-raising aspect of their work; as fund-raising is obviously the beginning of any charitable effort; and as it is a good rule to begin any story at the beginning it seems reasonable to begin this history by describing the administrative organisation of the Royal Infirmary as it was during the 1930s, including its fund-raising arrangements upon which the whole of its other work depended.

In 1929, and from then until 1948, there were three main organisations each playing a part in maintaining the Royal Infirmary. Two of these had existed from its earliest days; the third was of quite recent origin. First, there was the Court of Contributors which existed loosely and informally from 1728, though it seems not to have met between 1731 and 1736. From 1736 onwards this body, in a legal sense, *was* the Infirmary because in that year it was recognised by the Royal Charter granted by George II. The Charter, in its own words, 'Erected, Created and Incorporated . . . all and every the said contributors who have already contributed to the Infirmary and all such persons as shall hereafter contribute thereto, into one body corporate and politic, by the name of the Royal Infirmary of Edinburgh.' They were to meet as the 'General Court of Contributors' in January every year.

That large and somewhat vague body was modified by the Edinburgh Royal Infirmary Act of 1870, passed primarily to authorise the acquisition of the Lauriston Place site, but also dealing with other matters. Under that Act membership of the Court of Contributors was limited to those who had contributed to the funds not less than one donation of £5 or who, having made three consecutive annual donations of £1 each, continued to do so. The same Act also redefined the powers of the Court of Contributors, making it clear that they had no executive function in the management of the hospital but might 'from time to time make any suggestions or recommendations which to them may seem proper and the Managers shall consider and, if they think proper, may adopt any such suggestions or recommendations'. The Act also authorised the Court to alter the statutory rules of the Infirmary or to make new rules provided the altered or new rules were not inconsistent with the provisions of the Royal Charter.

Clearly, no institution could have been efficiently managed by such a numerous and amorphous body. A small group of managers had, in fact, looked after the Infirmary's affairs since 1730 and the need for such a body was recognised by the Royal Charter which included provision for the appointment of twenty managers 'for better accomplishing the ends . . . and managing the affairs of the Corporation'. By the Charter the Managers were to be appointed out of certain specified 'classes' of the citizens – physicians, surgeons, lawyers and others. They were the second of the three bodies concerned with the funding and administration of the Infirmary and by far the most important.

As modified by the Act of 1870, the Board of Managers were to have a membership of 21 made up as follows:

The Lord Provost of Edinburgh (*ex officio*) and one other member of the Town Council;

Two members chosen by the Royal College of Physicians of Edinburgh and two chosen by the Royal College of Surgeons of Edinburgh;

Two members chosen by the Senatus Academicus of the University of Edinburgh;

One member each, chosen by the Edinburgh Merchant Company, the Edinburgh Chamber of Commerce and Manufactures, the Judges of the Court of Session, the Faculty of Advocates, the Society of Writers to the Signet and the Society of Solicitors in the Supreme Courts;

The Managers themselves were to choose one member from among the Ministers of the Gospel in Edinburgh; and the Court of Contributors were to choose six members among whom two were to be selected from the subscribers to the funds of Convalescent House at Corstorphine, belonging to the Infirmary, which had been built in 1867.

Appointments were made annually and the maximum number of consecutive years for which a member was permitted to serve as representative of any one organisation was five, after which he was ineligible for one year for re-election by the same organisation. He might, however, be re-elected immediately by a different organisation. It will be seen that the constitution provided for the inclusion of members of the organisations which had participated in the founding of the hospital and ensured that there would always be at least four lawyers and four medical men on the board; but serving members of the Infirmary medical and surgical staff were never included.

That group of 21 citizens had remained the pattern of the Board of Managers until 1919. By then it had been recognised that miners and other manual workers who, more than most sections of the community, were prone to illness and accident, were not only heavily dependent on the services of the Infirmary but were considerable contributors to it through various works' funds and local subscription schemes. By means of a section of a local Act of Parliament then being promoted by Edinburgh Town Council, power was obtained to increase the number of Board Members from 21 to 26 by the addition of two representatives of the Edinburgh and District Trades and Labour Council and one representative each from the Miners Association of Fife and Kinross, the Miners Association of Midlothian and East Lothian and the Coal and Shale Miners Association of West Lothian. Thus, for the first time in 190 years, a share in the management of the Infirmary's affairs was given to those groups in the community who were likely to need its services most often.

Meanwhile, in 1918, the third of the three bodies mentioned had been formed, this one concerned only with the raising of funds. It was the League of Subscribers. It adopted as its slogan 'A League of all who Labour, in the Service of all who Suffer' and, as its statement of Objects, 'The raising of systematic voluntary contributions from all classes of wage-earners, officials and employees generally within the City of Edinburgh and Provincial Districts on behalf of the funds of the Royal Infirmary and of stimulating public interest in all matters affecting the welfare of the Institution.' By 1930 the League had carried on its work to such effect that it had raised an aggregate of £235,500, an annual average of £19,600 since its foundation.

On the strength of that record it was agreed that the League should be invited to be represented on the Board. So, again by means of a Section in an Act of

Parliament promoted by Edinburgh Town Council, power was obtained for the election to the Board of two League members. Thus the number on the Board became 28 at which it remained until the coming of the National Health Service in 1948.

Strangely, despite the rather elaborate form of the Board's statutory constitution, no provision was included for the appointment of a regular Chairman. The practice was that the Lord Provost of the day as a member *ex officio* would take the chair whenever he was able to be present. In his absence, the senior member among those appointed as hospital visitors for the month would preside. This arrangement was little designed to encourage continuity of interest or leadership unless the Lord Provost was one who happened to have a special interest in the well-being of the hospital; and even then his ability to attend meetings regularly was liable to be limited by his many other civic duties.

One who did take a keen interest in the Infirmary was the Right Hon. (later Sir) Thomas B. Whitson, DL, LLD, Lord Provost of the City from 1929 till 1932. He recognised the disadvantage of conducting the business of the Board with no regular chairman to take a close continuing interest in its work and at a Board meeting towards the end of his first year of office, in October 1930, he proposed that in future a Chairman should be appointed annually who would also be a member of all Committees of the Board, thus providing a continuity of interest in and knowledge of the Board's affairs; but no-one to be appointed for more than three successive years.

Sir Thomas's proposal was unanimously approved and, there being no legal obstacle to its adoption, a Chairman was immediately appointed, also unanimously. The choice fell upon Harriet, Lady Findlay, DBE, who had first been appointed to the Board in 1922. She was the widow of Sir John Findlay, Bt, of Aberlour, principal proprietor of *The Scotsman* newspaper who had died in April 1930. Both she and her husband had given generous financial support to many good causes including the Royal Infirmary. Despite her wide range of interests and activities which included work for the Queen's Institute of District Nursing, the Royal National Lifeboat Institution and other social welfare groups, she served enthusiastically and acceptably as Chairman of the Infirmary Board during the following three years. She retired from the Board in 1933 but served again as a Board Member, from 1936 until 1947 as a representative of the Court of Contributors.

By 1933 Sir Thomas Whitson's term as Lord Provost and therefore as *ex officio* Board member had come to an end. He was then appointed to the Board as representing the Edinburgh Chamber of Commerce and was immediately elected to the chairmanship. This, too, was a wise and popular choice. A successful chartered accountant and one-time President of the Society of Accountants in Edinburgh, he was well qualified to guide his fellow members of the Board and their officials through many of the financial problems they were facing during the depression of the 1930s; as a Town Council member from 1916 to 1932 he had gained varied administrative experience and was able to help in preserving good relations with the Town Council at a time when some apprehension was arising about the possible effects on the Infirmary of the development of the city's three municipal general hospitals; he was a Fellow of the Royal Society of Edinburgh and a man of cultured tastes; and he had wide sympathies, tact and—not least important—abundant commonsense.

The limit of three years service having been removed, Sir Thomas continued to serve as Chairman till he found it necessary to resign from that position in 1937 though continuing as a member for one more year. During his chairmanship the new pavilion for venereal diseases and skin diseases was completed and the foundation-stone of the Simpson Memorial Maternity Pavilion was laid.

The next elected Chairman was Mr. John R. Little in 1938. He had joined the Board as a representative of the Court of Contributors in 1934. His abilities and his interest in the Infirmary's affairs had quickly been recognised and his service as Chairman proved so acceptable that he continued in that position for ten years till the Board of Managers were disbanded on the coming of the National Health Service in 1948. During his 14 years membership he had represented the Court of Contributors for nine years and the Edinburgh Chamber of Commerce for five.

Mr. Little's career had been in insurance—as General Manager of the Century Insurance Company from 1920 until 1934 and afterwards as Director of the Company. Outside his profession he had many activities having been at different times Chairman of the Chamber of Commerce, a Governor of the George Heriot Trust, President of the Edinburgh Rotary Club and worker for Boys' Clubs. Like his predecessor he was a Fellow of the Royal Society of Edinburgh.

During his long period as Chairman of the Infirmary Board, Mr. Little and his colleagues had to face several exceptional circumstances. There were the financial and organisational problems connected with the completion and opening of the Simpson Memorial Maternity Pavilion, the difficulties and responsibilities of the war-time years and the problem during the immediate post-war years of coping with shortages and financial stringency while, at the same time, seeking to ensure that in July 1948 the Infirmary would be transferred to the new hospital authority as smoothly and efficiently as possible.

At the final meeting of the Board of Managers held in June 1948 Mr. Little was congratulated by the members 'on his many achievements as Chairman of the Board of which he had been an able and successful leader', and as one who 'had maintained the administration of the Royal Infirmary at the highest standard in the interests of the patients whom it was their privilege to serve'.

So in the 212 years since their recognition by Royal Charter, the Board of Managers of the Royal Infirmary as a voluntary hospital had had a formally elected Chairman for only 18 years during which time only three persons had held that office. Happily, all three had held it with distinction.

The relationship between the Board of Managers and the Court of Contributors is not without interest. The Court met annually in January and every year they received from the Managers a report on the work of the Infirmary during the previous year. From time to time in the past, the Court had also sought to exercise some supervision. Generally, however, the proceedings at meetings of the Court were formal. The practice was for the meeting to receive the Managers' report and statement of accounts and, almost automatically, to remit them to a committee of some 15 members who would read them and report with comments or suggestions to an adjourned meeting of the Court a few weeks later. If the Court then endorsed any suggestions the Committee had made, these were conveyed to the Managers who might, or might not, act upon them. But more often than not, the Court and their Committee did little more than give formal approval to the Managers' stewardship. The standard form of words adopted for several successive years in the 1930s was that 'as has been stated in previous reports the Committee are satisfied that it would scarcely be possible for any Institution to be managed with more efficiency than prevails in the case of the Royal Infirmary'.

In 1928 a proposal was made at a meeting of the Managers that the procedure of submitting report and accounts to the Court for examination by Committee was cumbersome and really unnecessary. This view was examined both by the Managers and by their Law Committee and the conclusion was reached that the practice was 'a long-established one consistently followed since 1738' and therefore 'it was conceivable that members of the Court of Contributors might consider any change as an interference with a wholesome practice'. So the procedure hallowed by 190 years of use continued for a further 20 years, until 1948. Happily for the patients, the Infirmary's physicians and surgeons, over the years, have been less reluctant to change their procedures with changing times.

Fund Raising

As has been said, in the voluntary hospital days the need to further the business of fund-raising made constant demands on the Managers and officials of the Infirmary. One long-standing source of funds on which they relied was the Court of Contributors, that body of citizens committed to making at least one £5 donation or three of £1 thereby qualifying to attend an annual meeting and, if so disposed, to criticise the Managers' activities.

In 1931 the Board of Managers decided to revise the list of members of the Court of Contributors which then contained more than 6,000 names. Of these, 3,630 were known to be active contributors. A letter of enquiry was sent to the others as a result of which, after deducting the names of those who had died, those whose letters had been returned by the Post Office and those who replied that they did not wish to continue as members, the roll was reduced to 3,900; by 1939 it had fallen to about 2,600. Of those numbers, however, only a very small proportion ever attended the annual meetings despite several attempts to find ways of increasing interest in what tended usually to be a brief and formal occasion.

At the January meetings in 1934 and 1935 minor sensations were caused by the Chairman, Sir Thomas Whitson, when he took the opportunity of rebuking the better-off citizens of Edinburgh for their failure to give sufficient support to the Infirmary. In 1934 under the heading 'Startling Edinburgh' the *Edinburgh Evening Dispatch* reported that Sir Thomas had sought to shock the citizens by quoting figures which 'seem incredible of a city like Edinburgh'. There were in the city, he had said, only 1,340 individuals or firms who subscribed £1 or more to the Infirmary, only 554 who subscribed ten shillings and only 1,200 who subscribed five shillings. 'Sir Thomas' said the *Dispatch* 'calls those figures startling. Frankly they are disgraceful. There are many thousands who could give yearly to the Infirmary a pound or more and never miss it.' Sir Thomas himself, the lists for those years disclose, made a practice of giving £5 : 5s annually.

A year later, at the meeting of the Court of Contributors in 1935, Sir Thomas Whitson returned to the attack. This time he made quite clear which group of citizens he was criticising for he began by praising the work of the League of Subscribers through which he said, many thousands of work-people willingly contributed by allowing a weekly deduction of one penny to be taken from their wages to help the funds. Compare that, he suggested, with the half-crown annually which far too many people in better positions thought they had done well by subscribing. He went on to tell of a door-to-door collecting campaign which had recently been undertaken in his own West End area of the city and he quoted some of the excuses given for not contributing. One collector, he said, had been told by a servant at a house at which he had called that the householder 'would give in his usual way, at the church'. 'But, of course', the servant added, 'that is just a put-off; he hasn't been to church for fifteen years'.

This time *The Scotsman* commented on the Chairman's remarks, but unlike its sister-paper the *Dispatch*, it did not give unqualified support to Sir Thomas. 'His criticism of the comparatively well-to-do for lack of response' the leader writer said 'was perhaps a trifle hard . . . If the work-people show greater alacrity in responding it may be partly because they are more conscious of the value of the institution. There are few working class families in Edinburgh and district which have not had direct experience of the benefits of the Royal Infirmary. The contributions of the wealthier classes are purely altruistic and on the whole they play their part nobly.'

The writer of that leader had obviously not read his own paper's report of the speech in which Sir Thomas had already answered the point by saying that 'without the work, the teaching and the experience afforded by the Infirmary, the skill upon which, sooner or later, all would have to depend in their own homes or elsewhere would be very much less. Therefore, rich or poor, all benefited directly or indirectly from the Infirmary. He wished people would realise it.'

Of course, as *The Scotsman* writer implied, many wealthy people (and some who were not so wealthy) made large donations and bequests to the Infirmary. Not all such donations were in cash; sometimes they were made in kind. In 1934, Mrs. M. D. Bonthron of Tonbridge, Kent, presented wireless sets to the ear, nose and throat wards. So greatly were the programmes enjoyed by the patients, that before the year ended she arranged for radio programmes to be made available throughout the hospital. Thirty-seven wards were equipped with 924 plug-in points, 428 headphones and 35 loudspeakers. The main receiving set had a selector switch for either national or regional programmes, the operation of which was controlled by the Lady Superintendent of Nurses. The installation, costing over £1,200, was given in memory of the donor's parents, Mr. and Mrs. James

Bryson, Mr. Bryson having been a well-known Edinburgh optician with premises at 60A Princes Street. When Sir Thomas Whitson, as Chairman, formally accepted the equipment on behalf of the Managers, the BBC broadcast a special message to the Infirmary patients. Thus began wireless in the wards which, along with such later developments as specially relayed football commentaries, radio programmes provided by the voluntary Edinburgh Hospital Broadcasting Service, religious services relayed from the Infirmary chapel and, finally, the provision of television sets has brought pleasure to generations of patients.

That is one example of many gifts. The benefits from others will appear as this story of fifty years continues. But such special gifts alone could not have kept the hospital going and, as for all voluntary hospitals, there existed the constant need to seek day-to-day support from many sources. So we come back to the League of Subscribers which, for thirty years, was one of the regular channels of such support.

Since 1906 the Board had had on their staff an Organising Secretary for Subscriptions. He was Mr. Russell Paton who had joined the Treasurer's staff in 1892, had become the first Organising Secretary in 1906 and continued enthusiastically in that post till he retired in 1942. His job had been, by publicity, lectures to associations, the organisation of collectors and other means to encourage the practice of systematically subscribing to the funds of the Infirmary.

Not the least part of his work from the outset had been to arrange for the collection of regular donations from work-people at their places of work. By 1918 some £10,000 was coming each year from that source but that sum included £7,000 from the coal and shale mines of the Lothians and Fife and it was thought that much more than £3,000 should be obtainable from other work-places if a more comprehensive collecting system could be devised.

The idea was supported by the Edinburgh and District Trades Council and other bodies and so in September 1918 a few weeks before the end of the Great War, a public meeting had been held in the Oddfellows Hall, Forrest Road—a stone's-throw from the Infirmary—presided over by the Chairman of the Trades Council, Mr. Andrew Eunson who later, as a member of the Board of Managers, took an active part in the administration of the Infirmary. At that inaugural meeting a letter was read from Mr. William Adamson, MP for West Fife in which he said 'The League is certainly on the right lines. Whatever national schemes for financing hospitals may eventually mature in the reconstruction year ahead of us, the workers meanwhile cannot afford to have the extensive benefits of our great infirmaries in any way curtailed through lack of funds.' The formation of the league was then unanimously approved and at that point in the proceedings Mr. W. B. Blaikie, LLD, who was the Board of Managers' representative, declared to the meeting: 'This is the happiest moment in my 18 years' connection with the Infirmary. Hitherto, there has not been much vital interest taken in the Institution by the citizens, but I believe we are on the eve of a burst of prosperity which will save the Infirmary in the long run.' This declaration having been cordially applauded, he continued: 'Perhaps it is not fully recognised how largely the Infirmary is financed by the dead who last year, through their legacies, contributed £38,900 while the living gave only £27,000.' With those words the

League of Subscribers was launched on its way, Mr. Russell Paton becoming Organising Secretary while still continuing in his Infirmary post.

The stage had thus been set for development of the scheme whereby employees, in ever-growing numbers, in offices, factories, schools and workshops throughout Edinburgh and a wide surrounding area were enabled through arrangements made with their employers to contribute regularly to the funds a minimum of one penny weekly from their wages. A penny-a-week may seem today a modest contribution and in 1934 it was, in fact, increased to two pence. But in the 1920s £2 was regarded as a good weekly wage and many were earning less. It is against that background that the contribution must be judged.

By 1929 the League's scheme for collection through deduction from wages or by works collection had been adopted in about 1400 workplaces and the amount collected in that year was £21,500. As the average cost to the Infirmary per in-patient treated during the year was quoted as £7 : 15s the League members' donations can be seen as having met the full cost of treating nearly 2,800 of the 19,600 in-patients recorded as having been 'treated to a conclusion'. Put another way, the League's contribution was sufficient to cover roughly, one seventh of the total ordinary annual expenditure which at that time was £151,765.

Another annual source of income had been introduced in 1920. It was organised by a voluntary committee, separate from the League of Subscribers but working in close association with it. This was the Royal Infirmary Pageant and throughout the nineteen twenties and thirties the pageant was held on a Saturday in May, the Infirmary's annual 'badge day'. The event was always eagerly looked forward to in Edinburgh as a great gala occasion. It is difficult, now, to recall the atmosphere of those days. True, the *Edinburgh Evening News* in 1979 in collaboration with the Edinburgh Festival Society and the organisers of the Infirmary's 250th anniversary celebrations, arranged a somewhat similar occasion with some success. But in these more sophisticated times they could not hope to recapture quite the old sensation of universal excitement and participation. In the twenties and thirties of this century there were many families in the city who could not afford to go away on holiday and to whom even a day in the country, except on a Sunday-school 'trip' or other charitable excursion, would have been an extravagance. To such families the sight of a long procession including many gaily adorned horses making its way through crowded, enthusiastic throngs, accompanied by a variety of bands and with hundreds of collectors in fancy dress cavorting alongside, was something not to be missed. It brought with it gaiety and a sense of holiday and despite the poverty of so many who watched there were few who would not spare a penny or two in response to the collectors' demands.

To convey some idea of these occasions and at the same time to glimpse a fragment of the city's social history, here are a few extracts from a press report of the first pageant, held in May 1920:

> All day, badge-sellers and collectors, many of whom wore fancy
> costume, rattled money-boxes before passengers in the streets, in the
> parks, in the railway stations—wherever, in fact, they could gain admission.
> In the evening a pageant and procession, almost two miles in length and

in which over 5,000 people took part, paraded the main streets of the
city. . . On the 200 lorries, both horse and motor, tradesmen were to be
seen at work—laundresses ironing, hospital nurses and doctors watching
over patients . . . Tableaux, ingenious in arrangement and pretty in setting
occupied other vehicles. . .

There were the Friendly Societies with gaily-coloured banners,
representatives of the trades with their craft emblems, butchers, bakers,
brass-finishers, coopers. The tableaux presented by the Edinburgh
Domestic Servants' Association . . . displayed a laundry, a kitchen, a
nursery, the children of course included.

Here the description of the procession gave way to a brief explanation that,
although this was probably the first time that the city's domestic servants had
appeared thus in public, 'they have always been generous to the Royal Infirmary.
So far back as 1879 they raised £543 to assist in furnishing two wards and they
have been regular contributors to the funds of the Institution.' That, considering
the level of servant's wages then, was a tribute of which they might well feel
proud. In those days domestic servants seem to have enjoyed some priority in admission to the Infirmary. This was not because of the generosity of their giving
but rather because resident medical officers were often instructed by their Chiefs
to be generous in admitting servants whose employers might find difficulty in
arranging medical and nursing care for them at home.

In the following 19 years the pageants took roughly the same pattern. In the
afternoon a long line of strangely transformed vehicles interspersed with brass
bands and pipers assembled in Holyrood Park where decorations and tableaux
were judged and prizes awarded. Some of the vehicles carried elaborate scenes of
daily life or of episodes in history or romance; others had taken on the shapes
of houses, ships, castles and curious monsters. Prominent in all the pageants were
the University students' displays. One memorable contribution was provided by
Indian students in national costume accompanying a gleaming model of the Taj
Mahal on a lorry drawn by six magnificent grey horses lent for the occasion by
a city brewery.

The pageant, although the principal feature of 'badge-day', was not the only
one. Other events took place in suburban districts and beyond. On the day of
the first annual pageant the combined proceeds amounted to £4,500 and in
following years, with variations due to weather and other circumstances, the
amounts collected were usually between £5,000 and £6,000. Then, in 1939, with
war approaching, the Infirmary Pageant was held for the last time and with it, a
minor but memorable bit of Edinburgh history came to an end. With it, too, ended
a useful source of income, though a modest one in relation to the total annual
running costs, then £188,000.
The main sources of income fell into five groups:

  (1) subscriptions and donations, including payments by grateful patients,
      and from Insurance Societies (of which increasingly, patients were
      members).
  (2) regular contributions through the League of Subscribers;
  (3) legacies of large and small amounts, some immediately available for

general purposes and others directed towards capital or for specified
purposes;

(4) interest and dividends;

(5) rents and feu duties from properties throughout the country which
had been given or bequeathed to the Infirmary from time to time
the management of which formed a material part of the duties of
the Secretary and Treasurer's Office.

Then there were a few payments, mainly from public authorities, for services
rendered and also fees from medical students for their 'hospital tickets' and from
nurses in connection with their training. One means of encouraging larger bequests
and donations which had been operated since the 1880s was the arrangement
whereby a bed or cot could be endowed and named in accordance with the donor's
wishes, in memory of an individual or group. The amounts qualifying for this in
1930 were, for an adult bed £2,000 and for a child's cot £1,000. In 1930 there
were 221 named beds and cots; by 1939 there were 312, including six transferred
from the former Royal Maternity Hospital to the new Simpson Pavilion.

To illustrate what has been said about the Board's money problems it may
be helpful to quote some statements from their annual report for the year 1937–38,
that being the last normal year of the voluntary system before it was affected by
special war-time arrangements and afterwards by the approach to the National
Health Service. Under the heading 'Finance' the report says:

The financial position as a result of the year's working reveals a position
which cannot be regarded otherwise than most unsatisfactory, especially
so as, in the coming year, the Managers will be faced with considerably
greater expenditure owing to the enlarged hospital. On the ordinary
account a deficiency of £46,976 was realised . . .

The total ordinary income for the year amounted to £140,882,
an advance over the previous year of £4,119 . . . The item under the
head of Badge Day which includes the Pageant effort, shows a decrease
of £1,384. This result is due to the fact that the weather on the day of
the Pageant was exceedingly bad which had a most unfortunate effect on
the attendance.

Legacies and special donations received during the year . . . are as
follows:

General Purposes—Royal Infirmary   £51,473
Endowment Purposes—Royal Infirmary   9,346
Donations for special puposes   2,049

The increase in ordinary expenditure [to £187,859] amounted to
£10,851—a truly alarming figure . . . This result is due primarily to the
larger scope of the Infirmary's activities and to the necessity in several
instances for renewing apparatus and machinery. There has also been in
many items a great advance in the price of materials.

Bearing these statements in mind, it is interesting to look at the following
entries taken from the Board of Managers' statistical tables and accounts in their
Report for the year 1937–38 (Column A) alongside corresponding figures included
among the Lothian Health Board's statistics for the year 1978–79 (Column B):

	A From Annual Report 1937-38	B From 'Scottish Health Service Costs'—(Scottish Home and Health Department) 1978-79
Royal Infirmary of Edinburgh:—		(excluding Simpson Pavilion)
Number of patients etc.,		
Bed Complement	1,141	978
In-patients	21,883	30,269
New out-patients	75,622	128,538
Out-patient attendances	393,695	516,360
Costs:—		
Net Hospital Running Costs	£187,859*	£17,767,000
In-patients: average weekly		
cost per patient	£2. 19s. 7d (£2.97)	£358.38
average total cost		
per patient	£7. 1s. 3d (£7.06)	£493.90
Out-patients: average cost		
per patient	8s. 6d (43p)	£14.14
average cost		
per attendance	1s. 9d (9p)	£5.46

* Equivalent purchasing power in 1979: £2,350,000 (approx.) (Based on Table in 'The Scottish Economy in Figures' issued by Lloyds Bank Plc in 1982).

These two sets of figures separated by forty years and now placed side by side may be astonishing but any attempt at a detailed analysis and comparison of them would be profitless, so many different factors would have to be assessed. The change from the old voluntary hospital system to the new and the effects of inflation; the vastly increased cost of every commodity used in hospital; the steady advance from almost unaided medical and nursing care to medical and nursing care supported by an array of costly drugs, expensive sophisticated equipment and scientific processes previously unknown; changes in accounting methods—all these and other factors would have to be evaluated before a valid cost-benefit comparison could be made. It is simpler to ask the question: How many patients of the nineteen-thirties who, though given every care and attention, could not be cured or could be only partially cured would have been fully restored to health and vigour if (at the same ages and with the same symptoms) they had been patients of the nineteen-seventies? The answer must be 'many thousands'; and in that answer, and the immense public benefit and personal happiness it represents, lies the comparison that counts.

The Infirmary as it was

The period from 1930 to 1939, the first decade of the Infirmary's third century, was also the last decade of the old order of things. The six war-time years that followed and, after them, the three years leading on to the National Health Service brought into being special financial arrangements for coping with the special problems of that time. Those nine years also saw many advances in medicine and surgery and associated sciences and techniques and so much change in the economic climate of the country and in attitudes to social welfare generally that a return to the old pattern of hospital provision, even if it had been wanted, would have been impossible. A new regime in one form or another was inevitable.

It would be wrong, however, to regard the decade of the thirties in the Infirmary simply as the last years of an old order ending abruptly in 1939. During those years many things were happening in the hospital world. In the Royal Infirmary, changes were taking place, new trends were beginning to appear and the Board of Managers were planning important improvements and extensions and working with energy and remarkable success to bring them about.

To understand the pattern of life in the Infirmary in those years and to appreciate also the size of the tasks which the Managers set themselves, it will be well to look first at the hospital lay-out and buildings as they were in the 1930s. The Infirmary consisted then principally of two large departments built just over fifty years earlier. There was the 'surgical house' beside Lauriston Place with long east-west corridors linking its six three-storey pavilions containing the wards and their associated operating theatres. In these wards, in 1930, 14,600 in-patients were treated. There was the 'medical house' with four ward pavilions running south towards the open space of the Meadows. In these wards 5,000 in-patients were dealt with in that year. In accordance with the best advice of his time, David Bryce had designed the lay-out of these two 'houses' and the individual ward-blocks within them so that they would stand well apart from each other to ensure sufficient ventilation and to reduce the risks of cross-infection. Off the main surgical corridor were the Board Room and administrative offices and, cleverly incorporated with the new building, were parts of the 1738 building and 1857 wings of the original George Watson's Hospital (later School) including its chapel which became the Infirmary Chapel. Other parts of the old school had been adapted as doctors' residency, living accommodation for the Lady Superintendent of Nurses and some nursing and domestic staff and also for the hospital kitchen. With the aim of avoiding the dangers of cross-infection which had bedevilled the former Infirmary buildings in the congested area between Cowgate and Drummond Street, the only enclosed link between the surgical and medical houses was the long curving corridor known to everyone then, as now, in suitable anatomical language, as the 'duodenum'. Elsewhere the wards were well insulated from one another by the open areas between them.

Encroachments on the open spaces of the original plan had, however, begun long before 1930. The first large addition occurred in 1892, only 13 years after the opening of the new Infirmary when the nurses' home, known as the 'Red Home' from its red brick construction, was built roughly midway between the surgical and medical departments. Then it was possible to leave a small open area of grass and trees beside it and this 'nurses garden' is still a quiet, green oasis among the crowded buildings.

Three other encroachments on open space had taken place before 1930. One was the building in 1904 of the surgical out-patient department theatre between the first two pavilions of the surgical house. The second was the building, in 1926, of the radiological department. It, however, was fitted so snugly against the duodenum that it seems scarcely to be there at all. The third was the construction at the eastern end of the medical house by Edinburgh University, with substantial help from the Rockefeller Foundation, of a clinical laboratory incorporating also two wards for patients requiring special diets. That extension, opened in 1928, encroached on part of the garden ground attached to the Medical Superintendent's house which, until 1967, stood close beside Middle Meadow Walk on the eastern edge of the Infirmary site.

Other additions to the hospital had been built mainly on the sites of demolished buildings immediately west of the original site and so had involved little or no sacrifice of open space. First were the gynaecological wards attached to the western end of the medical house and known as the 'Jubilee Pavilion' the building having been financed partly from funds contributed in celebration of Queen Victoria's Diamond Jubilee in 1897. It had been opened in 1900. As befitted a royal commemorative building, the Jubilee Pavilion was built in rich red Dumfriesshire stone, giving it a handsome appearance beside the drab grey Hailes stone of the main buildings. This, however, as Dr. Logan Turner recorded, came about by accident rather than design, the Hailes quarry having been unable to supply sufficient stone at the required time.

The Jubilee Pavilion was built over parts of the sites of the former Royal Hospital for Sick Children and Watson's Junior School for Boys. A short distance northwards from it, two other blocks were added in 1903. The nearer was the Ear, Nose and Throat block; the other, a little further north, was for the Eye Wards and it was named the 'Moray Pavilion' in acknowledgement of a gift of £50,000 from the 14th Earl of Moray in 1896. Both built of the familiar grey stone, they occupy part of the former junior school site and the site of other buildings in Lauriston Lane. North of these two blocks were the laundry, opened in 1896, the boilerhouse and workshops and the mortuary. Such, in broad outline, were the main Infirmary buildings in 1930, extending from Middle Meadow Walk on the east to the boundary wall of George Watson's Boys' College on the west. A year later the Infirmary Board acquired the College and on its site in due course the Simpson Memorial Maternity Pavilion and the Florence Nightingale Nurses Home were built. That, however, is a later story. For the time being the hospital boundary continued to be the George Watson's School playground wall a few yards to the west of the Jubilee Pavilion.

Within the main building the wards, which had been designed in accordance with the favourite advice available in the 1870s, that of Florence Nightingale, were mostly arranged in pairs—one for men and one for women—the number of beds in each varying from 20 to 30, augmented for many years by the addition of centre-beds along the middle of the floor. These centre-beds, long frowned upon but made necessary by demand constantly exceeding bed complement, were not finally officially dispensed with until 1961 and even now they have to be resorted to in times of stress. The open layout of the wards provided minimum privacy for patients but maximum facility for supervision by nurses and there is still a school of thought that prefers them to the modern sub-divided ward except for very ill patients. In the 1930s the large open ward was normal and no-one in the United Kingdom expected anything else. In those years too, patients still spent almost the whole of their hospital stay in bed and so the sparseness of toilet facilities mattered a good deal less than in later years when, increasingly, patients were encouraged to be up and about. The facilities provided were mainly in David Bryce's baronial turrets at the outer end of each ward block and so, in Royal Infirmary parlance, the word 'turret' came to mean bathroom, sluice-room or water-closet. As for 'day-room' accommodation, for the same reason a few chairs where space permitted in the ward were all that circumstances then re-quired. Some of the chairs would be grouped round the open fires which had to be supplied laboriously by porters wheeling coal-trolleys some of which had originally been moveable baths intended for use in 'outside bathrooms', off the ward corridors.

Within these wards the organisation whereby the skills of the honorary medical and surgical staff were brought to the patients followed a single pattern throughout the 1930s. It was a pattern which had existed for many years but which had then reached a new level of excellence, especially in the surgical house. In the main these were still the days of general surgery. Specialism existed in the field of problems of the eye and of the ear, nose and throat, for which, as we have seen, separate buildings had been provided for about thirty years. There were already, also, specialists in diseases of the skin and in venereal disease and for them, new up-to-date accommodation was soon to be provided. The development of other specialties, in such fields as radiotherapy, surgical neurology and orthopaedics had scarcely begun.

The system both on the surgical and the medical side was organised as a series of 'charges' each charge being the responsibility of a Chief, designated 'surgeon-in-ordinary' or 'physician-in-ordinary' most of whom on retiral were invited to become consulting physicians or surgeons. There were seven surgical charges. Associated with each surgeon-in-ordinary or Chief was an assistant surgeon ('junior chief'), a clinical tutor who would be a recently qualified Fellow of the Royal College of Surgeons of Edinburgh; and a house-surgeon, a recently-qualified doctor. Of these only the clinical tutor was paid a regular fee—an annual sum of £75 for his tutorial duties. The Chief and the junior chief received small honoraria from a 'clinical fund' in recognition of their clinical teaching duties. Otherwise they depended on their earnings from private practice—supplemented for those who were University professors by their professorial salaries, in those days far from princely sums. The house-surgeons, appointed then for six-monthly periods, gave their services in return for the valuable experience they received and the prestige gained from working in a famous hospital under a distinguished Chief. Their duties were arduous. They lived in the hospital residency in the heart of the hospital during their term of service and might be called upon at any time of the day or night. Yet there was no shortage of applicants for these demanding, unpaid posts.

The house-surgeons (residents) would usually have served an 'apprenticeship' as junior house officers who were students, unpaid and non-resident, one or more of whom were attached to each charge. These 'juniors' were required to maintain case-notes, to undertake 'side-room' work—blood counts, urine tests and other such checks and to apply certain dressings and carry out some treatments. They undertook the 'portering' of patients between ward and operating theatre and administered anaesthetics under supervision, usually on many more than the twelve occasions required by the General Medical Council as part of their training. In such ways they saw a great deal of the art and practice of surgery and of the ways of their Chief in dealing with complications and emergencies; experience which would equip them to deal confidently with most cases that might come their way in later days.

Each such team was responsible for the treatment and well-being of the patients in a pair of wards (one for men and one for women) and had the use of the operating theatre allocated to their wards. They were helped (and, it is said, sometimes guided) by the ward sister responsible for the nursing of their patients. Several former Chiefs, recalling those days, have praised the work of their ward sisters. Said one: 'They were wonderful women; they were the ones who knew what to do.' The ward sisters practically lived on the job, many having their own sitting-room and bedroom beside their wards. Many had spent years in charge of the same pair of wards, had become fully familiar with the Chief's methods and requirements and would have dealt with every aspect of nursing care and almost every emergency that could arise.

By the 1930s ward sisters had been relieved of theatre work, theatre sisters having recently come into being. Although the light blue of their uniform was more akin to that of a staff nurse than a sister, their status was recognised from their special frilled cap. Their usual domain has been described as 'a bothy-like arrangement hewn out from the cavern under the theatre's student gallery. Here, and in adjoining preparation and sterilising rooms, most of the surgical para-phernalia was prepared and sterilised in what must have been close to a twelve-hour day . . . On them depended the asepsis which, together with relatively light theatre-usage, maintained a freedom from infection unexcelled in later, more sophisticated days, with heavier theatre usage.'

The Chief of each charge was in complete clinical control of all the patients in his wards except occasionally when he might have made a proportion of beds available to a colleague. In some cases he would allow patients to be operated upon by his assistant surgeon who might also, by courtesy of the Chief, have some beds allotted to him. Until the mid-twenties the clinical tutor's duties had been restricted to the clinical instruction of students (though not including bedside teaching). Thereafter, by a decision of the Managers, they were allowed to undertake some operations, either in emergency or at the behest of their seniors, and to have continuing care of the patients on whom they had operated. A useful by-product of that arrangement, from the clinical tutor's point of view, was that he would then have the opportunity of writing to the patient's family doctor about the operation and the patient's progress, thus bringing himself to the notice of the doctor who might be sufficiently impressed to refer private patients to him later. His reputation and, therefore, his livelihood might depend on such referrals.

Each charge, in rotation, had a 'waiting day' on which they would have to admit all emergency cases requiring general surgical attention. These (by order of the Managers) included all patients on whose referral letter a general practitioner had written 'Please admit'. Such patients could be turned away only if the Chief so directed or if, after a telephone conversation, the doctor concerned agreed.

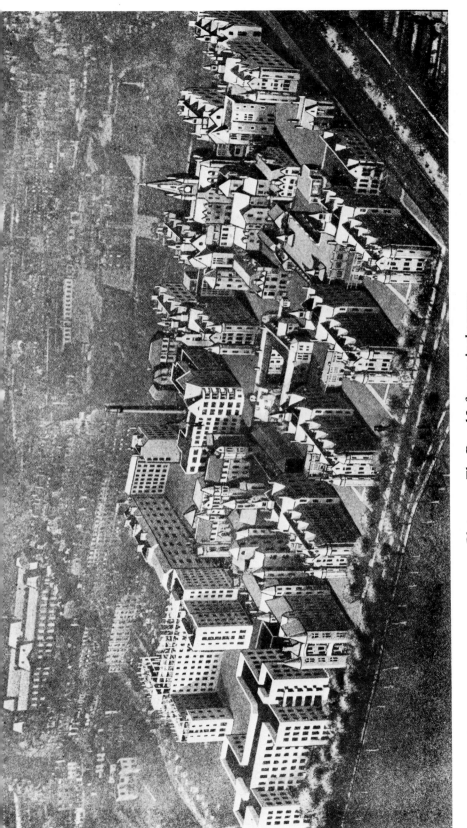

Plate 1   The Royal Infirmary in the 1930s

This sketch formed the centre spread of an appeal brochure issued by the Infirmary Managers in 1937. It shows, in outline, the Infirmary as it then was, with open spaces between its pavilions. The Simpson Pavilion, completed but not yet equipped, is on the left with the Florence Nightingale Nurses' Home under construction beyond (compare with Plate 35).

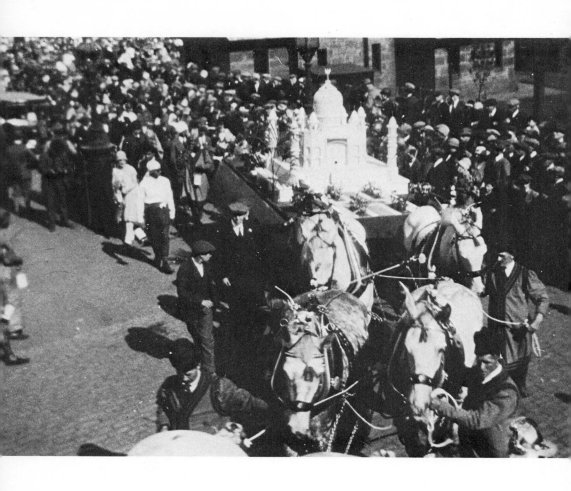

Plate 2   Royal Infirmary Pageant — about 1929

A model of the Taj Mahal, complete with its minarets and ornamental canal

Surgical out-patients were dealt with in two ways. Many, with letters from their doctors, would be seen on one day a week at the Chief's ward clinic held often in a ward corridor or a side room. Of those seen, some requiring admission would be placed on the waiting-list and some would be chosen as suitable cases for demonstration to students. The other arrangement for out-patients was through the surgical out-patient department (SOPD) at which patients arrived daily in large numbers either on referral by a doctor or as the result of an accident or on a return visit. There, they were dealt with by the two most recently appointed assistant surgeons. Many of those who were not urgent accident cases had to endure a long wait, often from 9.30 am. till noon or later. Patients who, on examination, were found to require admission would be transferred to the 'waiting ward' for that day; or after 1936, if only a one-night stay in hospital seemed necessary, to one of six beds introduced in that year for such cases. Some patients would be placed on the list for operation in the SOPD Theatre on one of its two operating days each week. Minor procedures of many kinds were carried out in the department. Its dressing-rooms were crowded every morning for the application of dressings to wounds and ulcers. These were done by nurses and students guided by notes on the patients' cards indicating which of an imposing range of lotions was to be used, for this was before the era of antibiotics. Few of the lotions they used survived into the new era.

A high proportion of the men and women awaiting attention in those days were of the poorest. Many of the women, from overcrowded closes in the old town or cottages in the city's still rural suburbs, would be wearing the traditional shawl around their shoulders from which they were known to the staff, affectionately, as 'shawleys'; the last of whom, it is said, were seen in the mid-1950s. They and all who were waiting were content to sit patiently in the knowledge that they would be seen sometime that day by a 'professor' of the Infirmary in whose ability to cure or alleviate their complaint they had a touching confidence. Although they were treated with kindness and courtesy (albeit sometimes masking an inability to help) patients and staff alike seem then to have accepted as a normal fact of life the inevitability of so many having to spend so long in such uncomfortable and, to the lay person, often distressing surroundings.

In the Medical House in the 1930s there were eight charges, each with a physician-in-ordinary (the Chief), an assistant physician, a clinical tutor, a resident house-physician and one or more juniors—the same pattern as on the surgical side of the hospital. Rules as to payment and non-payment were also the same. Here, however, in addition to consulting physicians there were then three highly distinguished 'physicians-consultant' who might be called upon when required for advice in their special fields.
They included:
   —for tuberculosis, until 1939, Sir Robert Philip, LLD, world-famous
      pioneer in the fight against that disease and founder, in Edinburgh,
      of the Royal Victoria Hospital Tuberculosis Trust;
   —for psychiatry, from 1933, Professor (later Sir) David K. Henderson
      practitioner and teacher of that branch of medicine, also
      world-renowned, who was Physician-Superintendent of the Royal

C

Edinburgh Hospital for Mental and Nervous Disorders from 1932 till
1954; and
—for diseases of tropical climates, Lt-Col E. D. W. Greig, CIE, until 1938
and thereafter Lt-Col E. H. Vere Hodge, CIE, each of whom had
acquired knowledge and expertise during a distinguished army
medical career in India.

Each medical charge was responsible for one ward plus half a ward for patients
of the opposite sex. The physician-in-ordinary might, but often did not, delegate
the care of some beds to his assistant physician. The assistant physician was responsible for seeing out-patients in the medical out-patient department from which
he would offer an opinion to any family doctor who referred a patient to him. He
would place on a waiting-list those who required non-emergency admission
and also might admit urgent cases.

The energies of the physicians were devoted to the diagnosis of disease and
treatment of acute diseases. Patients with chronic conditions were transferred to
their homes whenever possible or, if they were patients for whom a local authority
had statutory responsibility, to the care of that authority. Almost all the physicians
engaged in private practice as well as having consulting practices; they would,
however, refer patients with even minor surgical, gynaecological or obstetric
problems to appropriate colleagues, often to the clinical tutors or the private
assistants of these colleagues. As with the surgical side, all the chiefs and the assistant physicians took part in teaching especially, in their case, instruction in methods
of clinical examination and diagnosis of disease. Skill in diagnosis will no doubt
always involve a subtle mixture of art and science. For physicians in the thirties,
art still predominated and there were those among them who distrusted 'laboratory
medicine' beyond the level of the simple tests which had long been carried out,
with varying degrees of accuracy, in ward side-rooms.

All the members of the honorary staff, physicians and surgeons alike were
men of character. Many were autocrats within their own charges. As the time for
the Chief's ward rounds approached, great was the bustle of activity to ensure
that all was neat and tidy and no bed-cover ruffled; even, it is said, that the castors
on the legs of all the beds faced at the same angle lest any irregularity might spoil
the overall effect.

Walking in the hospital corridors in the 1930s, which of these men of character
might one have met? In the surgical house during that decade there were only three
changes among the surgeons-in-ordinary, the earliest taking place in 1937. The
scene was dominated by two outstanding figures, both of whom brought world-
wide renown to the Infirmary and to the University and each of whom was
beloved by his patients and admired by all Edinburgh. They were Professors
David Wilkie and John Fraser. David Wilkie had been Professor of Surgery since
1924. He was knighted in 1936. He it was who had developed the laboratory in
the medical school in Teviot Place in which valuable research was carried on by
a succession of 'Wilkie's young men' and which was named, after his death in 1938
(at the early age of 56) 'the Wilkie Laboratory'.

John Fraser had been Regius Professor of Clinical Surgery since 1925. He was
knighted in 1937 and awarded a baronetcy in 1943. In 1944 he became Principal

of the University of Edinburgh, an appointment which was universally acclaimed. His contribution to the conduct of University affairs was great, but sadly curtailed by his sudden death at the age of 62 as he was leaving the University after a meeting of the University Court in December 1947. Soon after his death a writer in the University of Edinburgh Journal said of these two great surgeons: 'Each a supreme master of the art of surgery and each a teacher of quite exceptional gifts, with strongly individual characters, they were yet strikingly alike in some of the finest human qualities—in perfect sincerity and unselfishness, in delicate courtesy and personal charm.' Until 1937, either of them might have been seen any day—Wilkie hurrying to his Wards 13 and 14, off the upper surgical corridor and Fraser, walking, seemingly with less haste, to his Wards 7 and 8 off the main corridor. One who knew them has pin-pointed their differences: 'Wilkie, bird-like and scientific; Fraser, broader and ebullient'. Both were gifted teachers and both were noted for their compassion and their power to inspire confidence in their patients.

At the time when Wilkie and Fraser flourished, the five other surgical Chiefs were George L. Chiene, James M. Graham, John W. Struthers, W. J. Stuart and Henry Wade. All were general surgeons but all had areas of special interest in which they developed special skills. They are among the many surgeons whose work and characteristics are fully described in Mr. James A. Ross's book—'The Edinburgh School of Surgery after Lister' (published in 1978). From the wealth of information in that book I have gleaned with his permission, a few short sentences to give a fleeting glimpse of each of the men who, as Chiefs along with Wilkie and Fraser, contributed so much to the fame of the Infirmary's surgical work in the 1930s.

George L. Chiene (1873-1951)—(Surgeon-in-Ordinary, 1922-1937, Wards 11/12) an excellent teacher, particularly of undergraduates, and an ingenious surgeon who devised several new procedures including operations on wryneck, inguinal hernia, ventral hernia and appendicitis. He also wrote a popular book of surgery.

James M. Graham (1882-1962)—(S-in-O 1928—1946, Wards 5/6) He made great original contributions to the development of blood transfusion and in particular to the surgery of the thyroid gland. He established this speciality on a sound basis and achieved results never previously obtained in Edinburgh.

John W. Struthers (1874-1953)—(S-in-O 1924-1939, Wards 9/10) Struthers became a very able general surgeon. He was a remarkably accurate diagnostician and as an operator he was sound and eminently safe rather than showy or brilliant [but] he could be bold when necessary . . . He was always a prominent and not infrequently a dominant member of any committee.

W. J. Stuart (1873-1959)—(S-in-O 1923-1938, Wards 17/18) 'Pussy' Stuart, to give him the nickname which he happily bore for seventy-six years, will long be remembered, not as a brilliant surgeon but as a surgeon who regarded both the welfare and peace of mind of each individual patient as by far the most important consideration.

(Sir) Henry Wade (1877-1955)—(S-in-O 1924-1939, Wards 15/16)
  In the years between the two world wars . . . Wade established a world reputation in urology, recording his work in some thirty-five papers . . . He was a great clinical teacher at a time when there were many outstanding teachers in the Edinburgh Medical School . . . He instilled immense confidence well borne out by the results obtained from his superlative skill.

In the Medical House, among the Physicians-in-Ordinary who had charge of wards in the 1930s, there were several well-known and highly-regarded men. As with the surgeons of the same period, two were outstanding; in this case, however, the two were not already in charge of wards at the opening of the decade but appeared in that capacity towards its close. They were Professor (later Sir) Derrick Dunlop (1902-1980) and Professor (later Sir) Stanley Davidson (1894-1981). In 1936 Dr. Derrick Dunlop was appointed Professor of Therapeutics at Edinburgh (in succession to Professor D. Murray Lyon) and Physician-in-Ordinary in the Infirmary where he had been an assistant physician since 1934. In 1938 Dr. Stanley Davidson who had been an assistant physician in the Infirmary briefly in the 1920s, returned from Aberdeen where he had occupied the chair of Medicine since 1930 to become Professor of Medicine in Edinburgh and a Physician-in-Ordinary at the Infirmary.

These two distinguished physicians whose work, though in different spheres nevertheless dove-tailed neatly, continued as leading members of the Infirmary's medical team until they retired—Sir Stanley in 1959 and Sir Derrick in 1962. Their interests ranged widely over the medical spectrum though, as will emerge in later chapters, Sir Stanley Davidson had a special interest in the science of haematology and diseases of the blood and Sir Derrick Dunlop in endocrine malfunction including diabetes and its treatment by diet and also in the scientific use of drugs. Both were eminent as teachers, a field in which Professor Dunlop's ability and technique were superb.

Earlier in the decade, two physicians were prominent. They were:

William T. Ritchie, OBE (1873-1945) a Physician-in-Ordinary in charge of wards from 1922 till 1938 and Professor of Medicine at Edinburgh from 1928 till 1938. His special interest lay in research into and treatment of heart disease at a time when the science of cardiology was still in an early stage of development; in this work he was followed by Dr. Rae Gilchrist who became a physician in charge of wards in 1939.

David Murray Lyon (1888-1956) who was Professor of Therapeutics from 1924 till 1936 and of Clinical Medicine from then until 1953. He had charge of wards in the Medical House from 1924 till 1935 and again from 1938 till 1953, the intervening years having been spent in helping to develop, as a teaching unit, the recently established municipal general hospitals in Edinburgh. His outstanding contribution to the work of the Royal

Infirmary lay in the early use of insulin for treatment of diabetes and in the sphere of dietetics, work in which Professor Dunlop collaborated and later developed.

Among the other physicians who had charge of wards in the Infirmary in the 1930s were Dr. Edwin Bramwell, Professor of Clinical Medicine from 1922 till 1934, who enjoyed a national reputation in neurology and was an elegant and popular teacher; Dr. John Eason, much concerned with thyroid disease and Dr. Alexander Goodall who did valuable work on diseases of the blood. Although these physicians each developed special interests they were first and foremost general physicians concerned with all aspects of medicine. The era of full specialisation was only beginning to dawn.

The Astley Ainslie Institution

Some welcome relief of pressure on beds in the Infirmary was provided in the late 1920s and early 1930s by the establishment of a new hospital in the city— the Astley Ainslie Institution (now Hospital). Although under separate management, it was designed specifically to accommodate convalescent patients from the Infirmary, almost doubling the facilities earmarked for such patients, who had previously been provided for only at the Infirmary's own Convalescent House at Corstorphine.

As narrated by Logan Turner, Mr. David Ainslie, a land-owner and well known sheep breeder of Costerton between Pathhead and Humbie, in Midlothian, had died in 1900 leaving instructions to his Trustees that the residue of his estate, after the lapse of fifteen years, was to be applied 'to the purpose of erecting, endowing and maintaining a hospital or institution to be called the Astley Ainslie Institution, for the relief and behoof of the convalescents of the Royal Infirmary of Edinburgh'.

For the new hospital, the Ainslie Trustees had acquired from their accumulated fund a magnificent site on the south side of the city consisting of four neighbouring mansion houses and their grounds. They were Millbank, Southbank, Canaan House and Canaan Park (to which Morelands and St. Roque's House and their grounds were added later). The properties formed a combined south-sloping area of parkland, gardens and woodland with fine views to the Blackford, Braid and Pentland Hills—an ideal setting in which to regain strength after illness.

An 'experimental' unit of 34 beds had been opened in 1923. In their Annual Report for 1928-29 the Royal Infirmary Managers recorded that 90 beds were available in the new Institution, that 30 more were expected to be available in 1930 and that the total accommodation would ultimately be 150 beds. Lest there should be doubt as to the respective uses of the Infirmary's own Convalescent House and the new Astley Ainslie Institution, it was early agreed that the former would be used mainly for patients requiring a short period of rest between illness and return to ordinary life while the latter would provide for those requiring longer care and supervision to fit them for normal activity and work. It was also agreed that the hospital might, in special cases, admit patients who were to undergo operations in the Infirmary but who needed a period of preliminary 'building up'.

It was made clear that beds at the Astley Ainslie Institution should not be used for patients suffering from chronic disabling illnesses or debility due to old age for whom a return to normal or nearly normal health and fitness could not reasonably be expected.

In pursuance of its aims the Institution grew from being a convalescent hospital to become a leading rehabilitation centre in which patients were actively taught to regain old abilities and skills or to acquire new ones. It became also a leading training school for occupational therapists. These functions were greatly developed after 1948 under the National Health Service; and especially after 1954 when it was linked with Edenhall Hospital, Musselburgh (a former Ministry of Pensions Hospital) under a single Board of Management. After the reorganisation of 1974, as one of the hospitals in the South Lothian District, the Astley Ainslie Hospital continued to expand, reaching by 1979 a capacity of 200 beds. Its main aim remained the same—to restore to the fullest possible activity patients disabled or incapacitated by accident or illness, in a more relaxed environment than that of a busy general hospital. Over the years its staff have developed increasingly sophisticated techniques for doing so. Though no longer attached exclusively to the Infirmary, it still provides, as it did in the 1930s, some relief from the constant pressure on accommodation there.

The Municipal Hospitals

During the 1930s a development occurred which had an important bearing on the future of the Infirmary and on hospital and health provision in Edinburgh as a whole. It was in a sense a prelude to the National Health Service. Had it not occurred then, hospital facilities in Edinburgh for the coming wartime emergency, for transfer to the health service in 1948 and as a base for future growth, would have been much less adequate than, in fact, they came to be. This development, which meant so much to the present-day hospital service in the city, was the coming of the municipal general hospitals.

Until 16 May 1930 (the day on which the Local Government (Scotland) Act 1929 became operative) people who were sick and in need of hospital care fell into three main groups. These were:

(1) the 'destitute sick' for whom the parish councils provided 'poor law hospitals' either as part of a poor house or in a separate building, the standards in which—with very few exceptions—were deplorably low;

(2) those who were able or whose families were able to pay for accommodation and treatment in a nursing home, many stretching their ability to do so to its limits and beyond;

(3) a large group, neither poor enough to qualify for parish care nor earning or owning enough to pay nursing home fees, and for this group, voluntary hospitals such as the Royal Infirmary with its ever-open door provided an essential and much appreciated service.

Cutting across all three groups were two other categories:

(a) persons suffering from infectious diseases for whom local health authorities were required to provide special hospitals without charge;

(b) persons injured in accidents or taken suddenly ill in a street or public place who would normally be taken to the nearest suitable voluntary hospital which, in Edinburgh, was almost always the Infirmary.

As part of a wider re-organisation of local government and with the object of removing the 'stigma' of the poor law, the Act of 1929 did two things. First, it discontinued the parish councils and transferred their poorhouses and poor-law hospitals to the counties and large burghs (including the four cities) in Scotland and secondly, it empowered these authorities to up-grade the former poor-law hospitals and make them available to the general public as part of the local authorities' public health provision. In their schemes for doing so they were required 'to have regard to any other facilities for treatment of sick persons, including those provided by any voluntary hospital or other institution'.

Edinburgh Town Council soon took advantage of these provisions. Among the former parish council institutions transferred to them were those at Craigleith and Seafield. In each of these and in East Pilton Hospital (Leith's former Fever Hospital) a scheme of renovation and improvement was begun, the aim being to equip and staff them as fully efficient teaching hospitals.

In view of the problems then facing the Royal Infirmary Managers in their efforts to reduce the growing waiting-list for beds and arising also from the large numbers of students who crowded into the wards for clinical teaching, one might have expected them to welcome eagerly any proposals that might help to solve these problems. But, though little of this was recorded in their minutes, there seems to have been some measure of doubt, or even suspicion, in the Managers' minds about this intrusion of local government into what had hitherto been the domain of the voluntary hospitals.

The Honorary Staff of the Infirmary, in February 1932, intimated that they were in favour of the Municipal Hospitals being available for teaching and after consultation among the three authorities—Town Council, University and Infirmary—the city's hospitals scheme went on. Craigleith poor-law hospital became the Western General Hospital with 280 beds, Pilton became the Northern General Hospital with 260 beds and Seafield became the Eastern General Hospital with 360 beds—a total of 900 beds. By agreement with the University and the Royal Colleges of Physicians and Surgeons they were designated as teaching hospitals and under an arrangement in which the Royal Infirmary co-operated four units were established within the three hospitals and placed under four Directors, three of whom already held honorary appointments in the Infirmary, as follows:

Medicine—Professor W. T. Ritchie of the Chair of Medicine and Physician-in-Ordinary in the Infirmary;

Surgery—Professor David Wilkie of the Chair of Surgery and Surgeon-in-Ordinary in the Infirmary;

Obstetrics and Gynaecology—Professor R. W. Johnstone of the Chair of Midwifery and Gynaecologist in the Infirmary;

Children—Professor Charles McNeil of the Chair of Child Life and Health and Honorary Paediatrician to the Simpson Memorial Maternity Hospital (later Paediatrician in the Obstetrical and Gynaecological Department in the Infirmary).

At the municipal hospitals, under these Directors, there were Assistants and resident medical officers payment of whom was shared by University and Town Council. The teaching of medical students soon came into operation and during 1933 a residence for 12 students was provided at the Western General. The training of nurses had at first to be arranged in collaboration with other hospitals but by 1933 the number and variety of cases dealt with were just sufficient to enable the three municipal hospitals to be recognised as a training school by the General Nursing Council for Scotland. In 1936 a nurses' home was built beside the Western General Hospital and a new kitchen and dietetic kitchen were also provided.

For the first three full years of operation of the municipal hospitals the numbers of patients treated, compared with those in the Infirmary, were as follows:

Municipal Hospitals		Royal Infirmary		
Year	Patients Treated	Year	Patients Treated	Waiting List
1933	5,280	1932/33	19,253	3006
1934	5,918	1933/34	18,955	'over 3000'
1935	6,425	1934/35	19,802	'about 3000'

These figures being for such a short period prove little but they do, perhaps, suggest that if there had been no municipal hospitals the Infirmary waiting-list, which had been growing steadily for years, would have continued to grow instead of remaining roughly level at about 3000.

At the Western General Hospital in 1935 the number of operations performed was 901, of which 550 were classed as 'major'; and 818 medical cases and 649 children were listed as in-patients during that year. Each year, however, throughout the thirties, the same complaint was voiced by the Medical Officers of Health who had overall administrative charge of the municipal hospitals—Dr. John Guy until 1938 and Dr. W. G. Clark thereafter. Their complaint was that far too high a proportion of the patients referred to the municipal hospitals were in the category of chronic sick and aged. This was partly accounted for by the fact that the Town Council had a statutory responsibility for patients receiving Public Assistance but there was more than a suspicion that long-term cases were being foisted on to the municipal hospitals and, while Dr. Guy was full of praise for the efficiency and kindness with which these patients were treated by the staff, he repeatedly had to point out that their presence in such numbers was making medical teaching and the recruitment and training of nurses exceedingly difficult.

There were three main reasons for this state of affairs. One was, undoubtedly, the reluctance of many general practitioners to refer their acutely ill patients to these newly-designated hospitals. Despite the improvements made, the modern equipment installed and the high quality of their consultant and other staffs, the aura of the old poor-law regime in the public mind still clung to the buildings. Then, many doctors in and around Edinburgh had affectionate memories of their student and resident days in the Infirmary and when their patients required hospital treatment, it was the hospital that came immediately to mind.

The third reason for the Infirmary to be so often preferred was the difficult problem of payment in the municipal hospitals. The Act of 1929, having authorised the provision of municipal general hospitals, went on to state that 'it shall be lawful for' the local authority to charge patients for their accommodation and treatment. The legal advice then given to Edinburgh Town Council and accepted by them was that the ability to charge, in this context, must be read as a duty to charge because it would be unfair to the ratepayers generally if the authority having been given the power to charge did not exercise that power. So charges for inpatients were fixed as follows: Edinburgh citizens—£1.5s (£1.25) weekly; patients from other areas—£2.12.6 (£2.62½) weekly; private patients (for whom some small rooms were available)—£3.3s (£3.15) weekly. It was competent, however, for the local authority to reduce the first two of these charges, or to waive them altogether, if their officials were satisfied that the patient's means were so limited as to make it unreasonable to enforce payment in full.

To the Town Council's credit it must be said that these provisions were usually generously interpreted. Nevertheless, the requirement that payment be made in full or a 'means test' imposed, however sympathetically that might be done, introduced a difficulty which did not arise in the Infirmary and which caused much concern, especially to the League of Subscribers. They considered it unfair that a member who had subscribed to the Infirmary for many years and then found himself in need of hospital treatment but unable to be admitted to the Infirmary without long delay should have to pay a weekly charge if he sought treatment in a municipal hospital. Year after year this problem was discussed with the Town Council and plans were suggested for forming a hospitals contributory scheme to cover both voluntary and municipal hospitals. Year after year these discussions and suggestions came to nought. It was not only the League who were concerned about this. The Committee of the Infirmary Court of Contributors, usually so blandly complimentary to the Managers, became highly critical on this point. They noted that at intervals since 1934, conferences to seek a solution of the difficulty had been held with the Town Council; and they noted also that the Infirmary Managers in referring to these conferences in their annual report for 1939 said only, 'it is to be hoped these will be continued'. On this the Contributors commented sternly: 'This is a very tepid statement and the Committee strongly recommend that the Managers should take up the matter with decision and press it to a conclusion'.

At last, in the Royal Infirmary Annual Report for 1945, the following paragraph appeared:

An agreement has been made and is in operation for an experimental
period, between Edinburgh Corporation and the Royal Infirmary,
whereby contributors to the League of Subscribers who are citizens of
Edinburgh and who may be on the waiting-list for admission, may, if
they so desire, be admitted to a municipal hospital for earlier treatment.
The Corporation makes no charge to the patient, whose maintenance is
paid for by the Royal Infirmary from funds provided by the League.

So far so good. After so many years, an experimental, partial scheme (for Edinburgh subscribers to the League only) had been devised; and then, a little more than two years later came the National Health Service, making any such scheme unnecessary.

For all these reasons—prejudice, inertia on the part of G.Ps and the problem of payment—positive co-operation between the Royal Infirmary and the municipal hospitals had been slow to develop during the 1930s, a curious state of affairs in view of the continuing size of the Infirmary's waiting-list. (In 1938 it was 3,235.) In October 1938 Dr. (later Sir) Stanley Davidson had returned from Aberdeen to Edinburgh to take up appointments as Professor of Medicine in the University, Physician-in-Ordinary in the Infirmary and Director of the Medical Unit in the Municipal Hospitals. In his inaugural lecture as Professor he had this to say:

> At 11 o'clock on the 1st of October 1938 I took over my wards in the
> Royal Infirmary and was informed that there were 81 sick persons
> awaiting admission to my wards. Many of these patients were suffering
> from serious illnesses, but nevertheless they could not be admitted for
> weeks or months. At 12 o'clock I took over the medical unit of the
> municipal hospitals where, at the Western General Hospital, I found 43
> beds vacant on the medical side and 33 on the surgical side, while 56 beds
> were vacant at the Eastern and 86 at the Northern Hospital . . . There are
> hundreds of cases awaiting admission to the surgical side of the Royal
> Infirmary who are suffering incapacity and loss of economic efficiency
> for periods of a year or longer while awaiting admission. At the Western
> General Hospital the surgical unit—staffed by three highly-skilled and
> scientific surgeons—continues to have year after year, large numbers of
> vacant beds . . .'

These numbers of vacant beds, he explained, did not include beds (of which there were then 120) necessarily vacant because of the shortage of nurses.

The Professor went on to explain two of the reasons, already stated above, to account for the under-use of the municipal hospitals—prejudice arising from their previous use and the problem of payment. He condemned the former 'since the services at the Western General Hospital bear no recognisable resemblance to those found in the former poor-law institutions'; and he made some suggestions as to how the payment difficulty might be overcome. He did not mention the other reason, the long-standing affection of general practitioners for the Infirmary.

Looking back now, it is difficult to believe that even all these reasons combined can have accounted for the existence of all the 218 empty municipal hospital beds to which the Professor referred; and one is tempted to the conclusion that the Infirmary authorities of that time, imbued with pride in their old and famous hospital, although not opposing the diversion of patients to the municipal hospitals, did not strive unduly hard to encourage it.

As the quotations from his lecture imply, Professor Stanley Davidson on his arrival in Edinburgh, set himself the objective of remedying this unsatisfactory situation. But almost immediately he found another urgent and onerous task thrust upon him. War was approaching and the Department of Health for Scotland were urgently planning the emergency medical services that would be necessary. Among their plans were proposals to provide emergency hospitals strategically placed throughout Scotland, away from centres of population, and they appointed

Professor Davidson along with their Chief Medical Officer and Professor T. J. Mackie, of the Chair of Bacteriology at Edinburgh to advise on the siting, construction and equipping of such hospitals. Work on this committee entailed much travelling and occupied much time in the months that followed. Combined with his other duties this left the Professor little time to devote to seeking a solution of the hospital admission problem. Then, within a year, war was declared and, as it continued, the whole system of admissions came to be regulated by the needs of the Emergency Medical Service. It can never be known, therefore, how effectively the Royal Infirmary as a voluntary hospital and the municipal hospitals might have worked together if normal times had continued and Professor Davidson had been able to encourage and develop their co-operation. What is certain is that during and after the war he played a leading part in the modernisation of his departments in the Royal Infirmary and also in bringing the municipal hospitals generally, and the Western General in particular, to the outstanding position they now hold, along with the Royal Infirmary, in the National Health Service.

New Buildings

Judged on the basis of stone and lime alone, as distinct from the installation of new medical, surgical and scientific apparatus, no decade in the first 100 years life of the present Infirmary saw such spectacular progress as did the ten years from 1930 to 1939. In those years, besides some lesser extensions and adaptations, three large and important additions were made to the Infirmary buildings, adding altogether some 250 beds to the total complement for patients which in 1939 reached 1,300 beds, and providing new accommodation for 280 nurses. The three buildings were the Dermatology and Venereal Diseases Pavilion opened in 1936 and the Simpson Memorial Maternity Pavilion and Florence Nightingale Nurses Home, both opened in 1939. The total cost of these schemes, including associated extensions to the boiler house, laundry and kitchens was over £500,000.

To have achieved all this in ten years was creditable enough. To have done so in a decade of national depression such as the 1930s demonstrates the enthusiasm and perseverance of the Managers and officials who carried the schemes through and the generosity of thousands of donors who responded to the Infirmary Extension Appeal, launched originally in connection with the bi-centenary celebrations of 1929 and renewed in 1937. But, if one individual more than any other is to be commended for the success of these projects, the choice must fall on Thomas W. Turnbull, Architect and Master of Works to the Infirmary who designed the buildings and supervised their erection while, at the same time, undertaking several lesser projects and, with his works department staff, being responsible for the day-to-day maintenance of the whole hospital.

Thomas W. Turnbull, FIAA, MISE, was Clerk of Works from 1920 until 1924, designated 'Master of Works' from then until 1929 and thereafter 'Architect and Master of Works' till his retiral in 1956. During his 36 years service there was scarcely an alteration or extension to the Infirmary fabric that was not devised and supervised by him. He lived for the hospital and became so accustomed to working closely with surgeons, physicians, scientific and nursing staffs that, when new accommodation, technical installations or alterations were called for, he could readily interpret and often anticipate their needs. As one former specialist put it—'With Turnbull, if you told him the object of the exercise, you didn't have to tell him all the details; you could be sure they would be right'. In 1943, with the consent of the Board of Management, he was appointed Honorary Consulting Architect to the Royal College of Surgeons of Edinburgh 'whom he had so often helped in the past'; and from time to time he was asked to advise other hospital authorities— in Dumfries, Elgin, Orkney and elsewhere. Undoubtedly, however, Thomas Turnbull's main achievements were those three buildings of the 1930s, the Dermatology and V.D. Block, the Simpson Pavilion and the Nurses' Home.

How did these three buildings come to be built at that inauspicious time? And how fortunate, in the light of later events, that they *were* built then!

Dermatology and Venereal Diseases Departments

The need for new accommodation for the dermatology and venereal diseases departments arose directly from the recognition, in the early 1930s, that provision for these departments was out-of-date and inadequate. The wards allocated to skin diseases were off the lower surgical corridor, with 8 beds for men and 14 for women. Both wards were overshadowed and dull and their ancillary consulting-rooms and X-ray and ultra-violet treatment room were ill-lit and ill-ventilated. As if skin diseases in themselves were not depressing enough to the sufferers the department was described as one of the most depressing areas in the whole hospital. In those insalubrious surroundings all beds were always occupied, with a long waiting-list, and there were at least 15,000 outpatient attendances each year with a queue of patients waiting in the uninviting corridor. Sir Norman Walker and Dr. Cranston Low, Consulting Physicians, Dr. Robert Aitken, Dr. (later Professor) G. H. Percival and Dr. Grant Peterkin among others struggled nobly, against the odds, to maintain in these unlikely surroundings the highest standards of treatment. Happily, better things lay ahead.

Conditions in the old Venereal Diseases Department were just as unsatisfactory. Male patients were accommodated in Ward 5A in the basement of the westmost surgical pavilion while women patients were in Ward 20, high in the clock tower. Since 1919, the Venereal Diseases Department had been operated as a joint venture with the Town Council of Edinburgh who had a statutory duty to ensure that such provision was made. Dr. David Lees, for 15 years the Physician-in-charge was also the Town Council's Venereal Diseases Medical Officer. In his annual report for 1933 he complained bitterly about conditions in the poorly-ventilated, cramped premises allocated to him, at a time when there were 84,000 male outpatient attendances and 22,000 female attendances annually in addition to the inpatient work. Clearly something had to be done quickly to improve facilities if for no other reason than to ensure that the Public Health department of the Town Council could properly fulfil their statutory duty.

With these two departments of the Infirmary in equally dire straits it was agreed that a joint remedy should be sought by providing a new building to house both departments but each quite independent of the other, with separate entrances. The Town Council agreed that, if the Infirmary Board met the whole capital cost of the building, the Public Health Department would pay an appropriate rent for the venereal diseases section and would continue to meet a share of that Department's running costs as before.

A site involving minimum interference with other buildings was selected to the north of the 1903 Eye Pavilion and, in collaboration with the medical staffs of both departments, Mr. Turnbull designed a modern five-story block incorporating the latest types of equipment. Dr. David Lees took a keen interest in the planning of the V.D. section and many of the new ideas there must certainly have been his but, sadly, he died suddenly in 1934 and so never had the advantage of working in the new surroundings to which he had so eagerly looked forward. That benefit was enjoyed by his successor, Dr. R. C. L. Batchelor. Dr. Mary Liston who for many years had looked after the women patients in Ward 20 retired in 1936 after only a brief sojourn in the new department. She died in 1978, at the age of 101, still remembered for her devotion to her patients so many years before.

On 5th June 1936 the new building was formally opened by Sir Norman Walker, LLD, Consulting Physician to the Dermatology Department and President of the General Medical Council. He was accompanied by Councillor Peter Given, Chairman of the Public Health Committee of the Town Council. The new building was of steel frame construction encased in concrete with external walls of artificial stone. As a well-mannered gesture towards the architecture of the older buildings by which it was so closely surrounded, the Architect included crow-stepped gables and a slated roof, and the south-eastern angle of the building was given curved balconies to soften the effect of the harsher straight lines elsewhere. It cost a total of £45,000, a modest sum even for those days, economy having been achieved through his ability to keep within expenditure limits set by the Board and produce a building which, although utilitarian, satisfactorily met their requirements. All contemporary descriptions of the new building praised its up-to-date specialised facilities and the appearance of brightness everywhere—in welcome contrast to the former dismal conditions.

The new venereal diseases department included an 'irrigation and dressing station' in which a novel feature was a system for supplying sterile hot water at a constant temperature, but within a year the old unpleasant form of treatment for which this was mainly required had begun to be superseded by the coming of chemotherapy and later antibiotic treatment. In 1937 Dr. Batchelor recorded his opinion of sulphanilamide and its derivatives as 'the finest chemotherapeutic agents yet evolved against the genococcus'; in 1938 it was reported in the British Medical Journal that about 90% of cases of gonorrhoea had been successfully treated in his department by use of the new 'M. & B. 693', sulpha-pyridine. So patients in the new building had the twin benefits of new facilities and new scientific methods of treatment.

Simpson Pavilion and the Nurses' Home

Apart from being a valuable addition to the Infirmary, construction of the new venereal and skin diseases building provided Thomas Turnbull with a useful 'trial run' for the much more ambitious projects of the Simpson Pavilion and the

Nurses' Home. Their story is longer and more complex. It starts in the 1920s and it had, in fact, two beginnings.

The first was the concern of the Infirmary Managers at the growing waiting-list of patients. An average monthly list of 950 names in 1920 had risen to more than 1800 in 1923. By 1929 it had reached 2,800, but already in 1923 the Managers were anxiously searching for some way of reducing it. Although emergencies were always dealt with promptly, the waiting-lists for other cases continued to grow as also did the Managers' concern and the distress of the League of Subscribers.

Other means having proved elusive, the Managers turned their attention to the possibility of expansion and in 1923 they said: 'as it is for hygienic reasons undesirable to increase the buildings upon a site already congested, expansion involves the acquisition of additional land'. So, for the fourth time in the history of the Infirmary, they fixed their eyes upon property belonging to the Edinburgh Merchant Company; the property, this time, being George Watson's Boys' College and its grounds of about three acres, immediately west of their site. The College, built in 1818 as the Merchant Maiden Hospital became George Watson's Boys' College in 1870 and had been enlarged in the 1880s. It was thus an out-of-date, much altered building and the Merchant Company might, quite possibly, welcome an incentive to remove the school to a modern building elsewhere.

Meanwhile the second reason for the Infirmary extension scheme was emerging only a short distance away at 79 Lauriston Place where the Directors of the Edinburgh Royal Maternity and Simpson Memorial Hospital had been facing an equally serious problem. Their hospital, like the Infirmary, had been opened on its Lauriston site in 1879. It was the direct descendant of the Edinburgh Lying-in Hospital, opened in 1793 which, fifty years later, had become the Edinburgh Royal Maternity Hospital and which had been closely associated with Sir James Y. Simpson. In its wards countless women had benefited from his recognition of the anaesthetic properties of chloroform. But it had never occupied purpose-built premises till, after seven removals in 80 years from one adapted building to another, it had finally come to rest in Lauriston Place, in its own building, erected nine years after Simpson's death as a memorial to him. The building had since been extended and much pioneering work, especially in the ante-natal field, had been done there but by the 1920s its accommodation was inadequate and its facilities were rapidly becoming obsolete—just how inadequate and obsolete will be seen later. Its Directors therefore turned their attention to the need for a new, larger and more modern hospital. Their funds, however, were limited and they were well aware that any appeal they might launch would be overshadowed in the public mind by appeals which they knew the Royal Infirmary Managers were likely to make in the near future for their contemplated extension.

In December 1923 the Directors of 'the Simpson' had called a meeting of interested organisations at which a Committee had been appointed 'to consider and report on the subject of a new Maternity Hospital generally, and specially as to suitable sites and the future relations of the Hospital and the Infirmary'. Some members of that Committee were also members of the Infirmary Board and thus were well aware of the Infirmary's thoughts of expansion. No doubt that influenced

the deliberations of the Committee in December 1923 when general agreement
was reached on the following points:

(1) That in providing a new Maternity Hospital it was essential that the
    name of Sir J. Y. Simpson should continue to be associated with it as a
    Memorial of his eminent service of humanity.

(2) That great advantages, scientific and administrative, would accrue if a
    site for the new Maternity Hospital were found in the closest possible
    proximity to the Infirmary.

(3) That some form of association or affiliation between the Hospital and
    the Infirmary in their obstetrical and gynaecological work was desirable
    in the interests of efficiency and economy.

In the letter officially informing the Infirmary Board of these points, two
questions were asked: 'Whether, in their knowledge, a site conforming with the
above description was likely to be available within a reasonable time?' and 'What
were their suggestions as to the form the desiderated association or affiliation
between the Maternity Hospital and the Infirmary might take?' Fifteen years and
two months later, as a direct result of those questions, the Simpson Maternity
Pavilion opened its doors for the first time, the doors of the old 'Simpson' were
closed and its Board of Directors were disbanded. Preliminary negotiations had
been difficult, involving first, a delicate approach by the Infirmary Board to the
Merchant Company as to whether they would be willing to transfer their school
to another place and sell the site to the Infirmary, followed by a prolonged discussion about price.

The Infirmary's original idea in deciding to seek additional ground had been
to build on it a new gynaecological department and a nurses' home. That would
have enabled the gynaecological wards in the 'Jubilee' pavilion to be made available
for general surgical cases thus enabling the waiting-list to be reduced. Following
the approach from the Maternity Hospital it was necessary to consider building a
maternity block as well and sketch-plans were called for to show how this could
be done. By March 1925 the Infirmary Board had become very doubtful about the
possibility of doing it at all and their Treasurer and Clerk, William Caw, wrote
to the Simpson Directors: 'As the situation has changed somewhat through increase in the pressure for bed and other accommodation it is possible that, even if
the Managers are successful in obtaining the site in question, they may not be in a
position to offer any portion of it as a site for a new Maternity Hospital'. Not
unnaturally, the Directors were upset to find that they were 'just where we were
two years ago'. They pointed out that 'what is done now will affect midwifery
for the next hundred years' and that the importance to the community of obstetrical
teaching of students and nurses and catering for the treatment of patients made it
essential that a thoroughly up-to-date Maternity Hospital should be provided.

Soon afterwards it seemed likely that the whole plan would collapse because
the Merchant Company, although willing to sell, were asking a price of £100,000
to help them to replace their school worthily on another site while the Infirmary
felt unable to offer more than £75,000. Then a benefactor who had helped the
Infirmary more than once before again stepped in. He was Sir John Findlay and he
announced that he would contribute £10,000 if the Infirmary would raise their

offer to £90,000. They did so and on that basis the matter was settled. But the problem remained—how to fit on to the site all that had been intended—gynaecological wards, maternity wards and nurses' home. It was a problem that gave much food for thought during the next few years and one that was destined never to be solved.

In the old Simpson Maternity Hospital there were 94 beds including those for ante-natal care and it was calculated in the light of the current trend towards more births taking place in hospital that at least 120 beds should be provided in the new building. A sketch-plan was considered by the Infirmary Board in May 1929 showing two blocks, with a connecting link (one with 153 maternity beds and the other with 98 gynaecological beds) and a home for some 300 nurses. The Board then agreed that while there was a certain conflict between the interests of the Maternity Hospital and the Royal Infirmary in this matter 'the needs of the Maternity Hospital (to which the Royal Infirmary owed a moral obligation) were imperative, whereas the Infirmary's requirements for nurses' accommodation were susceptible of being dealt with in stages by providing completely satisfactory quarters for a number of nurses on the Watson's College ground immediately and attending to the rest later'. They also agreed that the name 'Simpson' should be transferred to the new maternity block.

On the second question asked by the Maternity Hospital Directors—as to the form of association between the two bodies, the Infirmary Managers were in no doubt. 'The only satisfactory method of amalgamation' they said 'would be one of absorption as any idea of divided authority or management within the buildings of the Infirmary is not to be contemplated'. The capital funds of the Royal Maternity Hospital would be taken over and used towards meeting the cost of building the new blocks. For these purposes Parliamentary authority was required and, in due course, it was obtained in the Edinburgh Royal Maternity and Simpson Memorial Hospital Order Confirmation Act of 1932. Among the Act's provisions was the requirement that 'the name "Simpson" shall continue in all time coming to be associated with the new building or with any building or buildings which shall, in time to come, replace the new building or buildings'. The Act authorised the Infirmary to make charges for accommodation and services in the new pavilion 'the same as or as near as may be similar to those made by the Directors of the Maternity Hospital'.

All these matters having been agreed to by May 1929, the stage was set for the launching by the Infirmary Board of a massive Appeal for funds for the new extension. This they planned as part of their 1929 Bi-centenary commemoration but such an appeal, to be affective, must be thoroughly organised, involving much preparation and so it was not until October 1930 that it was formally launched. But it was given a preliminary boost four months earlier, on 13th June, by the Prince of Wales (later King Edward VIII) in course of a brief visit to Edinburgh during which he toured several wards of the Infirmary and planted a tree in the hospital grounds near the Meadows, between wards 31 and 34. Afterwards, in a speech at a civic lunch in the City Chambers, the Prince expressed his interest in the forth-coming Appeal and added: 'If my visit today can help to draw any attention to the needs of the Infirmary and to the Appeal which you are making later, I can only

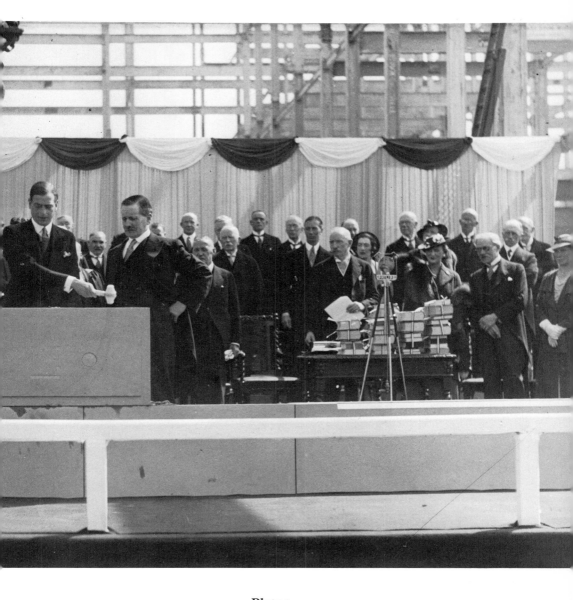

Plate 3

Simpson Memorial Maternity Pavilion, foundation stone ceremony — 22 May 1935

H.R.H. The Duke of Kent declares the stone 'well and truly laid'

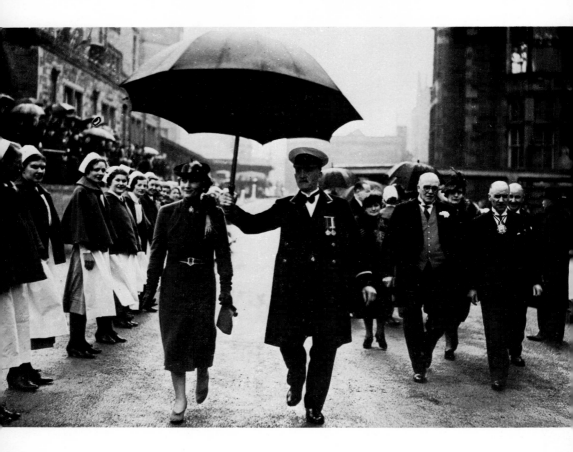

Plate 4   Simpson Memorial Maternity Pavilion — opening — 14 April 1939

Arrival of H.R.H. The Duchess of Gloucester to perform the opening ceremony. She is escorted by Mr. Alexander Strathdee, Chief Porter: on their left are Mr. J. R. Little, Chairman of Managers; Harriet Lady Findlay, former Chairman; Lord Provost Henry Steele and Lt-Col. A. D. Stewart, Superintendent.

say I am very happy indeed; and I sincerely hope you will get the funds you need for the extension for the good of the Infirmary and for this great city, the capital of Scotland'.

If that seems a brief and off-hand speech for such an occasion, it is only fair to explain that, in welcoming the Prince, the Lord Provost had forestalled him by including in his speech a detailed account of the Infirmary's extension plans and an appeal to all to contribute generously to the Fund. The Lord Provost of the day was the Rt. Hon. (later Sir) Thomas B. Whitson. No-one would have expected him to miss such an opportunity of boosting the Infirmary and his speech was given wide publicity.

When the Appeal was formally issued in October it was stated that at least £500,000 of which £80,000 had already been subscribed, would be needed to complete the new buildings, including the cost of the site. To help the Appeal, Walter McPhail, Editor of the *Edinburgh Evening News*, who was always a good friend of the Infirmary, inaugurated an 'Evening News Shilling Fund', asking readers to contribute as many, or as few, shillings as they could afford and daily lists of contributors' names were published including, even, the names of those who had given only one shilling. By the end of the first week he was able to announce that 10,192 shillings had been received. Seven years later the 'Shilling Fund' had reached more than £45,000—909,000 shillings. In acknowledgment of this help, a ward in the new Simpson Pavilion was named 'The McPhail Evening News Ward' (Ward 51).

In publicising their Appeal the Board explained that, in addition to re-housing the Simpson Memorial Maternity Hospital and providing accommodation for nurses, the new accommodation for gynaecology would release sufficient ward space in the existing Infirmary to enable an additional 2,000 patients to be treated annually. This, in turn, would effectively reduce the waiting-list which, it was said, 'bears an average of between 2,000 and 3,000 names, the majority being of patients requiring surgical treatment'. That solution of the waiting-list problem, however, turned out to be too simple to be true.

The way was now clear for the Board to instruct their Architect and Master of Works to prepare detailed plans of the new buildings, or so they believed. But it was not quite so. Before long the first of a series of difficulties arose. In July 1931 the Town Council's representative on the Board, Bailie Peter Given, suggested that the planning of such an important project should not be left to their own official but should be the subject of an open competition among qualified architects. This suggestion having been allowed to simmer in members' minds until November, twelve members then demonstrated their confidence in Thomas Turnbull by voting for him to proceed, against eight members who favoured a competition; but by way of compromise, it was then decided that an outside architect with hospital construction experience should be appointed as 'consultant and adviser'. This compromise arose in response to a protest by the Edinburgh Architectural Association who were of opinion that the design of such a project should be undertaken by a person with the full Royal Institute of British Architects' qualification (which Thomas Turnbull did not hold) and that a competition should have been arranged. The Association were only partly mollified by

D

the decision to appoint a consultant architect but did not further pursue their protest. In due course, Mr. James Miller, RSA, was appointed as consultant for the maternity and gynaecological blocks, but not for the nurses' home.

So the first difficulty was overcome, soon to be followed by a second and more far-reaching one. In February 1933 it began to be realised that, presumably because of the difficult time the country was going through, money was not being given to the main Appeal Fund as generously as had been hoped. This raised doubts as to whether the full scheme should proceed. There was also the problem of the limited area of the site although this had been slightly eased by the purchase of some houses at the south end of Archibald Place. The doubts were voiced at a Board Meeting by Lord Provost William Thomson who, showing due municipal caution and possibly having rather less personal enthusiasm for the Infirmary than his predecessor in office, expressed the view that 'it appeared to be a very dangerous policy for the Board to embark upon a large scheme of extension without any guarantee that funds would be forthcoming to maintain the enlarged hospital'.

This gave the Board members food for anxious thought. Because of their agreement with the Board of the Maternity Hospital, now sanctioned by Act of Parliament, they could not easily give up the idea of a maternity block. More accommodation for nurses was essential. So reluctantly, in April 1933, they abandoned the proposed gynaecological block and decided to proceed only with the maternity department and the nurses' home.

Where did this decision leave their much-vaunted plan to wipe out the general waiting-list? The answer was, in fact, 'nowhere'. The 'gynae' patients would have to remain in the Jubilee Pavilion which would therefore not become available for general surgery. The Board sought to put a good face on the situation by suggesting that 're-arrangements could be made within the existing buildings to provide increased accommodation for surgical patients'. No-one seems to have asked why, if that was possible now, it had not been possible three years earlier; so the coast was clear to proceed with the modified scheme with the added advantage of a little more 'breathing-space' on the site.

In consultation with Professor R. W. Johnstone who had been on the staff of the old Maternity Hospital since 1920 and knew its defects only too well, the architects made good progress with the preparation of their amended plans and in obtaining approval of them by the Infirmary Managers and the Directors of the Maternity Hospital. Then, in December 1933, an unexpected problem arose. The Edinburgh Master Builders Association had learned that it was intended to construct the outer walls of both buildings of artificial stone which was a material of which the Association did not wholly approve. A deputation from the Association received by the Managers in January 1934 alleged that artificial stone had not been sufficiently tested and was subject to 'crazing, cracking, shrinkage, discolouration and porousness'. They also said that 'it would not be in accordance with the dignity of the Infirmary or the City to erect a building on such a prominent position of anything but the best material'. Nevertheless, the Architect and Consultant Architect both pointed out that natural stone would be much more expensive and both were willing 'to stake their reputations' on the efficacy of artificial stone. On the strength of these assurances the Board decided by 18 votes to 7 that artificial stone should be used. That, however, was not the end of the matter.

The stage had been reached at which, under local building statutes, the plans had to be submitted for approval to the City of Edinburgh Dean of Guild Court, a quasi-judicial body of ancient lineage and formidable character (superseded in 1975 by the City of Edinburgh District Council Building Control Committee). The Court shared the Master Builders' dislike of artificial stone and, although usually mainly concerned with structural design and safety, they seem this time to have concentrated on appearance for, although prepared to accept artificial stone for the other elevations, they decreed 'that the character or appearance of the south eleva-tion [facing the Meadows] of the buildings proposed to be erected would be injurious to the amenity of the neighbourhood on account of the materials proposed to be used and . . . Therefore Order that the south elevation of the proposed buildings be constructed with natural stone'.

The argument continued for five months, the Infirmary Board invoking to the full the statutory appeal procedure available to them but without success. Under that procedure the final decision rested with the Town Council and in March 1935 that body, disregarding the views of their own Advisory Committee, upheld the Dean of Guild Court's decision and insisted on the use of natural stone for the south-facing front of the maternity block. There was no alternative but to comply and eventually stone brought from Blaxter quarry in Northumberland was used for the south front at an extra cost, compared with that for artificial stone, of £7,000. Later, at a meeting of Directors of the Maternity Hospital, their Chairman suggested that, as the City Fathers had been responsible for this extra expenditure, they should contribute a like amount to the building fund. There seems to be no evidence that they did so.

A sad postscript to that part of the Simpson Pavilion story is that in 1941, the Ministry of Home Security pointed out that the new buildings, seen from the air, offered too clear a target for enemy attack and must be coated overall with dark paint. This was done; and even today after 42 years, traces of that war-time camouflage still disfigure the buildings including the precious natural stone of the south front.

That dispute was not the last snag to hit the building scheme. In November 1936 the Scottish National Operative Plasterers Federal Union declared a strike. Despite strong pleas to them to exempt the Infirmary from strike action on humanitarian grounds, the Union withdrew their labour from the project, thus also holding up the work of other trades. It was not until June 1937 that the plasterers resumed work and then, for a further month, other tradesmen were on strike. In the end it was reported that a total of nearly nine months had been lost through these industrial disputes.

At last, in late February 1939, the Simpson Memorial Maternity Pavilion was ready to receive patients. From 1755 until 1793, when the Edinburgh Lying-in Hospital was opened, a few maternity beds had been provided in the old Infirmary. Now, 146 years later the Infirmary was once again ready to take responsibility for maternity care and teaching. On the first of March, under the guidance of Miss J. P. Ferlie, efficient and kindly Matron of the 'old Simpson' since 1935 who remained in charge of nursing at the Simpson Pavilion until her retiral in 1958, the patients were transferred. An article in *The Pelican*—the Infirmary nurses' magazine—described the occasion: 'It was a day of great excitement, for was not this the morning the new Pavilion was open for the admission of patients at 8 o'clock? At 2.30 a fleet of ambulances had been engaged to move the patients from the old hospital to the new; V.A.D.s helped this work and in exactly one hour and one minute, forty-nine mothers and their babes found themselves in their new surroundings. Nurses and patients were full of bewilderment and joy— large spacious wards, balcony doors open and the warm spring sunshine coming in. Tea was served to delighted patients many of whom had already donned ear-phones and were listening to the strains of soft music. The least concerned were the babies. Even air-conditioned nurseries were beneath their notice.'

Two days later more patients were transferred and the Superintendent reported that all had gone well and that there were now 84 mothers and 60 babies in the new building. The Board expressed thanks to all who had helped in the transfer, especially to the City Police who had lent four ambulances and the St. Andrew's Ambulance Association who had lent three—for there was then no comprehensive ambulance service, as there has been since 1948.

A doctor who worked in the old Maternity Hospital described it, in its last days, as 'obstetrically a slum'. At the front door a large handbell was provided which when rung by an approaching patient would bring a nurse scurrying to her assistance, the degree of urgency having been 'clearly indicated by the vigour with which the bell's clangour broke forth'. The labour ward contained five beds, inadequately screened and when an operation was necessary it was performed on an operating table brought into the centre of the ward, the other four beds with their patients having been wheeled temporarily to one end of the room. After such conditions, the patients transferred to the new Simpson might well have been 'full of bewilderment and joy'. The new building, five storeys high on the south and two storeys on the north, had 122 beds all in wards facing south some with balconies on to which (weather permitting) beds might be wheeled. No ward contained more than six beds and there were twelve single rooms. Nurseries, incubator rooms, milk preparation and other ancillary rooms were conveniently arranged and there were properly equipped labour and delivery rooms, an operating theatre and provision for students and pupil midwives to receive instruction. On the ground floor a welcoming reception area was provided (with no need for a hand-bell) and there were well planned rooms in which to carry on the ante-natal and post-natal clinics that had been pioneered in the old hospital.

A word must be said about that pioneering work, even though to do so involves a leap back in time. However shocking the primitive conditions in the old hospital may seem to us, there can be no denying the value of the devoted work carried on there by generations of physicians and midwives. Among the distinguished obstetricians who had served it in several capacities, medical and administrative, were Dr. J. W. Ballantyne, from 1884 to 1923 and Dr. Haig Ferguson from 1899 to 1927. As a result of Dr. Ferguson's experience of giving ante-natal care to unmarried mothers in the nearby Lauriston Home for Maternity Rescue Work (afterwards, 'The Haig Ferguson Memorial Maternity Home') these two doctors started an out-patient clinic for ante-natal attention and advice, which, by 1915, had become an important and busy department of the Simpson Memorial Hospital. Two years later the work of the clinic was integrated into the newly-established local authority maternity and child welfare scheme under which a network of such clinics came into being throughout the city. From these beginnings acceptance of the need for systematic ante-natal care grew and spread throughout the United Kingdom and across the world. In 1928 a post-natal out-patient baby clinic was started which quickly proved its worth and became an established feature of child care at the old hospital. Naturally, with such a background, the most up-to-date facilities possible for ante-natal and post-natal care were provided in the new Simpson Pavilion.

The foundation stone of the new pavilion had been laid on 22 May 1935 by the Duke of Kent (then Lord High Commissioner to the General Assembly of the Church of Scotland). He was accompanied by the Duchess who presented prizes 'to those of the nurses who had excelled in conduct and examination during their training'. On an afternoon of brilliant sunshine they had been watched by the Prime Minister (J. Ramsay Macdonald) and his daughter; the Duke and Duchess of Atholl; Sir Godfrey Collins, Secretary of State for Scotland; Sir Thomas Whitson, Chairman of the Board and a crowd of 4,000 people including 300 nurses in uniform and the choir of the High Kirk of St. Giles in their purple robes. 'Other onlookers' according to the next day's *Scotsman*, included 'workmen employed on erecting the new pavilion, the skeleton of which rose gaunt and high behind the platform. Perched on girders and scaffolding, these men in their working overalls had a bird's eye view of a scene which had colour as well as animation.'

The scene was different when the new Pavilion and the new nurses' home—which it had been decided to name the 'Florence Nightingale Home'—were formally opened on 14 April 1939 by Her Royal Highness The Duchess of Gloucester. Then, another distinguished gathering which included the Secretary of State for Scotland (Mr. John Colville), Lord Provost Henry Steele and Mr. J. R. Little, Chairman of the Board, sat in pouring rain under a roof of umbrellas while the Duchess, protected by a rain-drenched awning, declared the new Maternity Pavilion open. Later, in the greater comfort of the handsome recreation room of the new nurses' home, she declared that building open also. Explaining the choice of name for the Nurses' Home, Mr. J. W. Struthers, then the senior member of the Infirmary's honorary surgical staff, referred to Florence Nightingale's links with the Infirmary. She had visited the old Infirmary twice and the Lady Superintendent of Nurses had in her keeping a long letter from Miss Nightingale addressed to 'my dear nurses of the Edinburgh Infirmary'. That, coupled with the inspiration derived by nurses everywhere from Miss Nightingale's example, fully explained the choice.

Between the two ceremonies the Duchess toured the Simpson Pavilion in which, by this time, there were 122 mothers and 92 babies. Four babies, two boys and two girls, had been born that morning and the Chairman delightedly reported to the Duchess that, in honour of her and her husband, the girls were to be named Alice and the boys Henry.

Thus, on that Royal and rainy occasion, after 11 years of discussion and planning and five years of interrupted building, the Simpson Memorial Pavilion became officially a going concern. In *The Scotsman* of the following day, the Board of Managers announced that the whole scheme, including the Nurses' Home, and consequential additions to kitchen, laundry and other departments had cost over £500,000 to meet which a further £85,000 was still required. The opening of the new buildings, they said, would involve an extra annual expenditure of £30,000. 'But' they proudly added, the splendid new maternity pavilion 'is as up-to-date as medical science can make it and there is not a better equipped building in the world. Britain's greatest Voluntary Hospital still leads in this most important branch of service to humanity.'

George and Agnes Murray Home

The point we have now reached, at the climax of Thomas Turnbull's contributions to hospital building in the late nineteen-thirties, is perhaps a good one at which to recall one of the projects, on a much smaller scale, which he carried out for the Royal Infirmary Managers at the beginning of that decade—the design and building of the George and Agnes Murray Home.

Miss Helen Murray, formerly of Edinburgh, had died at Melrose in 1918, leaving to the Royal Infirmary the residue of her estate (£51,500) to found a home near the city for wounded and invalided British soldiers and sailors, the home to be named 'The George and Agnes Murray Home' in memory of her parents and her brother and sisters. Under her bequest the Home was fully endowed and she had expressed the hope that if the time came when it was no longer needed for its primary purpose, it could be used as a convalescent home for patients from the Royal Infirmary.

In 1923 the Managers bought (for £4,500) the mansionhouse and 24-acre estate of Moredun on the south of the city, near the village of Gilmerton. The intention of the Managers had been to convert the house to the new purpose. It was found, however, to be badly affected by dry rot and had to be demolished. In its place, Turnbull planned a two-storey building to accommodate twenty pensioners, each with a separate bedroom.

The Murray Home was opened by the Prince of Wales on 12 July 1930, the day on which he also visited the Infirmary and, in his speech at the civic lunch party, made his concise contribution to the launching of the Infirmary building fund. At the new Home he planted a tree and highly commended both the purpose of the Home and its design. The design included a small range of workshops in which some of the residents could indulge in various handicrafts. Others were encouraged to look after the grounds and gardens and to keep bees and poultry; the poultry-keeping being so successful that the Managers' Report for the year 1941 records that 700 dozen eggs had been supplied to the Infirmary 'which, in the existing stringency, have been most welcome'.

The Home continued to serve its valuable purpose for more than fifty years. Not being regarded as a hospital, it was not transferred to the National Health Service in 1948 but was afterwards administered separately by Trustees who initially included former members of the Infirmary Board. By 1978, however, rising costs of maintenance had inevitably outstripped the funds available to the Trustees from Miss Murray's bequest. They therefore submitted a petition to the Court of Session and, with the Court's consent, arrangements were made for the Home, still with some 20 residents, and its grounds (by then reduced to 14 acres) to be transferred to an organisation with somewhat similar aims, the Whitefoord House and Rosandael Scottish Naval, Military and Air Force Veterans' Residences. The continuing welfare of the Murray Home's residents was thus assured.

Radium and X-Rays

Until the 1920s, almost the only hope for the patient suffering from a malignant tumour was to have the tumour, if possible, removed by surgery; and many general surgical cases in the Infirmary were in that category. Then came X-rays and radium treatment and the position changed greatly—though surgery for such cases did not disappear. From, say, 1925 onwards cases of cancer fell into three categories—those best treated by surgery, those best treated by deep X-ray therapy and those best treated by the application of radium. These categories, of course, were not always mutually exclusive and it could be said that cases requiring a combination of two of these methods, or sometimes all three, formed a fourth group. That being so, it seems fairly obvious that an essential factor in ensuring the best treatment for a patient would be consultation and collaboration between surgeon and radio-therapist. In the early days of radium and radio-therapy treatments, however, such collaboration did not always take place and there was even, at times, a lack of contact between those who favoured the use of radium and those intent on exploiting fully the benefits of X-ray therapy. At one stage the type of treatment received might depend more on the preference of the practitioner to whom a patient was directed than on an objective assessment of his treatment needs.

The Royal Infirmary was early in the field with its use of X-rays, both for diagnostic purposes generally and for the treatment of cancer and also in its use of radium. The close relationship between radium treatment and deep X-ray therapy was soon recognised. The bringing together of surgeon and radio-therapist in full and equal association took a little longer, but, during the 1930s, that also was achieved and was one of the most important contributions to the efficiency of cancer treatment in the Infirmary during those years.

There had been a 'medical electrical department' in the Infirmary since 1898 when it was introduced, as if by an afterthought, as a corollary to the conversion of the hospital lighting system from gas to electricity. That was only one year after Wilhelm Röntgen, in Germany, had made his great discovery of X-rays and their power to enable matter to be 'seen through'.

As a result, by 1898, the Infirmary's first medical electrical department was established in cramped quarters formerly used as a splint store and a plumbers' workshop. In 1904, the Department moved to larger premises in the basement of the south-eastern ward block of the surgical house. By the 1920s, following the extension of the use of X-rays from photography for diagnostic purposes to their application to the treatment of cancer and other conditions, the equipment was soon out-dated and the accommodation quite insufficient. So it was decided to build and equip a new radiological department beside the 'duodenum', roughly midway between the surgical and medical houses where the department, much altered, is still situated.

On 9 October 1926 the new department was opened by the Duke of York (later King George VI). The building had been designed by Thomas Turnbull to meet the requirements of Dr. J. Woodburn Morison who was the Infirmary's Radiologist from 1925 till his resignation in 1930 to become Professor of Radiology at London University. The building was specially planned to accommodate the most up-to-date equipment of those days, much of which had been 'tailor-made'. Given the care that had gone into the planning of both building and equipment, it is not surprising that it was said of the department at the time that it was 'the largest and most completely equipped institution of its kind in Europe; indeed it is doubtful if its equal exists in any country. Moreover, it is also probably the only department of its kind which has been planned, built and equipped from start to finish, entirely for X-ray work and electro-medical treatment, which is the logical method of attaining the high degree of efficiency demanded in modern hospitals.' The cost of building and equipment was £52,000 towards which the Edinburgh Committee of the Scottish Branch of the British Red Cross Society had contributed £15,000.

An important feature in the planning of the new department had been the care taken to ensure protection against the dangers of too great or too frequent exposure to X-rays. These dangers in the past had not always been fully understood and the Infirmary, soon afterwards, had sad reason to be aware of them. Two of their electro-medical specialists are remembered as martyrs in the cause of radio-logical progress. They were Dr. Dawson Turner who had joined the electro-medical department in 1896 and Dr. Hope Fowler, CVO, who had joined in 1901. They retired in 1925 and 1926 respectively. Both suffered the effects of radiation for many years and both died as a result, Dawson Turner in 1928 and Hope Fowler in 1933. Along with John Spence, Dawson Turner's assistant from 1901 to 1907 and afterwards Radiologist at the Royal Hospital for Sick Children, they are commemorated on a memorial stone at St. George's Hospital, Hamburg, among 169 pioneers of radiology in many countries who lost their lives as a result of their work with X-rays; and in the Radiology Department of the Infirmary there is a plaque in memory of Dawson Turner: 'Pioneer and founder of Roentgen Ray and Radium Work in the Royal Infirmary'.

To ensure the safety of operators and others in the new building exhaustive experiments were undertaken as a result of which the walls of the Department were constructed of concrete slabs into which barium sulphate had been introduced in the proportion found to give the highest possible level of protection combined with sufficient strength. The walls were also coated on both sides with barium plaster. Radiographic screening rooms for diagnosis and treatment rooms for deep and superficial X-ray therapy were on the ground floor, along with a lecture room and ancillary accommodation; upstairs were rooms for electrical therapy and massage. The basement contained a machine-room with generators, trans-formers and switchboard.

Having established an up-to-date radio-therapy department, the Board of Managers turned their attention to improving and increasing the facilities for the use of radium in the treatment of cancer. For some years the Infirmary had owned a small quantity of radium contained in 'plaques' and 'needles'. These were stored in a specially protective safe and issued, as required, to wards where they were applied or implanted by the surgeon in charge. Radium was very expensive. (An anonymous donation of £5,000 was used for the purchase of about half a gramme in 1929). The effects of radium, where not intended, could be dangerous and the needles were tiny and slim. So the strictest instructions for its handling were issued. Despite that, in those early years, the minutes contain surprisingly frequent references to the loss of radium needles, such occasions setting in train dramatic and wide-ranging searches (not always successful) in wards, beds, cupboards, corridors and drains. Yet in 1931, Sir David Wallace, Consulting Surgeon, had assured the Board that their system for the care of radium 'had been accepted as a model for other centres and they might rest content that everything possible was being done in this connection'.

The system of issuing radium to whatever ward, at the time, had patients requiring its use was not altogether satisfactory. The number of beds available varied from time to time and control of admissions to ensure that the cases most urgently requiring, or most likely to benefit from radium treatment were given priority, was difficult or impossible to achieve. So the Board turned their attention to the possibility of allocating a number of beds specifically for the use of such patients.

It so happened that Lady Mary Anderson, widow of Sir George Anderson, Treasurer of the Bank of Scotland from 1898 to 1917, had bequeathed to the Infirmary their mansionhouse 'Beechmount' which he had built on the southern slope of Corstorphine Hill in 1900. It was a fine house about half a mile east of the Infirmary's 'Convalescent House' (now Corstorphine Hospital) with a wide open view towards the Pentland Hills and across the city. On Lady Anderson's death in 1926 it had come into the Infirmary's possession and had been let pending a decision on its use. On 17 December 1928 the Managers unanimously approved 'of the establishment of a Radium Institute for the treatment of patients suffering from Cancer and other conditions which are amenable to Radium; that the scheme to reconstruct "Beechmount" their property at Murrayfield for this purpose be adopted and that if necessary a sum of £40,000 be taken from the unrestricted funds of the Infirmary to be utilised to carry this out. That the Institute should be capable of accommodating 36 in-patients and should serve more especially Edinburgh and the South-eastern area of Scotland.' In the following year, however, this scheme was modified. Beechmount, instead of being developed as a full-scale 'radium institute' was adapted and enlarged at a cost of £11,000 for use, in effect, as a radium annexe to the Infirmary.

There had been for some time a widespread awareness of the need to encourage the development of all possible means of combating cancer and in 1929 *The Times* newspaper launched a nationwide appeal for funds for this purpose as a mark of thankfulness for the recent recovery of King George V from a serious illness. It had been decided that the fund should be used, in part, for the purchase of radium which could be distributed throughout the country. A Radium Trust and a National Radium Commission were established in London, the Trust to hold supplies of radium as it was purchased and the Commission to deal with its distribution and use, 'having regard to the advancement of knowledge, the treatment of the sick and economy of use'. In September 1929 the Commission held their first meeting and announced that in deciding which institutions should receive supplies of radium from them they would give preference 'in the first instance, to centres where radium therapy could be combined with teaching and research'. *The Times*, in commending this policy, explained that progress in radium treatment had hitherto been hindered by its faulty application by doctors with insufficient knowledge. The number of doctors suitably qualified was small and so supplies must be concentrated where it would be used most effectively for treatment and teaching.

The Commission divided the country into districts, each with a large teaching hospital at its centre and selected the Royal Infirmary as the Centre for South-east Scotland, a decision received with much satisfaction by the Managers; though not without a preliminary protest on finding that, in accordance with the Commission's general policy, communication between the Commission and the Board was to be conducted through the Dean of the Medical Faculty of Edinburgh University and not with the hospital direct. However, having recovered from that minor set-back to their self-esteem, the Managers, in March 1930, were glad to enter into a formal agreement under which the Commission, on the recommendation of the Faculty of Medicine, were to provide the Infirmary with a supply of radium on loan at a moderate rental plus the cost of its insurance and subject to certain conditions as to its use. Among these conditions was a stipulation that a scheme for the use of the radium for treatment, teaching and research would be drawn up jointly by the Infirmary and the University. Full records of treatment and 'follow-up' were to be maintained and the Infirmary were required 'to accept and to treat suitable and properly accredited patients from any source including such as come from rate-aided institutions, the selection of patients to be left to the discretion of the Hospital guided by the principle that the need and suitability of the patient for radium treatment shall be the sole determining factors in selection'.

By October 1931 the National Radium Commission were becoming impatient. The Infirmary had taken up only a small part of the radium allocated and the Commission were not wholly satisfied with the scheme for the use of Beechmount. However, after some tactful explanations had been given the Commission accepted the Beechmount plan on the understanding that it would be regarded as a temporary scheme, later to be extended and improved.

Beechmount was opened in October 1932 with 36 beds. At first many of the patients received treatment at the Infirmary and went to Beechmount for convalescence thus allowing a somewhat quicker 'turnover' of beds at the Infirmary but not really achieving what had been intended. Before long, however, this changed and most of the treatment was given at Beechmount though some patients there who required deep X-ray therapy had to endure the discomfort of repeated ambulance journeys between the two centres.

In 1934 history was made when Beechmount became the first hospital outside London to receive what was then known as a radium 'bomb'. This was a large concentration of radium element enclosed in a 'bomb-head' mechanism which enabled its effects to be directed towards an affected spot for a specified time. To house this safely, further adaptations had to be undertaken at Beechmount and to justify the holding of so large a supply of radium there, staffing and other arrangements were adapted to enable it to be used day and night.

The surgeon-in-charge and co-ordinator at Beechmount from the beginning was Mr. J. J. M. Shaw, then an Assistant Surgeon on the Infirmary's Honorary Staff. He had as his Assistant Dr. Margaret C. Tod, Associate Assistant Surgeon (Radium Therapy) who made an outstanding contribution to the pioneering work at Beechmount during her all too short stay there. She left in 1937 to become Assistant (later, Deputy) Director of the Holt Radium Institute in Manchester. Shaw was a highly skilled and greatly admired general surgeon who had come to have a particular interest in plastic surgery and in the application of X-rays and radium to cancer treatment. Having served with distinction in the first world war, he was again commissioned in 1939, becoming Consultant Surgeon to Army G.H.Q., Cairo. Tragically he died of disease contracted there, less than a year later, at the age of 54.

In addition to his professional skills, J. J. M. Shaw had a flair for administration and a deep interest in the advancement of any administrative arrangements designed to bring the benefits of such skills to those most requiring them. So it was not surprising that he was appointed a member of the National Radium Trust and the National Radium Commission. He also took a leading part in the setting-up in 1934 of the Cancer Control Organisation for Edinburgh and South East Scotland. This was a broadly based, pioneer body of influential citizens concerned to raise funds for the provision of facilities for treatment; to undertake publicity including propaganda against the all too common tendency to delay seeking treatment for cancer until cure became difficult or impossible; and to make grants to help patients to maintain regular attendance at treatment centres and follow-up departments. The Organisation gave valuable financial aid to the Infirmary including a sum of £1,400 to defray the cost of providing a new 'bomb-head' at Beechmount. The Organisation also played a pioneer part in the setting up of an efficient 'follow-up' organisation to assist in ensuring regular attendance of patients requiring further treatment and in the assessment of results; work which still forms an important part of the Health Board's arrangements for dealing with the problem of cancer.

Although Beechmount was established for the benefit of cancer patients, J. J. M. Shaw, well aware of the widespread fear of that disease, was anxious that it should not be branded in the public mind as being exclusively a 'cancer hospital'. He therefore arranged for it to be used from time to time for other purposes including some of his own plastic surgery operations. Miss M. C. Marshall, the first Matron of Beechmount (and later Lady Superintendent of Nurses at the Royal Infirmary) was also aware of the image of Beechmount that might arise in people's minds and, in a magazine article in 1935, she wrote: 'Many people seem to have the idea that Beechmount is a depressing place, but that is quite a mistake as the atmosphere is particularly cheerful. The results of radium treatment are encouraging, especially when the patients come early and even in later cases a good deal can be done to alleviate pain.'

By 1936, Mr. Shaw was able to report to the Managers that 'Treatment of malignant disease in certain situations such as the throat by means of the radium mass unit or "bomb" has surpassed anything previously known'. Beechmount continued to be used principally for treatment by radium until 1939 when, on the outbreak of war it became an auxiliary hospital and its radium was removed to the Infirmary for safe-keeping.

To return, now, to the radiology department in the Infirmary: following the resignation of Dr. Woodburn Morison in 1930, Dr. J. Duncan White from London was appointed in 1931 but he returned to London to take up a new appointment there in 1934. His successor, Dr. A. E. Barclay of Cambridge, set about introducing new equipment to the department and a Metropolitan-Vickers apparatus for deep X-ray was introduced at a cost of just over £5,000. Of this machine the Managers wrote in their report for 1936-37 that it 'had been specially designed and had the great advantage of lessening the period of treatment, enabling more patients to be dealt with'.

Dr. Barclay was dogged by ill-health as a result of which he had to resign in 1935. This change in control, coming so soon after the previous change, would have been particularly regrettable at that time when radiology was moving steadily from the stage of trial and experiment to become fully accepted as a scientific discipline; but, fortunately, Dr. Barclay's arrival had been accompanied by the appointment as a senior assistant radiologist of Dr. (later Professor) Robert McWhirter. He was a Fellow of the Royal College of Surgeons of Edinburgh, had been a Research Fellow of the Holt Radium Institute, had worked in radiology in the Mayo Clinic in Rochester, USA, and elsewhere, so it was not surprising that he was appointed to succeed Dr. Barclay as Radiologist to the Infirmary. Soon afterwards he was appointed by the University as a lecturer in radiology.

Dr. McWhirter's experience enabled him to take full advantage of recent rapid advances in technology and so to introduce more precise scientifically measured assessments and treatments than had previously been possible. To achieve this fully, he persuaded the Managers, in accordance with a National Radium Commission recommendation, to appoint a Physicist—Dr. C. A. Murison—to the department who would undertake the scientific calibration of the X-ray therapy tubes and of the radium 'bomb', advise on repairs to radium containers and tests for leakages and prepare other estimations thus ensuring continuous efficiency and reducing expense. Dr. Murison continued as a Physicist at the Infirmary until 1955, after which he was based at the Western General Hospital.

On the diagnostic side of the department's work—control of which had not yet been separated from that of radio-therapy—the practice had previously tended to be simply to point out on the X-ray film any abnormality, leaving its exact nature or cause to be identified by the surgeon in charge of the patient. The aim now was, whenever possible, to offer a more positive analysis of the condition revealed by the film.

Soon after his appointment, Dr. McWhirter submitted a comprehensive report on the state of the department, with plans for its improvement. It is a mark of the difference between the old and the new approaches that, while Dr. Duncan White, on leaving in 1934, had suggested that a sum of under £500 would bring the department sufficiently up-to-date, Dr. McWhirter's report in 1936 stated that 'all the old apparatus in the department is either out-of-date or useless and should be replaced by modern apparatus before satisfactory results can be achieved'. He therefore recommended the provision of additional items of modern equipment and extensive adaptation of the building. To their credit, the Managers accepted his recommendations and the improvements were put in hand in the hope, as they expressed it, 'that this special branch of the Infirmary's work will make a particular appeal and that the requisite funds will be forthcoming to meet the capital cost involved and also the large increase in maintenance expenses which will necessarily follow'. Four years later they reported that the work had been completed at a cost (including £5,000 for the new apparatus already installed) of £14,500 for equipment and £7,660 for reconstruction. The staff also had been greatly increased. By these means the Managers agreed 'a most important and beneficent work is being done—the results in many cases have been extremely gratifying'.

A year later they reported that the work of the Department, especially on the treatment side, had necessarily been interrupted by the outbreak of war 'but after a comparatively brief interval, a complete service was resumed and the department is now functioning at practically full pressure'.

Growth of Specialisation

Until the second quarter of this century few of the physicians and surgeons appointed to the general wards of the Royal Infirmary wished to be designated as specialists. Most preferred to be seen as being competent in all fields of either medicine or surgery. As explained earlier, however, there were several who within a wide range of practice took a particular interest, and developed skills, in one branch of their profession more than others—for example, in ear, nose and throat surgery and in ophthalmology, for both of which, as we have seen, special pavilions were built as early as 1903.

A prime example of a skilful general surgeon who became a distinguished specialist but remained a general surgeon at heart was Mr. (later Sir) Henry Wade. Between 1924 and his retiral in 1939 he took the leading part in developing, in Wards 15 and 16 and the diagnostic theatre what became in effect, if not in name, a department of urology; and there he acquired a world-wide reputation as specialist in that branch of surgery. Yet, until his retiral—and indeed to the end of his life in 1955—he preferred to regard himself as a general surgeon.

However, scientific and medical advances in the 1920s and 1930s were growing so rapidly that specialisation began to be the only practical means of keeping abreast of progress in certain fields. How some important specialties developed in the Infirmary during that period is the subject of the following sections.

Dietetics

Nowadays the profession of dietitian is one of several para-medical professions which play an important part in restoring and maintaining the health of hospital patients. Its practitioners work closely with physicians and nurses and, as part of their training, nurses are instructed in its theory and techniques. In the 1920s and 1930s dietetics had begun to emerge as a new medical specialty in the development of which a few physicians, aided by nurses with a special interest in the subject, led the way. In that development the Royal Infirmary played a pioneering role in this country. The practice of dietetics was begun in the Infirmary medical wards by Professor Jonathan Meakins, Professor of Therapeutics from 1919 until 1924 and it was enthusiastically continued by his successor in that Chair, Professor D. Murray Lyon, from 1924 until 1936 and by Professor (later Sir) Derrick Dunlop who occupied the Chair from 1936 until his retiral in 1962.

Although physicians had long taken an interest in their patients' food, prescribing for example a 'milk diet' or a 'light diet' for various ailments, the idea of the systematic control of diet adjusted to the individual patient and to the particular disease is of comparatively recent origin. In the Royal Infirmary it arose from the report of a committee appointed by the Board of Managers in 1920 to consider dietetic arrangements in the hospital. They recommended the appointment of a dietitian whose duties as well as being 'advisory and administrative in the general kitchen' would be 'educational and operative in directly providing or supervising the provision of special diets for individual patients'. Until then no-one on the staff had been given responsibilities of that kind and there were no trained dietitians in the country. Regulation of patients' diets in accordance with a physician's wishes, if any, was left to the ward sister concerned who might, or might not, have the appropriate knowledge or aptitude.

The Committee's recommendation was approved and Professor Meakins set about the task of introducing the practice of dietetics in Wards 25 and 26. There he had the eager co-operation of Sister Ruth Pybus, fully supported by the Lady Superintendent of Nurses, Miss Annie Warren Gill, whose interest in the subject is still recalled by the annual award of the Annie Warren Gill memorial prize for nurses proficient in dietetics. In 1925 Miss Pybus was awarded a Rockefeller Foundation scholarship, enabling her to study the work of dietitians in America. Back in Edinburgh, under the guidance of Professor Murray Lyon, she became one of the leading dietitians in this country.

In 1922 insulin, recently discovered, had been used in Canada for the first time in the treatment of diabetes and it was introduced to the wards of the Infirmary a year later. From then on the treatment of diabetic sufferers both by use of insulin and by the scientific regulation of their diets was pursued in the Infirmary with growing success. At first diabetic out-patients were interviewed in an alcove off the medical corridor near Ward 25 but in 1926 more suitable accommodation was found in the space below Ward 2 (then at the south-east end of the surgical house) which had been vacated by the removal of the 'medical electric department' to the new radiology building. From then on the clinic grew into one of the largest diabetic clinics in the country. A continuing problem of those days was that of ensuring that the diet prescribed could be consistently followed at home by patients, many of whom could not afford to buy the kind of food prescribed or supply themselves with scales for weighing the correct amounts. In such cases help was often given by the Infirmary almoner to out-patients and by the almoners of the Edinburgh Royal Infirmary Samaritan Society to in-patients returning home.

The co-operation of the successive Professors and Sister Pybus was often sought by the chiefs and sisters of other wards, surgical as well as medical, in dealing with diabetic patients, although in those early days there were some ward sisters who regarded the feeding of their patients as a matter for their own judgement and would accept no outside help. It seems, however, that such die-hards were, in time, won over by Sister Pybus's firm but friendly personality and her infectious enthusiasm.

When the clinical laboratory, funded largely by the Rockefeller Foundation was built in 1928 there were attached to it two research wards with six beds each, served by a dietetic kitchen. Designed to serve these twelve beds, it was soon called upon to provide special meals for many more patients. By 1938 it was grossly overloaded and Professor Dunlop found it necessary to send an impassioned plea to the Board of Managers for its extension or replacement. 'A kitchen designed to supply diets for twelve patients' he wrote 'now supplies them to forty or fifty a day and each case is an individual problem. In consequence, the accuracy of the work is suffering, the staff are becoming overstrained and the chaos in the kitchen at meal-times is considerable. Last month, for instance, there were 93 breakages, largely owing to the fact that there is only one sink in the kitchen and that it is becoming increasingly difficult to move about without treading on the trays perforce deposited on the floor.'

Despite the strength of that appeal—and partly because the outbreak of war brought other requirements to the fore—it was not found possible to do more than make minor improvements until, at last, in 1966 a new and up-to-date diet kitchen was provided. How, given such conditions, the department was able to become a leading dietetic centre and training school is difficult to understand but it did, partly because a large proportion of its work consisted not in providing meals but in giving advice on diets, but mainly because of the interest and enthusiasm of those who worked in it.

Treatment through diet, of course, was not confined to sufferers from diabetes. It was adopted also in dealing with other conditions including obesity, malnutrition and gastro-intestinal disorders. Already in 1931, Dr. Derrick Dunlop and a colleague had made a study of 523 cases of obesity and the effectiveness of the treatments, including diets, prescribed for them. In the following year they studied the records of 128 patients who had been treated for peptic ulcer in the medical wards and in the dietetic clinic. In thanking Professor Murray Lyon for his co-operation, the authors recorded also their appreciation of the willing and helpful way in which Sister Pybus had collaborated with them. Six years later, in 1938, a paper appeared in *The Edinburgh Medical Journal* on 'The Dietetic Treatment of the Average Diabetic' written jointly by Professor Dunlop and Sister Pybus. These were only three of many fruitful studies based on the work of the Infirmary Dietetic Clinic in the nineteen-thirties.

Sister Pybus had, as her senior assistant, an equally enthusiastic dietitian in Sister Anna Buchan who, in 1932, also gained a Rockefeller Scholarship enabling her to study in Columbia University, New York and to visit dietetic departments in hospitals in America and Canada. After her return and perhaps because of her report on training arrangements in those countries, the Managers decided to open a School of Dietetics in the Infirmary. The first formal training centre for dietitians in this country, it was opened in 1934 with provision for an 18-months diploma course suitable for state registered nurses, holders of domestic science diplomas and others. It was financed entirely from students' fees and so incurred no drain on the Infirmary's resources. Any loss of staff time during tuition was compensated by the contribution students could make to the work of the diet kitchen during their practical training. In the first session twenty students enrolled. They included seven nurses of whom four had come from Australia and only three from the Infirmary. Of the others, three held B.Sc. degrees and ten held diplomas in domestic science.

Between 20 and 25 students enrolled for the course in most later years but the school had to be closed for the 1939-40 session because of uncertainty about the likely effect of the war. Courses resumed, however, in 1940-41 and the school continued successfully until 1955. By then, for nurses, the practice of dietetics was an integral part of training and for others adequate training was available elsewhere. So the school was closed.

Such was the reputation of Sister Ruth Pybus that during the war years she was released for a time at the request of the Department of Health for Scotland, to act as consultant dietitian in connection with their emergency hospitals, and in 1945 she received the honour of OBE. The Infirmary's pioneering contribution to the science and practice of dietetic treatment is surely an outstanding early example of the progress that can be made by physician and trained nurse and, later, professional dietitian, working in a special field in close and equal collaboration.

Orthopaedics

As a specialty in its own right in the Royal Infirmary, orthopaedics dates from 1936, its chief exponents then being Mr. (later Sir) Walter Mercer, Honorary Assistant Surgeon to Professor (later Sir) John Fraser, in Wards 7/8 and Mr. William A. Cochrane, Associate Assistant Surgeon with Professor David Wilkie in Wards 13/14. Both were general surgeons who had had valuable orthopaedic experience and who were deeply interested in that work. Mercer had worked with the Ministry of Pensions in the care and treatment of first world war pensioners and Cochrane had worked with Sir Harold Stiles at Bangour Hospital when it was in use as a casualty hospital during and after that war; he had also served for a time on the staff of Massachusetts General Hospital, Boston, USA, dealing with orthopaedic cases.

One suspects, however, that the provision, at that time, of specialist facilities for orthopaedics in the Infirmary occurred mainly because of the great success of the Princess Margaret Rose Hospital for Crippled Children, as it was then called, at Fairmilehead, Edinburgh. In 1936 it had been in use for just four years and in its establishment William Cochrane had played a leading part.

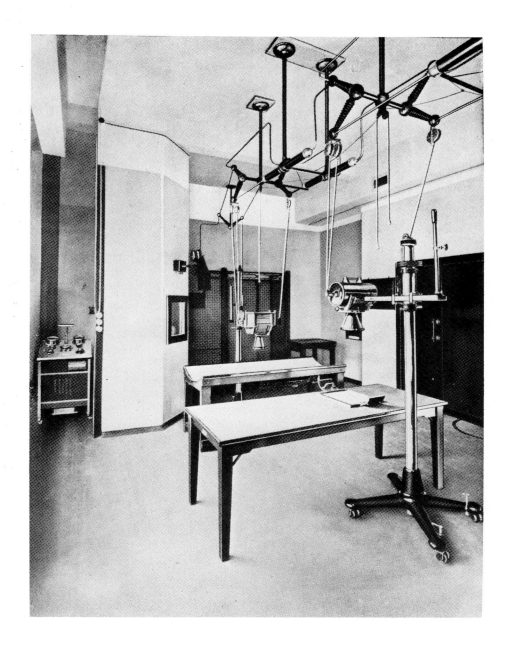

Plate 5   The latest radiology equipment in 1929

A room in the Infirmary Radiological Department, opened in
1926. The department was then described as 'the largest and
finest X-ray and electro-medical installation in existence'.

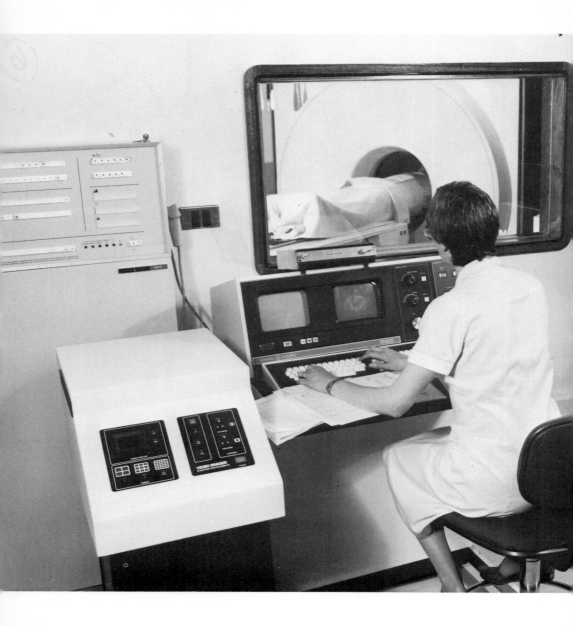

Plate 6   The latest radiology equipment in 1979
The computed tomography scanner, or 'whole body scanner' seen from its control room

It had long been recognised that facilities for treating children who were crippled either through disease or injury were gravely inadequate and in the 1920s, it was calculated that there were at least 1,000 children under 16 in South-east Scotland suffering from crippling conditions of one kind or another for whom less than 100 beds were available in the whole area. As orthopaedic treatment usually involves a long stay in hospital, that number of beds was very far from being enough and, in any case, they were scattered and unco-ordinated. So Cochrane, with the backing of a dedicated committee of voluntary workers who included Harriet, Lady Findlay and the Rev. T. Ratcliffe Barnet of Greenbank Church, Edinburgh, energetically set about raising funds to finance the building of a hospital for crippled children on a magnificent hillside site on the south side of the city. It received its first patients in June 1932. Two years later, as befitting a hospital for children, and with the gracious consent of the Duke and Duchess of York, it was named after Princess Margaret Rose, then just four years old. It had 125 beds in five wards with operating theatres and all other necessary facilities. William A. Cochrane, while still remaining on the Honorary Staff of the Infirmary, was appointed its first surgeon-in-charge. The new hospital served as the key-point in a scheme under which children could be referred to it from local authority child welfare clinics throughout the south-eastern area, each of which had a trained orthopaedic nurse in attendance and each of which was visited regularly by an orthopaedic surgeon from the hospital. In those days, still within the memory of many, vitamin deficiency and under-nourishment were common causes of rickets and other crippling diseases in children which, now, are almost never seen. So such a scheme was very necessary and through it a great deal of good work was done.

By contrast with that comprehensive, modern provision for children, the provision for adults requiring orthopaedic attention was totally inadequate, in fact almost non-existent, as they simply had to take their place in the general wards. Apart from those suffering from crippling diseases, the number injured in road traffic and industrial accidents was steadily increasing.

Any prospect of providing facilities at the Royal Infirmary for adults to match those at Fairmilehead for children was obviously too remote to be considered, because of both cost and lack of space. So it was decided to make the best possible provision in part of the accommodation which had been vacated in June 1936 when the dermatology patients had been moved to their new pavilion. Accordingly the main part of Ward 2 was re-floored, repainted and equipped to accommodate 12 male patients and a side ward was adapted to take four beds for women. Side rooms were fitted out for use as plaster room, examination room and records storage. The maintenance of records is important in any hospital department but particularly so in a specialty like orthopaedics where effects are long-term and results of operation or treatment can be assessed only over many years. The system of recording such cases had been far from adequate under the old regime where the patients had been scattered among several wards. Now, although it was still not possible for all orthopaedic cases to be kept together, an attempt was made to introduce a records system which would be of long-term value in treatment, follow-up and research.

E

The new department had no operating theatre of its own. Operations were performed, in the afternoons only, in the theatre attached to Wards 7 and 8. For that reason, as well as others, it was regarded at the time as being no more than 'a reasonably complete unit . . . the nucleus from which further development will spring'.

The department was opened on 5 November 1936 by Sir Thomas Whitson. 'The work of the department', he said, 'will be carried on by specially trained members of the surgical staff and all the medical men in the Infirmary have been most enthusiastic in their support of the project'. He referred to the great work for children being done in the hospital at Fairmilehead and expressed the hope that a similarly co-ordinated scheme might be developed for adults with the new department at its centre. This led him to what was then his favourite theme—the need for co-operation among all hospitals in the area—but, he admitted sadly, nothing so far had come from his efforts to bring that about. Hospitals, he added, were right to be proud of their own work; but it was essential for them to over-come the prejudice of insularity and to work together. He hoped a step in that direction might soon be achieved in the field of orthopaedics.

The new ward, under the general supervision of Professor John Fraser, knighted early in 1937, was in charge of Mr. Walter Mercer and Mr. William Cochrane. Their clinical tutors were Ian Smillie, transferred from the surgical out-patient department and William V. Anderson who had been clinical tutor to Mr. Henry Wade. Four years later, Smillie went on to the Emergency Medical Service hospital at Larbert to set up a war-time orthopaedic unit there. The department team was later joined by R. I. Stirling who, during the 1920s, had done original work on bone grafting and had performed what was probably the first leg lengthening operation. This was a technique which he, along with W. V. Anderson, later brought to the highest level of success in the world, at the Princess Margaret Rose Hospital.

Soon after 1948, with the coming of the National Health Service, the ortho-paedics team moved to larger and better accommodation in Wards 5 and 6 at the west end of the surgical block and the old ward beneath Ward 5 was altered and extended to form an orthopaedic out-patient department. Until then, they had to remain content with the limited accommodation and facilities at Ward 2. There, with a minimum of supporting staff, they successfully ran an enormous orthopaedic service.

Surgical Neurology

Should it be 'surgical neurology' or 'neurological surgery'? The names seem to be interchangeable and Professor Norman Dott, its first great exponent in the Infirmary used them indiscriminately. But it has been said that he preferred the term 'surgical neurology' because of its implication that neurology, the study and treatment of the central nervous system, is a single discipline with two related branches, the surgical and the medical; so that is the name I shall adopt except in quotations in which the other has been used. This section, then, is about surgical neurology and its development in the Royal Infirmary during the 1930s; and that story is primarily the story of Norman McOmish Dott. It is a story that illustrates dramatically how an unpleasant chance occurrence can sometimes, long afterwards, be found to have been the first in a chain of events bringing results totally unexpected and far-reaching in their benefits to mankind.

Here are excerpts from two newspaper reports separated by almost fifty years:

Edinburgh Evening News—30 August 1913. Norman Dott, 16 years of age . . . met with a serious accident in Lothian Road yesterday. He was riding a motor-cycle along the street there when, overtaking a horse and lorry, he made to pass it but unfortunately his machine came in contact with a motor taxi which was going in the opposite direction. The cyclist was thrown on to the street and severely injured and the motor-cycle and taxi-cab suffered severely as the result of the collision. The injured youth was conveyed to Edinburgh Royal Infirmary . . .

Scotsman—7 July 1962. Professor Norman Dott . . . yesterday became a Freeman of Edinburgh for his services to medicine. Making the presentation, the Lord Provost, Sir John Greig Dunbar said . . . 'Through his skill and knowledge he has restored to health many people who had been grievously afflicted. We in Edinburgh bask in the reflected glory of his achievements.'

When the young Norman Dott arrived at the Infirmary in 1913 the records show that he was found to have a compound fracture of the tibia and a fracture of the neck of the femur of his left leg. From the effects of these injuries he suffered, sometimes severely, for the rest of his life. He was taken to Ward 12 where he was attended to by Mr. (later Sir) Henry Wade, then an Assistant Surgeon. Dott remained in the ward for eight weeks, taking a keen interest in the comings and goings around him of surgeons, nurses and medical students. Their activities so impressed him that he gave up his former intention of becoming an engineer and there and then decided to embark on the study of medicine. In 1919, he graduated MB, ChB at Edinburgh and became a resident house officer at the Infirmary. There followed a period as assistant surgeon in other hospitals and of experimental work in physiology and the study of the pituitary gland—a gland connected to the under-surface of the brain and affecting many aspects of growth and metabolism in ways less fully understood then than they are now.

Having become a Fellow of the Royal College of Surgeons of Edinburgh in 1923, Dott was awarded a Rockefeller Foundation travelling fellowship which enabled him to work for a year in Boston, USA with Dr. Harvey Cushing, American pioneer of surgical neurology, then widely recognised as the world's greatest brain surgeon. Back in Edinburgh he was, as he himself put it, 'fired with missionary zeal to establish Harvey Cushing's neurological surgery in Edinburgh'. For a while he undertook his highly-specialised surgery in Edinburgh nursing-homes, travelling to them with an operating-table of his own design strapped to the roof of his car. That operating-table may not have been the first item of surgical equipment designed by him; it was certainly not the last, for throughout his career, he invented or improved many appliances and precision instruments to meet the exacting requirements of his work. In that, his early interest in engineering stood him in good stead.

At the Infirmary 'cranial surgery' mainly in the field of head injuries and their complications had been practised by Sir Joseph Cotterill (Surgeon—1897 to 1912) and Alexander Miles (Surgeon—1910 to 1924) and others. 'They were great surgeons', Dott wrote, 'but better known in other aspects of surgery'. It was in 1930 that the members of the Infirmary's Honorary Staff suggested to the Board 'that a neurological surgeon should be appointed and that the position should be offered to Mr. Norman Dott'. This was agreed to and in March 1931 he was appointed as 'Associate Neurological Surgeon' for five years in the first instance. He was given the use of four beds in Professor (later Sir) David Wilkie's Wards (Nos. 13 & 14) with the use of the operating theatre. In the following year, Dott was appointed to a lectureship in his specialty at the University. Thus, in that small way the Infirmary Department of Surgical Neurology began; and there, in 1933, a brain artery aneurysm (local dilatation of a blood vessel) was treated surgically, for the first time in the world, by Norman Dott. Many years later, Dott wrote that 'for surgical neurology in Edinburgh the Royal Infirmary provided, as it were, a cradle from 1924 and a cot from 1938' but that was too modest. With such a surgical 'first' to its credit, it had surely outgrown the 'cradle' by 1933 and, as will be seen, it was not long after 1938 that it also outgrew the 'cot'.

In 1936, after the removal of the venereal disease patients to their new building, Ward 20 in the clock tower became vacant, and it was allocated to Mr. Dott. The accommodation there, however, was neither spacious enough nor in a fit condition to meet the requirements of such a highly sophisticated specialty as surgical neurology and much work was needed before it could be used by him. It was found possible to add a small wing at each side of the central tower without adversely affecting the skyline of the building, and by that means, space for twenty beds was provided, with operating theatre, ophthalmic room, staff-room and out-patient facilities. This was the Infirmary's most important development of the year—perhaps for many years—and so it is worth quoting the account of it given in the annual report for 1938:

> The most notable feature of the internal administration of the Infirmary during the year has been the opening of Ward 20 for the reception of patients under the care of the Neurological Surgeon. This ward has been entirely reconstructed and many novel features have been introduced, including a very special arrangement for the lighting and air conditioning of the theatre. Arrangements have also been made to allow the admission of private patients to this Ward. The cost of reconstruction will be in the region of £12,000 and towards this cost special contributions amounting to £7,306 have been received or promised.

The 'very special' arrangements in the theatre included an ellipsoidal stainless steel lighting dome imported from Paris because no effective alternative could be obtained nearer home and a sound-proof viewing gallery with a polarised glass 'one-way' viewing window so that neither sound nor sight of watching students would disturb the concentration of the surgeon during his delicate painstaking work. For necessary communication between operator and observers a microphone system was provided.

The reference to paying-patients is of interest because this was the first occasion, at least in modern times, that charging patients for treatment (as distinct from inviting voluntary donations) had been authorised in the Infirmary. Indeed, in 1932, a proposal to obtain statutory powers to introduce charges for a proportion of beds had met with such vigorous opposition that it had been dropped. In this case, however, the circumstances were different. Those concerned were Dott's private patients and he had pointed out that, with the increasing technical requirements of his specialty, facilities matching up to the exacting standards he demanded were not available elsewhere. So his request to admit paying patients was agreed to, but only for surgical investigation and operation (convalescence to be at a private nursing home) and only on condition that no ordinary Infirmary patient requiring such treatment would thereby be denied admission to Ward 20.

Towards the cost of the elliptical dome, Mr. Dott himself and friends contributed £600. The annual reports from 1936 to 1940 show that Sir Alexander Grant, Bt, of Glen Moriston (and of McVitie & Price Ltd., biscuit manufacturers) donated some £3,300 most of which was received after his death from the Trustees for his estate; and that 57 other donors together gave nearly £6,000. Through the University various items of equipment were supplied from a grant made by the Rockefeller Foundation whose Travelling Fellowship, fifteen years before, had started Norman Dott on his outstanding career.

In October 1938, the first patients were admitted to the Department. It was formally opened by Lady Grant whose late husband had so generously contributed towards its establishment. In his new Department, Mr. Dott was ably assisted by highly professional colleagues, including Mr. George Alexander (who had worked with him since 1931), and they soon developed a close working relationship with such other Infirmary departments as those of ophthalmology, otolaryngology and radio-therapy. The Department however, was no more than getting into its stride when war was declared in September 1939. With the apprehension of air-raids on city centres, it had been decided that the main work of the department should be transferred to a brain injuries unit, established as part of the Emergency Hospital Service in and adjoining Bangour Mental Hospital, some 15 miles west of Edinburgh. At Bangour, a unit of 80 beds, with two temporary operating-theatres was quickly provided and there, again with the help of a Rockefeller Foundation grant 'for the promotion of neuro-psychiatry, including surgical neurology', a highly skilled specialist staff was built up, eventually to a total of fifteen. At Bangour, under Dott's leadership, the treatment of both civilian and military patients was undertaken throughout the war while at the Infirmary Ward 20 continued in use mainly for out-patient work and immediate attention to accident cases.

In that way the foundations were laid for the development of a modern comprehensive surgical neurology service to provide clinical care for patients, teaching and research.

Anaesthetics

'Medicine's greatest single gift to suffering humanity' is how the physician, Sir William Osler (1849-1919) once described the knowledge and practice of

anaesthesia. None, surely, would quarrel with that view after a moment's consideration of the horror of undergoing the simplest operation in pre-anaesthetic
days compared with conditions today when even lengthy surgical procedures can
be carried out without any pain being felt by the patient. The benefits go far
beyond the relief of pain, important though that is. Because absence of pain and
technical advances in anaesthesia give the surgeon time, many conditions that
would formerly have proved fatal or permanently disabling can now be dealt
with by the surgeon, and the patient restored to health.

Credit for the first use of ether anaesthesia in Britain is claimed by Dumfries
and Galloway Infirmary for an amputation undertaken on 19 December 1846,
two days before Robert Liston's more widely publicised first painless operation at
University College Hospital, London. Almost eleven months later came James Y.
Simpson's famous experiment in his home at 52 Queen Street, Edinburgh and in
November 1847 he was able to write: 'I have had an opportunity of trying the
effects of the inhalation of chloroform today in three cases in the Royal Infirmary
of Edinburgh'. The first of those three patients was a five-year-old boy and
Simpson reported that the boy had 'awakened about half-an-hour after the
operation with a clear, merry eye and placid expression of countenance wholly
unlike what is found to obtain after ordinary etherisation'. So, if Edinburgh's
Royal Infirmary was not the first in Britain to introduce painless surgery it was,
as befitted the principal hospital in Simpson's own city, the first to use chloroform,
an agent the after-effects of which were found to be a good deal less unpleasant
than those of ether. Appropriately, the Infirmary was long known for its devotion
to chloroform on which it continued to rely (perhaps from loyalty to Simpson)
after many hospitals had adopted other means of anaesthesia.

Here, until the 1930s, the practice of anaesthetics seems to have been regarded
as an important ancillary to surgical science but not a branch of scientific study in
its own right. It would, perhaps, be unfair to say that, until the 1930s the old 'rag
and bottle method' or, to put it more kindly, the 'open-mask chloroform-ether
sequence' was the only method used but certainly by 1930, techniques had not
advanced much beyond that state and Boyle's anaesthetic machine was only then
being brought into use. The Board minutes for December 1944 contain an
illuminating tribute to an anaesthetist who had won the admiration of the Infirmary
surgeons in the period just before the introduction of these technical aids. In that
month, the death had occurred of Dr. M. H. Jones (affectionately known to all as
'Daddy Jones') who had served as anaesthetist for a period of 24 years. Of him
Mr. W. J. Stuart said: 'He began in the epoch before the existence of complicated
anaesthetic machines. That these have added to the safety of the patient is indis-
putable, but it was an education to see Dr. Jones secure perfect anaesthesia by the
most simple methods; and he deserved the highest testimony that can be given to
an anaesthetist—that the surgeon forgot he was there . . .'

By 1930 each 'charge' in the surgical house had a doctor attached to it as
part-time honorary anaesthetist and as supervisor of anaesthetics but the law still
allowed any qualified resident physician or surgeon to administer anaesthetics.
Students were also permitted and, indeed, required to do so, under supervision,
as part of their training.

In December 1931, the Board received a letter from the Lord Advocate emphasising that medical students should never be allowed to administer anaesthetics except under qualified supervision and a case was cited where 'such supervision had been merely nominal, a medical man not being present at the time'. The Board replied that the rules of the Infirmary required two medical men to be present and 'in order to stress the importance of the administration of anaesthetics', they instructed that a copy of the Crown Office letter be sent to each member of the Senior Honorary Surgical Staff.

In September 1941 an event took place which prompted *The Scotsman* to state that 'the Royal Infirmary of Edinburgh has now been brought as up-to-date as any hospital can be in regard to the administration of anaesthetics in the operating theatres and of oxygen to patients requiring it either in the medical or surgical wards'. This referred to the newly-completed installation of copper pipe-lines to carry oxygen and nitrous oxide from a battery of cylinders in a central supply store to 342 outlet points which replaced the former laborious system of providing individual cylinders throughout the Infirmary. The installation, which it was said might have cost about £7,000 on a commercial basis, had been given by Colonel S. J. L. Hardie of Ballathie, in Perthshire, who was Chairman of the British Oxygen Company whose experts had designed and installed the system. In formally handing it over Colonel Hardie said that Edinburgh now led the world with such an installation which he hoped would be the forerunner of many others. A member of the medical staff described it as a 'Godsend' and said that besides its value in operating theatres, it would enable results to be achieved in the treatment of pneumonia which could never be produced before.

At the time much was said about the potential value of the installation in facilitating the administration of oxygen to victims of a war-time gas attack—a test to which, mercifully, it never had to be put. It was, however, of great benefit to Dr. John Gillies in his successful efforts to modernise the methods of administering anaesthetics in the Infirmary.

Blood Transfusion

As long ago as 1666, as one may read in Samuel Pepys' diary, the Royal Society witnessed an experiment in which blood was transferred from one dog to another 'with very good success' and soon afterwards a man, for a fee of 20 shillings, allowed a small quantity of sheep's blood to be introduced into his bloodstream, 'and finds himself much better since, and as a new man'! Two crude experiments, crudely conducted, they were not followed by any practice of blood transfer from one human being to another until, in the early nineteenth century, the procedure was used in London with some successes in obstetrical emergencies. During the Franco-Prussian war of 1870-71 it was used to a limited extent in the treatment of casualties; in the 1914-18 war it was used more extensively and with greater success.

Among surgeons who took a special interest in blood transfusion before and during the Great War was Mr. James M. Graham who was appointed an assistant surgeon in the Royal Infirmary in 1919 and became surgeon-in-charge of Wards

5 and 6 in 1928. He remained at the Infirmary until his retiral in 1946 and throughout that time and beyond it, he maintained his interest in blood transfusion and
in the extension and refinement of its processes.

When a transfusion was required for a patient in the Infirmary in the 1920s
it was carried out at the bedside direct from donor to patient, after the donor's
blood group had been checked for compatability. Speed of transfer was essential
as measures against coagulation had not then been fully developed. Usually the
donor was a member of the patient's family or a friend. If no such donor was
available other volunteers would be sought. Medical students were encouraged
to volunteer because, the Board said, 'from the nature of their training they are
aware of the dangers involved' but requests for donors were also made further
afield. On one occasion the press announced that 'the authorities are particularly
anxious to enlist Rover Scouts on account of the healthy lives they lead and the
fine type of young manhood they represent'—as if it was thought that their blood
might carry with it other virtues besides restored health.

The fact remained that donors were few, so few in fact that in November
1930 it was stated that there were only ten names on the hospital's voluntary list
and a permanent list of 160 was required. By that time, however, one man had
resolved that action must be taken to ensure that whenever blood was needed to
save a patient's life, it would be available. From his decision to do something
about it the whole elaborate organisation of volunteer blood donors in Edinburgh
and throughout Scotland began.

The man was John R. Copland, a dentist who lived and practised in Gilmore
Place, Edinburgh. In 1929 the wife of one of his close friends had died in the
Royal Infirmary because her husband's blood was not of the required blood-group
and no other suitable donor could be found in time to save her. This so shocked
John Copland that with the help of his family and some members of the Holyrood
Conclave of Crusaders, a small voluntary welfare group with which he was
associated, he set up a miniature transfusion service with a panel of voluntary
donors organised from his home. Their help was gratefully accepted by the
Infirmary Managers who arranged for the blood-testing and grouping of
volunteers' blood to be done in the hospital laboratory under the direction of Dr.
C. P. Stewart, the Infirmary Bio-chemist. So, from the end of 1930 when his
scheme began to operate fully, John Copland kept a telephone at his bedside and
undertook to answer calls at any time of the day or night, to find a suitable member
of his panel and whenever necessary (as it frequently was) to go in his own car to
collect the donor and drive him to the Infirmary or other hospital where blood
was needed. When necessary, he himself would be the donor.

The Crusaders had their own journal and in the issue for October 1931 they
reported that 'during the last ten days, eight donors were called upon to give
blood and three stand-by calls were received. The Edinburgh Royal Infirmary
have nothing but praise for the way in which this service has been organised. One
recipient received blood ten minutes after the call had been made for a donor.'
Some six months later, the same journal reported: 'During the past month,
twelve calls have been made and in each case we have been able to supply a donor.
It is interesting to note that the record number of transfusions have been given by

a Crusader who has given his services on no less than seven occasions and his family have given, in all, eleven transfusions . . . Since the inception of this service a little over a year ago, about 80 calls have been received from the various hospitals and nursing homes throughout the city and on no occasion has the Service failed to supply a donor.'

From such reports it is clear that, in those early days, the precaution of limiting donations by any one donor to about six-monthly intervals had not yet been adopted and the strain of giving more frequent donations may have been one reason why, after about five years, the interest of the original Crusaders began to wane. For the time being, however, the scheme went from strength to strength.

Although the work was voluntary some administration expenses were incurred and funds had to be found. In January 1934 a 'Grand Concert' was held in the King's Theatre to raise money for the cause and in this several Scottish singers and comedians took part, including two who were much loved at that time, Tommy Lorne and Harry Gordon. A note on the concert programme, after telling the story of the Crusaders and their blood transfusion service, enthusiastically added: 'These modern Crusaders [are] more worthy of the ideals of chivalry in their aid to the weak and suffering than any mail-clad hero of olden times'. The note then went on to explain that, in $3\frac{1}{2}$ years, more than 600 calls had been answered by the service.

John R. Copland did not confine himself to operating the service. He was active in fund-raising too. He was a keen amateur singer and actor and in July 1935 he played the part of 'Frederick, the Duke's brother' in an open-air performance of 'As You Like It' staged in the bandstand in Princes Street Gardens— the first time a play had been performed there. The weather was perfect and this seems to have been a successful event, despite the sound of steam trains passing to and fro detracting from the actors' efforts to sustain the arcadian atmosphere of the Forest of Arden.

With ever-increasing demands for blood and the slow evaporation of the Crusaders' interest, John Copland began to find that the task of organiser which he had set himself had grown beyond the scope of one man. In 1936, therefore, he had to announce that he could no longer continue the scheme in its original form. So, in June of that year a meeting was called by Lord Provost Louis S. Gumley and held in the City Chambers. It was attended by Mr. W. J. Stuart, FRCSE, representing the honorary staff of the Royal Infirmary, Professor W. T. Ritchie and Mr. Henry Wade, Presidents, respectively, of the Royal College of Physicians and the Royal College of Surgeons, of Edinburgh and over sixty other distinguished citizens from many walks of life. All were loud in their praise of Mr. Copland and the service he had initiated and carried on, and all were agreed that he could not be expected to continue to provide it on his own responsibility. More than 1,100 transfusions had been given in Edinburgh during the last year. They were given in many different kinds of case—severe shock after accidents, serious operations, complicated confinements, blood poisoning, anaemia and various forms of haemorrhage, medical and surgical were stated as examples. With such demands growing steadily it was readily accepted that a fully organised blood transfusion service was overdue.

Any suggestion that such a service should be organised on some kind of commercial basis was demolished, before it could even be made, by Mr. Henry Wade who said that the blood given 'must be the free-will offering of men who love their fellow-mortals'. On his motion it was agreed that a Committee should be formed at once to organise the service. Thus was born the Edinburgh Blood Transfusion Service. Mr. Charles Gumley, WS, son of the Lord Provost, became Hon. Secretary and John Copland continued as Organiser, but now with an assistant, Miss Helen M. White. The object of the Service was defined as being 'to provide to any Hospital, Institution or Nursing Home in Edinburgh or district, at any time of day or night, an adequate number of Voluntary Blood-Donors in response to calls, and to meet the entire cost of the Blood-Donors. No fees are paid to the Blood-Donors whose services are given absolutely voluntarily, and no charge is made against any Hospital, Institution, Nursing Home or private patient.'

Under the new arrangement the Service, though continuing as an independent voluntary body, was based on the Royal Infirmary. Messages were received there and provision was made to take donors to out-lying hospitals and nursing homes when necessary; but the cost of these services was met, not by the Infirmary, but by the Blood Transfusion Service.

After the Munich crisis of 1938, the Government realised that war was imminent and that, among many other necessary measures, something must be done to ensure adequate supplies of blood, not only for military casualties, but also for civilian air-raid victims and the general public. So, at the beginning of 1939, the Department of Health for Scotland set up a special Sub-Committee of members of the Department's Scientific Advisory Committee with Sir John Fraser as Sub-Committee Chairman 'to investigate existing facilities for trans-fusion; to consider the possibility of improving these facilities, especially in smaller centres and in country areas; and to advise on the storage of blood in selected centres'.

The Sub-Committee found that arrangements for blood transfusion varied widely throughout Scotland. In several areas there were no standing arrangements, each case in which blood was required being dealt with specially as the need arose. Only in the Edinburgh area was there an organised regional service.

It was clear from the report that the need for a national scheme was urgent and, on the initiative of the Department of Health for Scotland, the Scottish National Blood Transfusion Association was formed at a meeting in St. Andrew's House, Edinburgh on 9 February 1940. The Earl of Rosebery was President and Dr. C. P. Stewart, Royal Infirmary Bio-chemist, was Vice-President. Because of their experience, Mr. Charles S. Gumley became National Secretary and Mr. John R. Copland, National Organiser. Among 27 Council members the Royal Infirmary was represented by Mr. John R. Little, Professor Sir John Fraser and Mr. W. J. Stuart.

The Association set up five regional blood transfusion services, organised by five regional committees centred on Edinburgh, Glasgow, Dundee, Aberdeen and Inverness, each of which enjoyed a large measure of autonomy. The Edinburgh Blood Transfusion Service, already recruiting donors from a wide south-eastern area, was affiliated as the South-east Scotland Blood Transfusion Service. Its Director was Dr. C. P. Stewart, (doubling that role with the office of National Vice President) and Miss Helen M. White was appointed Regional Organising Secretary.

At the first meeting of the National Council it was estimated that the annual cost of the Scottish Service would be £10,000 towards which it was stated that the Chancellor of the Exchequer would contribute £5,000, a level of contribution which would continue to be met, as civil defence expenditure, 'during the period of war emergency'. Thereafter, it was expected that 'peace-time needs would be effectively met under voluntary auspices'. In fact, with rising costs and the greatly extended use of blood transfusion in the post-war years, the proportion of government contribution had to be steadily raised. Since 1974 the full cost has been met by the National Health Service through the Common Services Agency. Throughout its history, however, the Service both nationally and regionally has retained its character as a voluntary organisation, the voluntary aspect of the work being amply represented by the many thousands of donors who regularly give their blood.

An important recommendation by Sir John Fraser's Sub-Committee of 1939 was that blood-storage centres should be established. Already, progress had been made in the techniques of storing blood and plasma, thus enabling the giving of blood to be organised through attendance at regular sessions, quite separate from the process of transfusion to the patient. Before his Sub-Committee's report had been published, Sir John had already suggested to the Royal Infirmary Board that a blood store should be established and in July 1939 the Board agreed to this, a refrigerator in the central instrument department being ear-marked for the purpose. Only two months later it was agreed to extend this provision and to put the storage facilities on a permanent basis, with standby equipment which would enable refrigeration to continue even during a power failure. So when the National Association decided in 1941 to set up two central blood depots, one in Glasgow and one in Edinburgh, storage facilities for the East of Scotland were already well established in the Royal Infirmary. Thus the Infirmary played its part in the growth of an embryo blood transfusion organisation into a fully developed Scottish service in time to meet the demand of war-time.

2

Wartime and Approach to the N.H.S.

The War Years—1939 to 1945

In the minute books of the Royal Infirmary Managers, the first reference to the approach of war appears on 24 January 1938 when a letter from the Department of Health for Scotland was submitted intimating that the Government were considering what arrangements should be made to deal with civilian casualties in the event of a national emergency. To help in their examination of this problem the Department had decided to make a rapid survey of all hospital facilities in Scotland and they asked the Managers if they would allow their Superintendent, Lt-Col A. D. Stewart, I.M.S., to work with the Department's own officers 'in this matter of first-class national importance and of extreme urgency'; a request to which the Managers readily agreed.

At the time, war seemed to many to be almost immediately imminent. But seven months later, in September 1938, the Prime Minister, Neville Chamberlain, returned from Munich having secured, not peace in our time as he hoped but, at least, a respite of eleven months before war was declared. During those eighteen months of 1938 and 1939 the hospital survey was carried out and the Department of Health, acting for the Secretary of State for Scotland under his powers in the Civil Defence Act of 1939, were able to complete their arrangements for ensuring, so far as could be judged, that hospital beds would be available for casualties of enemy attack as well as for the essential needs of the general public.

How formidable this task was is evident from the fact that, before the emergency arose, there was in Scotland an estimated deficiency of 3,600 hospital beds below even peace-time requirements. The survey showed that, in Scotland as a whole, there were 475 hospitals with some 35,000 beds. Of these, 92 hospitals with 7,300 beds were in the south-east, by far the largest hospital in that area being the Royal Infirmary with 1,140 beds. It was estimated that, by restricting admissions to the most serious cases, by sending home all patients whose condition and home circumstances allowed, by transferring others from fully equipped surgical hospitals to less fully equipped auxiliary hospitals and by introducing additional beds where space permitted, about 11,000 beds could be kept available for casualties in Scotland, 3,000 of these being in the south-east. The Government decided to build seven new hospitals, with a total of some 7,000 beds, strategically placed away from large centres of population, and to provide a further 8,500 beds in annexes to be attached to several existing hospitals, also in country districts. In addition three large hotels were converted and numerous country houses were ear-marked for use as convalescent or auxiliary hospitals. The whole of the new building programme was completed by the middle of 1941 by which time a total of some 30,000 beds were available in fully equipped general hospitals in Scotland.

For purposes of administration of the emergency scheme Scotland was divided into the five regions which were previously regarded as appropriate for any hospital co-ordination scheme that might develop and which were later adopted for the National Health Service. Of these, the south-eastern region, from Fife to the Border, coincided almost exactly with the Infirmary's main 'catchment' area.

Only one of the new hospitals (at Peel, Selkirkshire, with 400 beds) and one large annexe (at Bangour, West Lothian, with 1,500 beds) were within the south-eastern region. It was at first suggested that Peel Hospital should be administered by the Royal Infirmary Board, a suggestion with which the Board were willing to agree. It was decided, however, that all seven new hospitals as well as the hotels and country houses should be under the direct control of the Department of Health. All other hospitals, including annexes where these had been added, were to continue under their existing voluntary or local authority management but would be subject to a measure of direction from the Department and would receive financial assistance towards the provision they were making to meet war-time needs. The financial assistance consisted largely of payments in respect of beds kept empty but ready to receive casualties if required and, under that heading in the first year of the war, the Infirmary received £49,000 with an additional £2,000 for Convalescent House and Beechmount Hospital. The Department also helped with the upgrading of facilities and the supply of items of equipment required to meet special war-time needs.

It was with the planning of the seven new hospitals and the annexes that, as mentioned earlier, Professors Stanley Davidson and T. J. Mackie had been invited to help. It is a tribute to them and to all who were involved in the setting-up of these hospitals that, although the hospitals were designed on the simplest 'hutment' lines and hastily erected to meet an urgent need, six of them (albeit renovated and improved) are still, after 40 years, making a useful contribution to the National Health Service; that it is still necessary for them to do so is less commendable.

Ready at All Times

Such, then, is the general background of hospital provision in Scotland against which the Royal Infirmary's contribution to war-time hospital provision should be seen. On 27 September 1938 an Emergency Committee of four members of the Board was set up to act promptly whenever emergency measures were necessary. The first major event the Committee had to arrange was the evacuation of patients in accordance with instructions issued by the Department of Health, so as to free as many beds as possible for the reception of service or air-raid casualties.

The mass removal of patients was thoroughly prepared. Ward Sisters, after consultation with the senior physicians and surgeons concerned, made lists of patients in three categories showing those able to go home, those fit to be moved to less central and less fully equipped hospitals and those too ill to be moved. The second of these categories included patients operated upon only two or three days before, many of whom at that time, would normally have expected to stay in hospital for at least fourteen days, probably ten of them in bed.

The transfers took place on the day on which some thousands of school children left the city for the safety of rural areas—Thursday, 31 August 1939, three days before the declaration of war. On that day great activity was seen in Lauriston Place, outside the Infirmary. Buses, from which seats had been removed to make room for stretchers, ambulances and a long line of private cars made available and driven by their volunteer owners were drawn up. Under the direction of Lt-Col A. D. Stewart, Superintendent, and guided by Miss E. D. Smaill, Lady Superintendent of Nurses and Miss M. C. Marshall, then her Senior Assistant, the entire staff of porters, many nurses and others helped to bring patients to the bus or car that would take them to their allotted destination. A nurse who took part wrote, many years later 'It was a great day to remember and those at the top were excellent organisers. Not so much "Organisation and Method" talked of in those days, but they had the know-how.'

Abour 400 patients went to their own homes. Some made their own transport arrangements, but (families with cars being far fewer then than now) many took advantage of the cars provided whose drivers cheerfully took them as far afield as Berwickshire and the other Border counties. Forty patients from surgical wards were transferred to Convalescent House and thirty to Beechmount which thus entered upon their war-time function as auxiliary hospitals no longer specifically allocated to convalescent and cancer patients.

Approximately 100 patients from medical wards went to the Town Council's Craiglockhart Hospital (now Greenlea Old People's Home) on the southern outskirts of the city. Built in the 1870s as a large parochial board poorhouse, it had become in 1930 a home for the aged and infirm for whom the Council's Public Assistance Committee were responsible. In 1939, as part of the emergency hospital arrangements, its residents were transferred to the smaller Northern General Hospital which became the Public Assistance Home while Craiglockhart was upgraded and, for the duration of the war, became the Southern General Hospital. On 31 August 1939 it was not yet functioning fully and the sudden influx of so many patients from the Infirmary made it necessary for the Medical Officer of Health to ask urgently for nursing help. To this the Emergency Committee immediately agreed and 20 nurses were seconded to Craiglockhart. The request also prompted that Committee to authorise the Lady Superintendent to send nurses to any other hospital in which Royal Infirmary patients might, later, be looked after. Similar assistance was given in February 1940 when 20 Infirmary nurses went to the Eastern General Hospital and 10 to the Western to help to look after some 60 seamen from the German prison ship *Altmark* who had been rescued and brought into Leith Docks by H.M.S. *Cossack*.

On completion of the evacuation some wards in the Infirmary were empty and in others only a few beds were occupied. The staff, too, were depleted because several of the Honorary Medical Staff, clinical tutors and junior doctors, as well as other staff, had left to join the Services. In addition, a number of doctors had transferred, under the Emergency Hospitals Scheme, to posts in other hospitals. This made things difficult for those who remained at the Infirmary to deal with urgent admissions and to be in readiness for any sudden influx of air-raid casualties. To help fill the gaps some Consultants—retired members of the Honorary Staff—returned to undertake ward duties. They included Professor W. T. Ritchie and Mr. W. J. Stuart; Mr. J. W. Struthers who undertook holiday relief duty; and Professor-Emeritus Edwin Matthew and Mr. George Chiene who acted as visiting physician and visiting surgeon for Convalescent House and Beechmount auxiliary hospitals.

A difficult problem arose in the first weeks of the war from the financial situation of junior members of the Honorary Medical Staff who suddenly found that their income from private work on which they depended had greatly diminished or entirely disappeared. It was pointed out that the services of these doctors were essential to the Infirmary and that the level to which their numbers had been reduced was the lowest which could be accepted. The Board recognised that the financial position of these doctors contrasted unfavourably with those who had left for service with the Forces or in the Department of Health's emergency hospitals, where salaries were paid. It was considered that this was a matter with which the Department should help and, after some negotiation, the Department agreed, in December 1939, to make annual grants of 200 guineas to 'junior specialists' and 100 guineas to clinical tutors who remained in the Infirmary.

The nursing situation changed little during the war years, the number of nurses on the staff recorded annually varying between 527 and 547. But, from September 1939, the Lady Superintendent of Nurses had to manage without the help of her Senior Assistant, Miss M. C. Marshall. At the request of the Department of Health, Miss Marshall was released from the Infirmary to become Principal Matron of the Scottish Emergency Hospitals and of the Civil Nursing Reserve. In that capacity she had the daunting task of ensuring that nurses, trained and in training and volunteers recruited to the Nursing Reserve, were effectively distributed among the principal new hospitals and allocated to the numerous large country houses which had been earmarked for use as auxiliary hospitals. While, generally, the fullest co-operation was willingly given by the owners of these houses, many of whom had elected to remain in residence, a high degree of tact was sometimes required to convince such owners that any old attic or basement room was not necessarily suitable as nurses' sleeping quarters and that the use of a house for hospital purposes did not automatically mean that the house-owner should act as matron-in-charge. These and many other more professional and technical difficulties were so successfully dealt with by her that, in 1942, Miss Marshall was appointed to the newly-created post of Chief Nursing Officer of the Department of Health for Scotland. This was regarded as an honour not to her alone but to the Royal Infirmary where, in the 1920s, she had trained as a nurse and had since held ever more responsible posts. Miss Marshall remained in her new post until 1944 when, on the retiral of Miss Smaill, she returned to the Infirmary as Lady Superintendent of Nurses.

As the first weeks of the war passed and the country was spared the ordeal of bombing raids, there were many who were puzzled as to what arrangements, if any, existed for the admission of patients other than those requiring urgent attention. So, in the Managers' Annual Report for the year to September 1939, the following explanation was given:

> Shortly before the outbreak of war, at the request of the Government all patients who could be removed were transferred either to their own homes or to other Institutions, and after this evacuation the number of available beds for the ordinary civilian sick was only about 300. Later in the month of September, however, arrangements were made to increase this number to just over 700 beds . . . It will thus be seen that (including the beds at Convalescent House and Beechmount) the provision for the civilian sick and injured is over 800 beds and these beds are all occupied at the present time.
>
> With regard to the provision for potential air raid casualties, the Managers are keeping vacant 400 beds of the normal complement and in addition 300 extra beds have been installed throughout the various wards all fully equipped.

After dealing with the bed position in the Infirmary, the Managers' Report for 1939 went on to state that, in addition to planning for the reception of casualties while, at the same time, seeking to make some provision for the ordinary sick, an immense amount of work had been undertaken, in collaboration with the local authority air-raid precautions organisation (ARP) to ensure, as far as possible, the safety of patients, staff and visitors in the event of an air-raid occurring. ARP arrangements had, in fact, been in preparation in the city since the mid-1930s. These included the establishment of a network of 'first-aid posts' throughout the city and the provision in part of the University Medical School building in Teviot Place, close to the Infirmary, of a large casualty-receiving station in which the injured could be classified and given preliminary attention before being passed on to the Infirmary, sent to some other hospital or allowed to go home or to other accommodation.

The Managers also explained that: 'An elaborate scheme of protection of the Infirmary buildings has been undertaken and air-raid shelters to accommodate over 3,000 persons have been provided throughout the large basements under the buildings, both in the main block and in the Maternity Pavilion'; and, they added, 'Something of the difficulties of effecting a black-out of the Infirmary buildings will be appreciated from the fact that there are over 10,000 windows in the Infirmary . . .' Those 10,000 windows of many shapes and sizes must indeed have created problems, not only in making and fitting the 'blackout' equipment but in ensuring that it was used on every window, every night.

Precautions against possible gas attack were also taken. Gas masks were kept in readiness for use by staff and patients who, contrary to the instructions given to all members of the public, might not have brought their own. Special protective arrangements were made for babies in the Simpson Pavilion. Under the local authority's civil defence arrangements, part of the venereal diseases out-patient department was converted into a reception station for stretcher gas casualties and the staff there were trained into a team proficient in anti-gas technique.

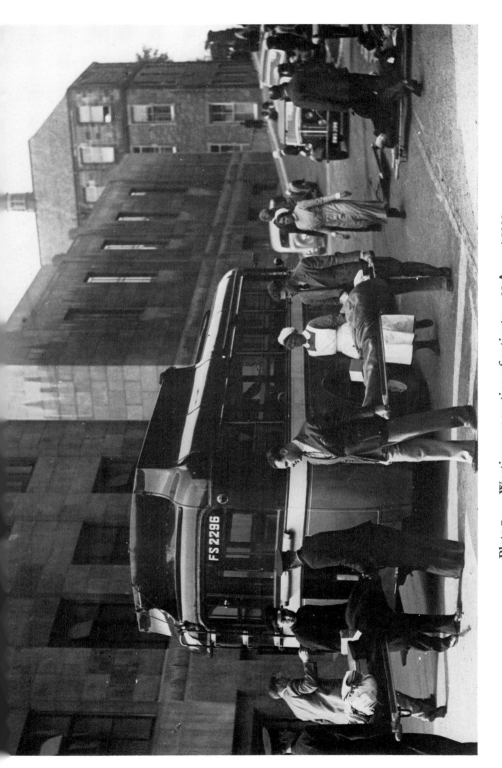

Plate 7   Wartime evacuation of patients — 31 August 1939

Stretcher-cases are being placed in an adapted bus while cars with volunteer drivers wait to pick up patients

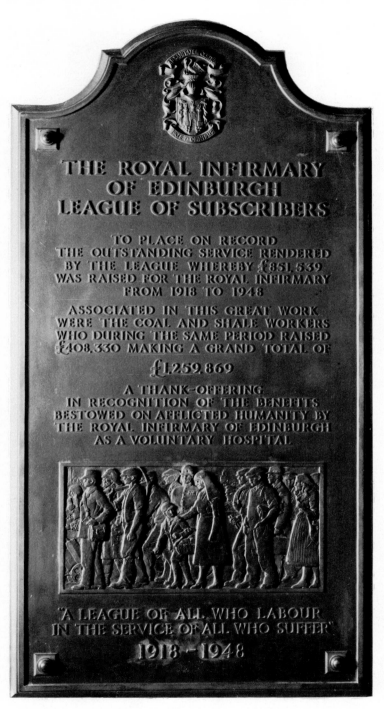

Plate 8   League of Subscribers commemorative plaque
erected in the main surgical corridor in 1950

Much thought was given to the safety of the Infirmary's supply of radium which, in an air-raid, might be dispersed and contaminate the area around it. The radium was stored in a basement in a specially constructed safe which the Radiologist, the Architect and the Board considered would give sufficient protection. The National Radium Commission, however, were of opinion that such supplies must be stored, during the war, at the foot of a shaft at least 50 feet deep. Argument continued for some time, but the Commission were adamant and so steps were about to be taken to sink a shaft of the prescribed depth in the Infirmary grounds. But just then, on 2 October 1939, it was reported to the Board that the Infirmary gardener had discovered (or had remembered) that a shaft already existed within the grounds of the hospital, close to Lauriston Place. This was, in fact, a 60-foot deep ventilation shaft connected with the 'Crawley tunnel' which had been constructed in the 1820s to accommodate pipes (which are still in use) carrying water to the city from the Crawley Springs and Glencorse Reservoir in the Pentland Hills. With little difficulty and at minimum expense a pulley-system was installed whereby the radium could be stored in the shaft in a protective container at the prescribed depth and could be retrieved whenever required. The small concrete chamber constructed above the shaft to house and protect the pulley mechanism can still be seen near the Infirmary west gate.

The various plans described had been made and put into operation on the assumption that Edinburgh and its surrounding area might, at any time, be the target of severe aerial attack. As things turned out, Edinburgh was exceedingly fortunate throughout the war. In contrast to the devastating loss of life, injuries and damage suffered in London, on Clydeside and in many other places in Britain, Edinburgh escaped almost unscathed. The official report by the Chief Constable of the City in 1946 put the situation in a nutshell. During the six wartime years there had been 105 'alert' warnings but only 15 air attacks during which two land-mines, 47 high explosive bombs and something over 600 incendiary bombs had been dropped. In course of the raids 20 people had been killed and 210 injured.

While these figures represent tragedy and distress for the victims and their families, they are nearly negligible when compared with the experience of other cities. So the Infirmary's main contribution, and that of the other hospitals in the area, to the civil defence arrangements was that of being ready at all times and thus giving confidence to the citizens that the best possible attention would be available whenever the need arose.

With many beds remaining empty and the number on the waiting-list of ordinary patients remaining high, the Managers in 1940 decided to take an immediate practical step to reduce the list of waiting patients 'whose complaints, while not acute, interfere either with the full enjoyment of life or with their ability to work'. They arranged to admit to two spare wards containing 25 beds, patients 'who are suffering from such conditions as hernia in various forms, deranged knee joints, haemorrhoids, chronic appendicitis, etc . . . All members of the surgical staff have willingly offered to undertake a share of the extra work involved.'

At the same time, the Department of Health were evolving a scheme for admission to vacant accommodation in their emergency hospitals. By mid-1940 twenty categories of persons were accepted as being eligible for admission to

F

these hospitals—the categories being defined mainly in recognition of the contribution to the war effort and to industry the patient could make when restored to
health. Then, early in 1941, the use of vacant emergency hospital beds was extended
further, enabling any patients on the waiting-list of voluntary hospitals to be
admitted to emergency hospitals, the voluntary hospital paying a flat rate of
£1. 10s (£1.50) in respect of each such patient and the patient paying nothing.
This scheme worked well and many patients unable to be accommodated in the
Infirmary received the necessary treatment at Bangour Hospital or one of the
other emergency hospitals. Those, however, who obtained their treatment in
municipal hospital beds not reserved for emergency scheme cases were still
required to pay the prescribed charge, unless they could prove their inability to
do so, an anomaly which, as already explained, continued until 1945.

Penicillin Appears

Although the Infirmary, thankfully, was not called upon to deal with great
numbers of local casualties it again played a useful wartime role by providing
accommodation and treatment for a total of 5,860 Emergency Hospital Scheme
patients including 2,512 Service patients, 220 Ministry of Pensions cases and 195
evacuees. More than 1,260 of these were wounded Servicemen brought from the
south of England in the months after the D-Day landings in France in 1944 and
the evacuees included 176 hospital patients transferred from London at the time
of the flying-bomb attacks in the same year. After the end of the war a letter was
received from the Secretary of State for Scotland passing on a formal resolution
by London County Council expressing appreciation of the care given to the
evacuees and concluding: 'London is very grateful for the welcome given to the
London patients'.

In June 1944 about 500 servicemen had been received from the south and,
after the end of the war in Europe, some information was included in the Board
Minutes about the arrangements which had been made for them. Quoting an
article by Professor J. R. Learmonth and Dr. (now Professor) J. P. Duguid which
had appeared in the 21st Army Group Medical Gazette, entitled 'Convoys in the
Royal Infirmary of Edinburgh after D-Day', the Secretary and Treasurer read
the following paragraph to the meeting:

> When it was decided that the Royal Infirmary was to receive convoys
> arriving by hospital train, the Superintendent set aside the medical wards
> on the ground floor for their reception, each ward being under the care
> of a surgeon-in-ordinary. This arrangement worked very well; patients
> could be quickly assigned to wards and rapidly put to bed and they were
> adjacent to the X-ray department and to the clinical laboratory. If
> operation was necessary it was carried out in the Theatre of the surgeon
> concerned and the patient returned to the medical ward unless his wounds
> were of such a nature that he needed special surgical nursing or such
> facilities as a suction apparatus. The sisters and nurses on the medical side
> seemed to take this revolution in their lives in their stride.

The minute of the meeting at which that account was read to the members by the
Secretary continues:

It was stated that the rest of the paper gave an interesting account of the treatment of the cases received from France, particularly the bacteriological findings which are important in view of the extensive use of penicillin and sulphanilamide, two drugs which are new since the last Great War. The use of these drugs produced a great change in the condition of war wounds and allowed of surgical methods which, in many cases, hastened recovery to an astonishing degree. The Managers received this report with much interest.

Not the least of their interest would be centred on the reference to penicillin and the details given in the article of its effects in aiding the rapid healing of injuries, for the Infirmary had already participated in very early trials of its use. Although penicillin had been discovered by Alexander Fleming as long before as 1928, no clinical use had been made of it until Howard Florey and his team at Oxford tried it successfully on six patients in 1941. In Edinburgh, Professor J. R. Learmonth, as a member of the Medical Research Council, knew of their trials before the results had been published and early in 1941 he had aroused the interest of his final year students in the possibilities of penicillin in a lecture in which he had described its properties and its therapeutic prospects. In 1942 he arranged with Professor T. J. Mackie for some penicillin to be produced in the laboratory of the University Bacteriology Department. Its production, however, was then a long and laborious process and by the middle of 1943 only one million units of concentrated penicillin had been produced—enough to treat one patient. After full consultation a seriously ill patient in the Infirmary was selected for treatment but, although some improvement was seen at first, the supply of penicillin proved insufficient and, later, the patient died.

In the autumn of 1943 a small supply of American penicillin became available for purposes of clinical trial and it was used by Dr. (later Sir) Ian F. W. McAdam, Clinical Tutor in Professor Learmonth's wards, to treat 40 patients (some in the Infirmary and others in the Sick Children's Hospital) who were suffering from staphylococcal osteomyelitis, a condition which had not responded well to sulphonamide drugs. The results of that trial showed a remarkable improvement as compared with other forms of treatment and many of these patients were saved who might otherwise have died.

By 1944, the issue of penicillin, still in short supply and expensive, was controlled by the Department of Health and its use was limited to the treatment of Service patients. In July the Infirmary Board were informed that the Department had asked that a member of the surgical staff should act as penicillin officer and take charge of Service casualties who might require such treatment. Dr. Ian McAdam, because of his earlier experience, had been selected for this work and had been undertaking it since the arrival of the hospital trains in June, 'the duties entailing a great deal of special work and knowledge and taking up a large amount of his time in addition to his ordinary duties'. It was therefore agreed to appoint him as 'penicillin officer' and to pay him £100 a year for this extra work. In January 1945 he was given an assistant who received an annual payment of £75.

Until the end of 1944 the dispensing of penicillin for use in the wards was done for the Infirmary by the University Department of Bacteriology. By that time, however, the process had become sufficiently straightforward for the Professor of Bacteriology, T. J. Mackie, to recommend its transfer to the Infirmary Pharmacy and it was then agreed that, from January 1945, an Assistant Pharmacist be paid an extra 15/- per week to undertake the work as an addition to her other duties. In March, a boy was engaged at a weekly wage of 37/6d to fetch and carry the penicillin between the pharmacy and the wards. In those early days of its use, penicillin was supplied free of charge by the Government. This continued until May 1946 when the Department intimated that the free issue would cease and hospitals would have to make their own arrangements through normal trade channels, although the price would be subject to Government control. At the same time, the Superintendent stated that the use of penicillin had now become so well known that it was unnecessary to continue to employ a penicillin officer. It was agreed, therefore, that the appointment should be terminated. Later, penicillin was prepared for ward use by a group of 'penicillin girls' working in a penicillin room in the Pharmacy under the direct supervision of the Chief Pharmacist. Thus, as with so many advances in medicine and other spheres, the use of penicillin, introduced in wartime, became a regular and widespread means of treatment, bringing immeasurable benefit and relief to the public at large.

Polish Medical School

From 1941 onwards the Royal Infirmary played an important part in the arrangements made by the University of Edinburgh for the formation and conduct of a Polish school of medicine in Edinburgh. After the German occupation of Poland in 1939 many members of the Polish forces who had fled from Poland formed a new Polish army in France; then, on the collapse of France, they were evacuated to England and later to Scotland. Among them were several eminent medical specialists from Polish medical schools and they were soon in touch with members of the Faculty of Medicine in Edinburgh. This was at a time when Universities in Poland were being closed and scientific life there was being destroyed. In course of discussions between the Polish professors and their Edinburgh counterparts—especially Professor Crew of the Chair of Public Health (then in charge of the military hospital at Edinburgh Castle) and Professor Sydney Smith of the Chair of Forensic Medicine, who was Dean of the Faculty of Medicine—it was recognised that the Polish Forces included a number of medical students and the idea emerged of forming a Polish Medical School here. The outcome was that, on 24 February 1941, the President of the Polish Republic, then in exile with his Government in London, issued a Decree officially instituting the Polish School of Medicine and, on the same day, an Agreement between the University of Edinburgh and the Polish Government was signed.

A detailed Constitution was drawn up for the Faculty complying, so far as appropriate, with the requirements of the University and also with those of the Acts on Academic Schools which had been in force in Poland before the war. Professor Antoni Jurasz, a distinguished Professor of Surgery from Poznan University, was appointed Dean of the School and it was formally inaugurated on 22 March 1941 at a ceremony in the McEwan Hall attended by the President of the Polish Republic who was welcomed by Sir Thomas Holland, Principal and Vice-Chancellor of the University. By arrangement with the Town Council part of the Western General Hospital, with 120 beds, was set apart as a Polish Hospital, named the 'Paderewski Hospital', with Professor Jurasz as Superintendent; but most of the medical and surgical teaching of the Polish School took place in the lecture theatres and wards of the Royal Infirmary. There were 13 Chairs within the new Faculty and it was found possible to appoint Polish professors to six of these. For the other seven Chairs, the teaching was undertaken by Edinburgh professors already associated with the Infirmary. They, and the subjects they taught in the Polish School, were—Professors Stanley Davidson (Medicine), Sydney Smith (Forensic Medicine), R. W. Johnstone (Obstetrics and Gynaecology), Charles McNeil (Paediatrics), Alexander Drennan (Pathology), T. J. Mackie (Bacteriology) and G. F. Marrian (Chemistry). The teaching in seven other specialties including ophthalmology and ear, nose and throat, skin and venereal diseases was in the hands of Polish staff on grades equivalent to Readers and Lecturers.

More than 330 students passed through the School of whom 227 graduated and 38 left to continue their studies elsewhere. By 1948 the numbers of students and staff had much diminished and in March 1949 the School was officially closed. In recognition of their work for the School, the President of Poland conferred the Honour of Commander of the Order of Polonia Restituta on Sir Thomas Holland, Professor Sydney Smith and Professor F. A. E. Crew in 1943 and on Sir John Fraser, Professor Stanley Davidson and Mr. W. A. Fleming (Secretary of the University) in 1945. On 15th November 1949 a commemorative plaque was unveiled by Professor Rostowski in the quadrangle of the University medical building in Teviot Place, expressing gratitude to the University 'for the part it played in the preservation of Polish science and learning . . . 1941-1949'. That tribute was one in which the Infirmary could also take pride as partner with the University in providing facilities for the Polish School.

Thirty years later, in October 1979, the Royal Infirmary's share in the success achieved by the project was formally recognised when a plaque, presented by the Polish Medical School, was placed in the main surgical corridor, close to the central entrance to the hospital. Beneath a shield bearing the crest of the Polish School is the following inscription:

> This is the emblem of the Polish School of Medicine at the University of Edinburgh which was founded in the second world war. It was in the Royal Infirmary that clinical instruction was conducted for the Polish soldier-students of whom 227 graduated in the years 1941-49. Presented on the 250th anniversary of the foundation of the Royal Infirmary.

Interregnum—1945 to 1948

The period between the end of the war in 1945 and the transfer of hospitals to the National Health Service in 1948 was a difficult one for the Board of Managers. In presenting their report for 1945 they had written that they did so 'in a spirit of profound thankfulness that the year has brought an end to hostilities . . . and that the vast amount of effort and energy which has in the past six years been directed to the prosecution of war can now be applied in more peaceful and profitable

ways'. The Board's own effort and energy were now applied to finding means of
carrying out improvements and repairs which had had to be left undone in recent
years. These were becoming increasingly urgent and important but, in seeking to
tackle them, the Managers were faced with three kinds of difficulty. There was
the psychological difficulty caused by the knowledge that any major project upon
which they might embark would not be completed by them but would have to
be handed on to a new management who might have different ideas; there was
the fact, affecting large and small projects alike, that stringent restrictions on the
use of building materials were still in force and would remain for several years;
and there was the universal problem of rising costs.

For 1946 the Managers' report ruefully pointed out that their total wages
bill, which in 1938 had been £73,700 had now reached the figure of £162,440
and that the annual cost per occupied bed which had been £257 in 1945 was now
£330. (In 1938 it had been shown as £188.) But the report showed also that
subscriptions and donations, perhaps surprisingly, in view of the uncertain future,
were only slightly reduced, to £124,000 and that this included £54,000 from the
League of Subscribers. Legacies and donations for general purposes in 1946
totalled £80,130 and, for permanent capital £13,700. In 1945 there had been 'one
particularly munificent bequest, a legacy of £40,000 by the late Mr. John Cowan,
WS, to endow a ward in memory of his father, the late Lord Cowan'; and,
despite their general concern about rising costs, the Managers were able to conclude the Finance section of their 1946 report with the words: 'Nevertheless it is
gratifying to note that the Royal Infirmary is still in a relatively strong position
financially, since the balance sheet shows that the total of invested funds falls not
very far short of one and a half million pounds'.

During the war years the Infirmary had been receiving regular payments
from the Department of Health for Scotland in respect of services to the Emergency
Hospital Scheme including the retention of a quota of empty beds in readiness for
emergency use. In 1944 these payments had reached a peak of £66,000 which
dropped to £12,380 in 1946. Concern had been felt about the possible effects of
the 'running down' of the Emergency Hospital Scheme and so it was with some
relief that the Board received two circulars from the Department of Health in
June 1946. The first of these explained that it had been decided 'that it would be
necessary to continue the essential functions of the Emergency Hospital Scheme
until a national health service is brought into being'. This meant that some beds
in the Royal Infirmary would still have to be reserved for a few continuing
categories of patients for whose treatment the Department of Health would go on
paying. The other circular explained that the Department's own emergency
hospitals would continue to be administered by the Department and that they
would still accept ordinary civilian patients, including patients from voluntary
hospital waiting-lists, but that the voluntary hospitals concerned would no longer
be required to pay the former fee of £1. 10s (£1.50) in respect of each such
patient. A note in the Board's minutes suggests that this, so far as the Infirmary
was concerned, chiefly affected patients from the orthopaedic waiting-list sent to
Peel Hospital in Selkirkshire where there was a special unit for orthopaedics.

During the war Gogarburn Hospital for mentally defective patients, on the western outskirts of the city, had been evacuated and transformed into an emergency hospital. There, in 1941 in collaboration with the Medical Research Council, a peripheral nerve injuries clinic was established under the care of Professor Learmonth to investigate and treat injuries sustained by services personnel. As these injuries were often associated with damage to blood vessels, the scope of the unit was extended. It became a peripheral nerve and vascular unit and it was opened to civilian as well as service patients. Several important research papers based on the work at Gogarburn were published and the unit acquired a considerable reputation.

By 1946 Gogarburn Hospital was returning to its normal function and the work of the peripheral vascular unit was therefore transferred to the Infirmary where a clinic with full investigative facilities was established in the clinical surgery laboratory above the theatre of wards 7 and 8. Being the first clinic of its kind in Britain and as it was associated with the Medical Research Council in physiological investigations and therapeutic trials, it attracted many research workers and visitors. The unit's situation at the top of a flight of stairs was an unsuitable one but it was not until 1958 that it was found possible to move it to more convenient accommodation close to Ward 4. There, under the administrative charge of Professor Woodruff, the work of the clinic, in some years involving 500 new patient visits and nearly 2,000 return visits, was carried on mainly by Dr. Catherine C. Burt until her retiral in 1967.

Meanwhile important developments were taking place in the University Faculty of Medicine in readiness for the expected increased demand for places and in order to keep abreast—or, preferably, in the forefront—of modern trends. Several of these developments affected the Infirmary. The first to do so was the decision in 1946 to merge the Chairs of Systematic Surgery and Clinical Surgery. These two Chairs had been held for many years by the two giants (albeit gentle giants) among Edinburgh surgeons, well-known and well-loved in the wards and clinics of the Royal Infirmary—Sir David Wilkie who held the Chair of Systematic Surgery from 1924 until his death in 1938; and Sir John Fraser, Professor of Clinical Surgery from 1925 until his resignation on being appointed Principal of Edinburgh University in 1944. In 1939, Professor (later Sir) James R. Learmonth had become Professor of Systematic Surgery, with charge of some 40 beds in wards 13 and 14. On Sir John Fraser's resignation from the clinical Chair in 1944, that Chair had not been immediately filled and responsibility for his charge of 40 beds in wards 7 and 8 had been undertaken, temporarily, by Mr. J. M. Graham, then the senior member of the Infirmary surgical staff. During 1944 and 1945 discussions about the future of the Clinical Surgery Chair took place between the University (with Sir John Fraser as Principal playing a prominent part) and the Infirmary; the Town Council also participating because of their municipal hospitals interest. For the University it was argued that neither of the charges in the Infirmary allocated to these Chairs provided facilities that were 'fully in keeping with the status of professorial office' and that co-ordination between the courses of clinical and systematic surgery was not so effective as might be wished. They suggested, therefore, that the two Chairs should be occupied by one person, thus broadening his scope for study and teaching and facilitating full co-ordination between the two approaches to the subject. The Managers of the Infirmary, while not denying the importance of teaching had, of course, to consider carefully the effect of any such change on the care of patients and it was not until November 1945 that they gave their qualified consent to the proposal specifying that the position should be reviewed after five years and that their own responsibilities in relation to both teaching facilities and treatment would be fully preserved. On that basis agreement was reached and, in 1946, Professor Learmonth was appointed to the Chair of Clinical Surgery while still retaining his earlier appointment. In the event, he held the double appointment not for five years, but for ten—until his retiral in 1956.

The change had been made at a time when the whole medical curriculum was being re-adjusted and it no doubt played a useful part in that re-adjustment. After Professor Learmonth's retiral, however, separate appointments were again made, but on a slightly different basis. Mr. (later Sir) John Bruce who, since 1947 had been surgeon-in-charge at the Western General Hospital, became Professor of Clinical Surgery with responsibility for undergraduate teaching of both clinical and systematic surgery, and with clinical charge of Infirmary Wards 7 and 8. Professor (later Sir) Michael Woodruff who had been Professor of Surgery at the University of Otago, New Zealand was appointed to the other Chair, re-named 'Surgical Science', with clinical charge of Wards 13 and 14 and responsibility for the University's Surgical Research Department, based on the 'Wilkie Laboratory' which had been initiated by Sir David Wilkie some 30 years earlier. Explaining in his inaugural lecture, the difference between the two Chairs, Professor Woodruff said it was one of emphasis. Both would be concerned with teaching and research and both would be charged with the care of patients which, he said, was every surgeon's duty and birthright.

During the post-war, pre-National Health Service period, four new Chairs were founded in the Medical Faculty of the University, the appointments to which brought distinction to the Royal Infirmary. First of these was the Grant Chair of Dermatology (the first such Chair in Great Britain) for the foundation of which Sir Robert McVitie Grant had given a large sum of money in 1944. In making that gift he had expressed the hope that the clinical activities related to the Chair would be associated with the Royal Infirmary and, at the same time, he had given £10,000 to the Infirmary to assist in meeting any necessary additional expense thereby incurred. In 1946 Dr. George H. Percival was appointed Professor. He had been, first, an assistant physician and, since 1936, Physician in the dermatology wards of the Infirmary. During that time he had undertaken and encouraged research in his specialty. He brought distinction to the new Chair, establishing a department of dermatological histology for the undergraduate and post-graduate study of the minute structure of tissues. Professor Percival continued in the Chair and at the Infirmary until his retiral in 1967.

The three other new Chairs were created in 1947. They were the Forbes Chair of Medical Radiology, the Forbes Chair of Surgical Neurology and the George Harrison Law Chair of Orthopaedic Surgery. The first two were in large part endowed from the bequest of £100,000 by Daniel Mackintosh Forbes, an East India merchant, which had been received by the University in 1916. The new

Orthopaedic Surgery Chair was funded from a bequest by George Harrison Law, one of the proprietors of *The Scotsman* who had died in 1944.

In 1946 the Infirmary Board had decided, because of the continuing increase in the work of their Radiological Department, that its two sections, for radio-therapy and radio-diagnosis, must be reorganised and placed under separate control. So, in October 1946, Dr. Robert McWhirter who had been Chief Radiologist (supervising both branches) since 1934, became Director of Radio-therapy and Dr. W. S. Shearer was appointed Director of Radio-diagnosis. In May 1947, the University Court announced the appointment of Dr. McWhirter as Professor of Medical Radiology, his appointment to be 'whole-time as between his duties in the Royal Infirmary and in the University'. The appointment was fitting recognition of the work which Dr. McWhirter had done in building up the Infirmary's radiological department into a highly sophisticated, scientific unit.

At this time demands for diagnosis and treatment were growing, partly because the Cancer Act of 1939, which had been in abeyance during the war, was being brought into operation. Under it, county and town councils were required to secure that adequate facilities for treatment of cancer were provided for their area. Already, in 1946, schemes had been introduced under which the Infirmary undertook, on agreed payments, to treat patients on behalf of Kirkcaldy and Edinburgh Town Councils, thus adding to pressure on both diagnostic and treatment facilities.

At that time there were in the radio-therapy department five sets of equipment the most powerful of which had a capacity of 250,000 volts and all were being grossly overworked. The problem of increasing provision, however, was one of those which had to be passed on to the National Health Service for solution; it was not solved until the new radio-therapy institute with its four-million volt linear accelerator came into operation in 1955 at the Western General Hospital where, still under Professor McWhirter's direction, a new era in the treatment of cancer began.

The appointment of Mr. Norman Dott as Professor of Neurological Surgery took effect in October 1947. Having introduced his specialty in 1931, with the use of a few 'borrowed' beds in the surgical house, he had developed it in the 1940s into a two-pronged department, with a rapidly growing reputation, which had beds at Bangour Hospital where he and his team dealt mainly with elective surgery and pioneered new methods of rehabilitation and in his Infirmary Ward 20 which had come to be used chiefly for accident and emergency cases and as a head and spinal injuries research unit. Now, his appointment as Professor had brought him, and his department, full academic recognition.

To the Chair of Orthopaedic Surgery founded in 1947, Mr. Walter Mercer was appointed with effect in October 1948. At the same time, he became the first Director of a new Orthopaedic Scheme for South-east Scotland to the establish-ment of which he had eagerly looked forward since the early 1930s and which he energetically set about organising although it was with regret that he gave up his work as general surgeon.

Anaesthesia was yet another discipline in the development of which the

Infirmary and the University collaborated in the immediate post-war period. The 1930s and early 1940s had seen a growing awareness of the need for improved arrangements for the administration of anaesthetics which had led Dr. John Gillies to organise a methodical system of training in the Infirmary. By the end of 1945 the Managers had come to realise the benefit that would be gained by giving one experienced member of their staff authority 'to control and be responsible for this most important subject'. They had learned, also, that the University contemplated the establishment of a lectureship (with prospects of advancement to Readership) in anaesthetics. So discussions were begun and on 1 October 1946 Dr. John Gillies was appointed, jointly, as Director of Anaesthetics within the Infirmary Department of Surgery and first holder of the 'Simpson Lectureship in Anaesthetics' in the University—that title having been chosen in anticipation of the centenary in 1947, of Sir James Young Simpson's first use of chloroform for anaesthetic purposes. These advances in the status of anaesthetics in hospital and medical school stemmed from several factors, including the introduction of new anaesthetic agents and more complex techniques and the return from army service and emergency hospitals of several young doctors who had had some training and experience in anaesthesia and resuscitation.

The year 1946 was an important one, also, for the Bio-chemistry Laboratory. In that year Dr. C. P. Stewart who had been in charge of the laboratory and also University lecturer in bio-chemistry since 1926 was promoted to become Reader; and the laboratory became a separate University department of Clinical Chemistry, still housed in the 'Rockefeller' building at the east end of the medical house, originally in three rooms and a basement store, but gradually expanding into other parts of the building. Expansion could not keep pace for long with requirements as the analyses called for by clinicians steadily increased. The number of analyses undertaken yearly doubled, from nearly 5,000 in 1930 to around 10,000 in 1946. The increase was accompanied by a growing variety and complexity in the tests asked for and the increasing importance of the research programmes undertaken. Accommodation became steadily more crowded and working conditions more difficult; yet fourteen more years elapsed before the laboratory was at last able to move into new premises designed and equipped to meet modern requirements, by which time the annual number of analyses was nearing 100,000.

As a matter of policy during the war years (as also in world war I) the Managers had made no appointments to the staff, their object being to ensure that young serving physicians and surgeons suffered no disadvantage on their return. Now, for the period after the end of the war, they had to consider the need for payment of members of the medical staff who had formerly given their services free. In the changing conditions of the day—for example, the closing of nursing homes on which many had depended for fees—most were in financial difficulties of varying degree. There were still some members of the Board who, even at this eleventh hour, were reluctant to agree to any breach of the voluntary principle. Some physicians and surgeons declined to accept any payment for themselves. It was plain, however, that many were in real difficulty and payments were therefore offered, though at first only to those who had returned from war service and were finding the problem specially acute; a limitation which raised strong protest from some other members of staff who had been required to remain at the Infirmary to enable it to function during the war. Temporary arrangements having been introduced and operated for the year to 30 September 1947, a final settlement was eventually made to cover the nine months from then until 4 July 1948. For that period, the Board authorised their Secretary and Treasurer to raise the sum of £25,000 by the sale of investments. From that sum it was agreed that the following honoraria should be paid:

£500 each to 25 physicians and surgeons
   335 each to 31 assistant physicians and assistant surgeons
   265 each to 5 junior assistant surgeons
   135 each to 2 dental surgeons
    70 each to 2 assistant dental surgeons
    25 each to 10 clinical tutors.

Even bearing in mind the greater value of money at that time, the payments seem less than lavish; but, in that way, one gap between the old and new regimes was bridged.

The Coming of the National Health Service

The wartime emergency hospital arrangements, controlled by the Department of Health for Scotland, provided some practical preparation for the coming of the National Health Service; but long before the emergency brought those hastily improvised arrangements into being the need for a fully organised and integrated hospital service had been considered, discussed and reported upon many times. In Scotland, as long before as 1920, a Consultative Council on Medical and Allied Services under the chairmanship of Sir Donald MacAlister, Principal of Glasgow University, had recommended that 'a complete and adequate medical service should be brought within the reach of every member of the community'; in England, in 1921, a Voluntary Hospitals Committee chaired by Lord Cave, Lord of Appeal, had advocated the introduction of some form of machinery to co-ordinate the work and finances of voluntary hospitals and that idea had been pursued, both north and south of the Border, by the British Hospitals Association, though with little practical result. In 1933 the Department of Health for Scotland published a Report on Hospital Services by a Consultative Council on Medical and Allied Services chaired by Sir Norman Walker, then Consulting Physician to the Edinburgh Infirmary Department of Diseases of the Skin and having among its members Professor T. J. Mackie, Honorary Bacteriologist to the Edinburgh Infirmary and Mr. Alexander Miles, Consulting Surgeon who had been a surgeon-in-ordinary there from 1909 until 1924. That Committee advocated the closest co-operation between voluntary and local authority hospitals with complete freedom of transfer of patients between them where circumstances so required.

    Several other reports made similar recommendations varying only in detail and emphasis. For Scotland, by far the most comprehensive report was the one published in 1936 by the Department of Health's Committee on Scottish Health Services of which the Chairman was Professor E. P. Cathcart of the Chair of

Physiology at Glasgow University and among the 18 members of which, again, was Alexander ('Sandy') Miles.

The Cathcart Report ranged far and wide over all aspects of health and hygiene in Scotland and, in its section on Hospital Services, it drew attention sharply to the overall shortage of hospital beds and urged the development of hospital services by the closest possible co-operation between the voluntary and local authority sectors, with exchequer help for voluntary hospitals. It suggested, however, that the main responsibility for making good the deficiencies should rest with the local authorities. The Committee also considered it essential that the voluntary hospitals should 'accept a measure of supervision and guidance from the Department of Health'.

It appears that the Infirmary Board did not give evidence to the Cathcart Committee on their own account, although Sandy Miles, with his forceful personality, no doubt found opportunities from time to time to put forward his own views and those of the Honorary Staff. The Board, however, did participate in the preparation of evidence to the Committee by the Scottish Branch of the British Hospitals Association. The Board's Chairman, Sir Thomas Whitson and their Secretary, Mr. Henry Maw, were among those who appeared before the Committee on behalf of the Branch. At the hearing they were asked for their views on the means by which co-ordination of hospital services might be achieved and on the place the Department of Health should hold in any scheme of co-ordination, particularly to prevent overlapping. Their answers are recorded in the Report:

> *Mr. Maw:* As is done in London, no new hospital is started or extension made, without the consent of the King Edward Hospital Fund.
>
> *Sir Thomas Whitson:* I think there should be some control.

Brief and cautious these replies seem to be, suggesting that the need for control was accepted, but without much enthusiasm. The view almost certainly held by many members of the Honorary Staff and the Board of Managers of the Infirmary at that time was: 'Co-ordination, yes; but direction, no'. In their annual report for 1936-37, however, the Managers made only brief reference to the recommendations of the Cathcart Report. They expressed full agreement with the need for better co-ordination of all hospital services and on the subject of exchequer help for voluntary hospitals they commented: 'Hospitals in these days do so much work of national importance both in regard to treatment of patients and teaching of students and nurses that it is felt that any inherited disinclination to accept money from the State should disappear'.

In the years that followed, before and during the war, the debate continued about the form a future hospital service should take. In January 1942, the Secretary of State for Scotland (then Thomas Johnston) appointed a Committee on 'Post-war Hospital Problems in Scotland' with Sir Hector J. W. Hetherington, Principal and Vice-Chancellor of Glasgow University, as their Chairman. Of the ten other members of that Committee, three were closely connected with the Royal Infirmary of Edinburgh. First of these was Sir John Fraser, KCVO (his Baronetcy was conferred a few months later) who was then Surgeon-in-Ordinary and, at the height of his reputation as surgeon and teacher, much in demand also as a member of medical advisory bodies. The other two were legal members of the Board of Managers, Mr. J. M. Vallance, WS, and Mr. David Robertson, SSC, former Town Clerk of Edinburgh. The Hetherington Committee reported in August 1943. They recommended that, after the war, the new emergency hospitals should be transferred to the local authorities for the areas in which they were situated; that local authority and voluntary hospitals should continue under their existing ownership and management, subject to a measure of control by the Secretary of State who should be advised by a Regional Council for each Region; and that these Councils should also have 'certain minor but important administrative duties' in connection with such matters as the admission of patients, the co-ordination of ambulances and the maintenance of central records. The Committee rejected any method of payment that would involve assessment and recovery of charges from patients at or near the time of treatment as then operated in the municipal general hospitals. They recommended that hospital costs should be met partly by local authorities, partly by government grants, partly from the voluntary hospitals' resources and partly through a compulsory contributory scheme which would entitle everyone to free treatment and maintenance while in hospital.

The Hetherington Report was only six months old when, in February 1944, the Coalition Government issued their White Paper: 'A National Health Service'. It also recognised the need for a comprehensive health service for everybody in the country and envisaged a dual hospital service with local authority and voluntary hospitals each continuing under their old management but subject to a system of central and local control. Central control would be by the Secretary of State advised by a Central Health Services Council and by five Regional Hospitals Advisory Councils. Local control would be through Joint Hospitals Boards formed by combinations of local authorities which would administer their hospitals and enter into arrangements with voluntary hospitals for the provision of services. Treatment and maintenance in hospital were to be free. Costs would be met partly from statutory social insurance contributions and partly from other central and local public funds but, in the words of the White Paper, 'the voluntary hospitals would still be dependent on voluntary resources for a substantial part of the income necessary to balance their expenditure'.

Whether such a hybrid scheme would have worked in practice is doubtful. The British Hospitals Association disliked it and in their criticism of it they were supported by the Royal Infirmary Board. The Board's minute of March 1944 records their concurrence in the wording of a resolution of the Association which expressed sympathy with the Government's aim to improve co-ordination, and gratitude for their tribute to the value of voluntary hospitals, but complained that the proposed form of administration fell short of the full partnership between local authorities and voluntary hospitals which, it was said, had been the avowed intention of successive Ministers; and complained also, that the financial proposals were 'inconsistent and unacceptable'. These were harsh criticisms and during 1944 and part of 1945 steps were taken to bring them to the notice of the Secretary of

State for Scotland and, by means of press publicity, to the notice of the general public.

What the outcome might have been if the coalition government's plan, modified to meet some of these criticisms had become operative cannot now be known for it became an academic question when in August 1945, the post-war Labour Government came into office with a large majority and their health service plans began to be prepared.

It would not be relevant here to summarise all the discussions and arguments that followed, or the long negotiations between Aneurin Bevan, as Minister of Health wholly dedicated to the ideal of a comprehensive health service for all, and the British Medical Association and other bodies until, in November 1946, the National Health Service Act for England and Wales and, in May 1947 the corresponding Scottish Act, received Royal Assent and became law. It remained, then, for the Minister in England and the Secretary of State for Scotland, jointly, to fix an 'Appointed Day' on which all hospitals (with a few special exceptions) would be transferred to them.

The day fixed was 5 July 1948. On that day the National Health Service came into being and the Royal Infirmary of Edinburgh, in the 220th year of its age, became vested in the Secretary of State for Scotland, to be administered on his behalf for the public benefit. No longer would the Royal Infirmary or any other hospital have to depend for support and progress almost entirely on charitable gifts, bequests and subscriptions and the rattling of collecting-boxes. The slogan of the League of Subscribers: 'A League of all who Labour, in the Service of all who Suffer' had been overtaken by the principle that everyone, through taxes and statutory contributions, would henceforth accept a share of responsibility for the provision, as of right and not as charity, of medical care and hospital treatment for all who need them. No longer would distinguished physicians and surgeons be expected, however willingly they had done so in the past, to give their skills and services without receiving payment. In future, all of them would be paid professional fees for their professional work.

At a service of thanksgiving in Edinburgh's Usher Hall on 4 July 1948, the eve of transfer of the hospitals, 3,000 people gave thanks and praise for the Infirmary's long record of voluntary service. The Lord Provost (Rt. Hon. Andrew H. A. Murray) presided, accompanied by members of the Town Council. The officiating clergy were the Rev. Irvine Pirie, B.D., Clerk of Edinburgh Presbytery, and the Rev. William B. Taylor, Infirmary Chaplain. Lord Blades, the principal speaker, said in the course of his address: 'Tomorrow the sun will rise on the famous buildings in Lauriston Place just as it has risen there for the last 70 years. The staff will go about their duties just the same; but the voluntary effort is ended and the hospital becomes a unit—but an important unit—in the great State medical service.'

Mr. Little, the Board's Chairman, also spoke. Characteristically, he took a realistic, practical view of the situation. Having expressed regret at the ending of an era and satisfaction that the hospital would be handed over well equipped, well staffed and well administered, he went on: 'Those of us who grieve most must confess we could not carry on very much longer as a purely voluntary institution.

The rise in costs in the last few years has been really staggering. In 1937, upkeep costs were £230,000; in 1947 they were £565,000, a rise of 150 per cent. Sooner or later we should have had to press for State assistance. Even those, like myself, whose hearts have been with the voluntary system feel it is probably the best thing to do, to hand it over with a good grace and wish them Godspeed.'

3

National Health Service — The First Decade

The New Administration

The form of administration laid down by the Scottish Act provided for the appointment by the Secretary of State for Scotland of a Regional Hospital Board for each of the five Scottish Regions, each Board to be responsible (under the supervision of the Secretary of State acting through the Department of Health for Scotland) for the planning, organisation and general administration of the hospitals in the Region. Within each Region there were to be Boards of Management appointed by the Regional Board each of which was to be responsible (under the supervision of the Regional Board) for the detailed, day-to-day administration of a group of hospitals, or one large hospital, within the Region. The Secretary of State, before appointing members to Regional Boards, was required to consult with local authorities and other interested organisations within the Region. Regional Boards, before appointing Boards of Management, had to undertake similar consultations and Boards with teaching hospitals in their Groups were required to include among the members of such Groups, persons nominated by the University concerned. Among first appointments, each Regional Board was required to include persons appointed after consultation with organisations representing governing bodies of voluntary hospitals in the Region; and Boards of Management were to include persons appointed after consultation with the governing body of each voluntary hospital within the group for which the Board was about to become responsible.

As a result of the consultations required by the Act, the Secretary of State's appointments to the South-Eastern Regional Hospital Board, Scotland, which had 27 members, included two members of the former Royal Infirmary Board of Managers and five former members of the honorary staff of the Infirmary and also the Lady Superintendent of Nurses. In consequence of these appointments it could reasonably be assumed that the interests of the Infirmary would not be neglected despite the Regional Board's wide responsibilities which embraced some 90 hospitals and clinics from Fife to the Border, with a total of more than 13,000 beds.

To allow time for their preliminary duties to be completed, the Regional Boards had been appointed eight months before the 'Appointed Day'. The

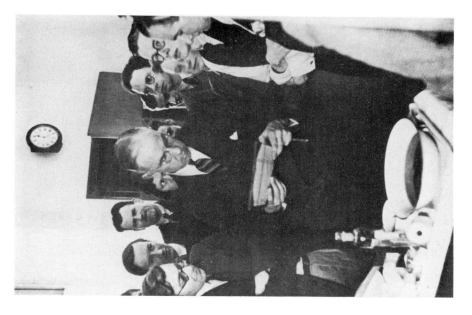

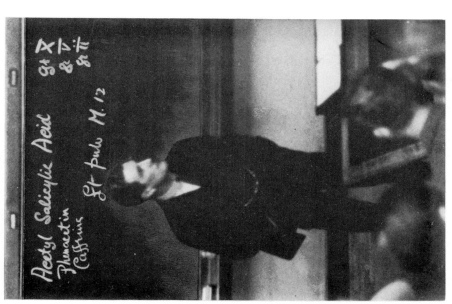

Plate 9   Medical teaching in the 1930s

Professor Derrick Dunlop (Therapeutics)

Professor Stanley Davidson (Medicine)

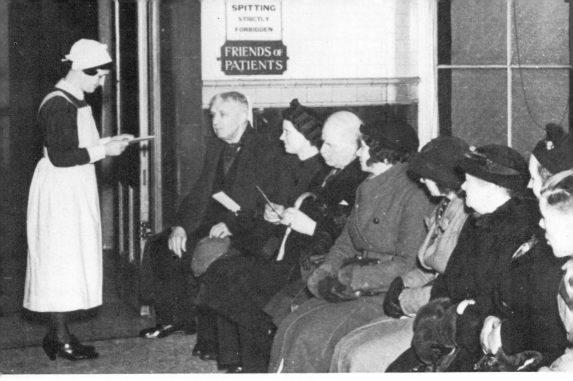

Plate 10   Surgical out-patient Department waiting room in the 1940s

The nurse is Sister Margaret Dewar, a well-known figure
in the Department for 25 years (1928–53)

Plate 11   Medical out-patient Department in 1950

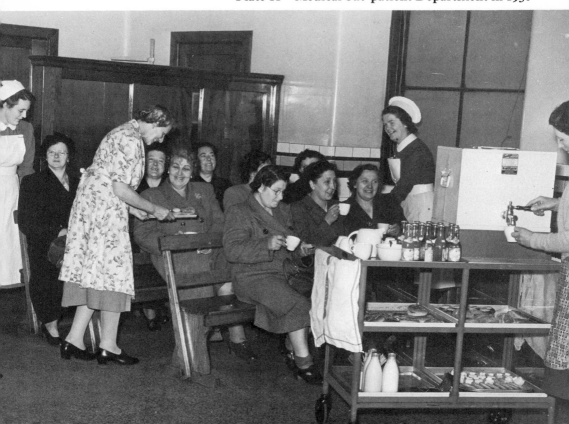

inaugural meeting of the South-Eastern Board was held on 10 November 1947. There, Sir George Henderson, KBE, CB, Secretary of the Department of Health for Scotland (who, from 1955 to 1958, was Chairman of the Royal Infirmary Board of Management) offered good wishes on behalf of the Secretary of State and said that the Board's main task would be 'to weld together a heterogeneous collection of hospital systems' but, at that time of post-war austerity, he was careful to add that 'new buildings or large-scale alterations to existing buildings will be impossible'.

The first Chairman of the Regional Board, appointed by the Secretary of State, was Dr. James R. C. Greenlees, DSO. He was a man of considerable medical and hospital experience having been for many years on the medical staffs of the Western Infirmary, Glasgow and the Glasgow Sick Children's Hospital and, from 1945 until 1948, Chairman of Directors of the Royal Edinburgh Hospital for Sick Children. His experience, however, had not been only medical. For nearly 20 years (1926 to 1945) he had been Headmaster of Loretto School, Musselburgh and the qualities of leadership seen in that appointment were just the kind needed in the Board's initial efforts to weld together their heterogeneous hospitals. Sadly, he died only three years later, before the fruits of those early efforts could be fully seen.

The Regional Board had two important preliminary tasks to perform before the appointed day—first, to arrange all the hospitals and clinics in the Region in manageable groups and then, having gone through the prescribed process of consultation, to appoint a Board of Management for each group. Under their Scheme, approved by the Secretary of State, they formed 16 hospital groups in the Region, the grouping being partly on a functional basis and partly geographical. Eight of the groups included hospitals in the city of Edinburgh. Of these, the group including the Royal Infirmary had the largest number of beds under its control. Named the 'Royal Infirmary of Edinburgh and Associated Hospitals', it consisted principally of the Infirmary (at that time with 1,146 beds) and its already related hospitals, the Simpson Memorial Maternity Pavilion (169 beds) Convalescent House (80 beds) and Beechmount (46 beds) and it included, also, such ancillary properties as Woodburn House, then a night nurses' home, at Canaan Lane, about 1½ miles from the Infirmary. To these were now added the Edinburgh Dental Hospital and School at 31 Chambers Street, with no beds but with an important teaching role in association with the University of Edinburgh; the Eye, Ear and Throat Infirmary of Edinburgh at 6 Cambridge Street, mainly for out-patients but with eight beds for in-patients; and two venereal diseases clinics formerly operated by the City Public Health Department in close association with the venereal diseases wards at the Infirmary—The Seamen's Dispensary in Leith (discontinued in 1970) and a clinic at 29 Windsor Street, Edinburgh which, in 1960, became a child welfare clinic (now child health centre).

The Dental Hospital and School had, historically, a link with the Infirmary. It had grown out of the Edinburgh Dental Dispensary opened in 1860 in Drummond Street, close to the old Infirmary, by John Smith, dentist and pioneer teacher of dental surgery, and three friends. After the passing of the Dentists Act

G

in 1878, the Dispensary became the Dental Hospital and School and moved to premises at the west end of Chambers Street. From 1889 until 1893 it occupied property in Lauriston Lane belonging to the Royal Infirmary and during those years provided free dental treatment for Infirmary patients and conducted short courses in dentistry there for advanced medical students. In 1894 the Dental Hospital and School removed to its old premises and an adjoining building in Chambers Street and that arrangement with the Infirmary ceased. In 1892, it had become an incorporated body with a Board of 15 Governors whose successors continued to direct its affairs until 1948.

The Eye, Ear and Throat Infirmary was conducted by a voluntary organisation (with its origins in the Edinburgh Eye Dispensary of 1822) which was founded as the 'Edinburgh Eye Infirmary' by Dr. Alexander Watson in 1834 'for the relief of persons labouring under diseases of the eye and to afford instruction to medical students'. In 1883 it expanded to deal also with ear and throat conditions. For many years it had occupied two upper flats in a three-storey and attic block of terraced houses at 6 Cambridge Street where patients were attended by visiting consulting surgeons in accommodation which was cramped and quite unsuitable for modern hospital use. Within a year of its transfer to the National Health Service the decision was taken to discontinue its use for in-patients (who could be more suitably cared for in the Infirmary) and to adapt the premises as an Ophthalmic Clinic and Hearing Aid Centre.

For reasons which were no doubt cogent at the time but are now difficult to imagine, two voluntary hospitals situated close to the Royal Infirmary were allocated to another Group despite representations made by the Infirmary Managers in April 1948 that they should be associated with the Infirmary. One of these was Chalmers Hospital, which then had 52 beds, in Lauriston Place about 250 yards from the Infirmary west gate. It had been built in 1864, using funds left by George Chalmers, a plumber in Canongate, to found 'an Infirmary or Sick and Hurt Hospital' and, under the terms of his bequest, it was managed by the Faculty of Advocates until 1948 when it was allocated to the Edinburgh Central Hospitals Board whose main hospital was the Royal Edinburgh Hospital for Sick Children in Sciennes Road. In 1970 on the discontinuance of the Edinburgh Central Hospitals Board of Management, Chalmers Hospital was at last added to the Royal Infirmary Group.

The other nearby hospital was the Hospital for Diseases of Women, with 40 beds, which occupied former dwelling-houses in Archibald Place, almost within the precincts of the Infirmary. Opened about 1900 as a private hospital, it had been managed since 1910 by a voluntary organisation and in 1948 it also was allocated to the Edinburgh Central Hospitals Board. From 1953 until its demolition in 1968 to make way for Infirmary extension it was administered as an annexe of Chalmers Hospital.

The Regional Board completed the appointment of members to the Royal Infirmary and Associated Hospitals Board of Management in time for their formal inaugural meeting to be held in the Royal Infirmary Board Room on 18 June 1948. There were 24 members on the new Board. Eight had been members of the former Board of Managers. They were:

Professor J. C. Brash, Professor of Anatomy ⎤ University members of the
Professor R. W. Johnstone, CBE, retired ⎱ former Board, again
   Professor of Midwifery ⎰ nominated by the
                                          ⎦ University.

Mr. A. Wallace Cowan, a former Chamber of Commerce member.
Mr. Peter Herd, a former League of Subscribers member
Mr. John R. Little ⎫ former Court of Contributors members
Mr. R. H. Munro ⎭
Mr. John Moffat, a former Trades Council member
Mr. J. M. Vallance, formerly appointed by the Writers to the Signet.

On the Board of Management there were five other members who had previously been among the honorary staff of the Infirmary, three of them Professors who under the new arrangements were nominees of the University. The five were:

Professor Emeritus D. Murray Lyon, retired Professor of Therapeutics
Professor R. J. Kellar, Professor of Obstetrics and Gynaecology
Professor G. H. Percival, Professor of Dermatology
Mr. F. E. Jardine, Surgeon
Dr. E. Chalmers Fahmy, Obstetrician and Gynaecologist.

From these names it will be seen that, with 13 of the 24 members of the new Board having had previous connections with the Infirmary, the need for continuity of thought in preserving its special qualities and traditions had not been overlooked by the Regional Board. A new feature was the inclusion on the Board of Management of some current members of the medical staff of the Infirmary. No such appointments had been made to the former Board of Managers.

The first Chairman of the Board of Management, elected by the Board, was Professor R. W. Johnstone with Mr. John R. Little as Vice Chairman. Professor Johnstone had been for many years a member of the Infirmary's Honorary Staff. Having held junior medical posts there in the early years of the century he became an Assistant Gynaecologist in 1922 and Gynaecologist in 1926. Over roughly the same periods he had held honorary Assistant Physician and Physician appointments in the Simpson Memorial Maternity Hospital, and when it was superseded by the Simpson Pavilion in 1939 he became an Obstetrician and Gynaecologist on the honorary staff of the Infirmary. He was Professor of Midwifery in the University from 1926 until his retiral in 1946 (when the name of the Chair was changed to 'Obstetrics and Gynaecology'). That recital of posts, however, is far from being complete, for he held many other appointments in connection with the branches of medicine in which he specialised.

In April 1953 Professor Johnstone resigned from the Board and was succeeded as Chairman by Mr. A. Wallace Cowan. A Justice of the Peace and former Managing Director of Redpath Brown & Co. Ltd., structural steel engineers, he had been a member of the Board of Management since 1948 and of the former Royal Infirmary Board for a total of 16 years between 1927 and 1947. He took the Chair, therefore, with a considerable knowledge of the Infirmary and its problems, including those inherited from its past.

Mr. Cowan remained as Chairman for only two years. In April 1955 his place was taken by Sir George Henderson, KBE, CB, whose background and experience were of a very different kind. Sir George had been appointed to the Board of Management after retiring from the post of Secretary of the Department of Health for Scotland in 1953. In that capacity he had played an important part in the shaping of the National Health Service plan for hospitals in Scotland (which differed in several respects from the English plan) and had also been in charge of the preliminary arrangements made to ensure a smooth transfer from the old service to the new. He was therefore singularly well qualified to give a lead in pursuing the development of the Royal Infirmary in its role as a unit in the new pattern of hospital provision. Unhappily, after less than four years in the Chair, Sir George was forced by failing health to intimate his intention to resign from the Board and he died suddenly a few months before the date in April 1959 on which his resignation was to have taken effect.

Sir George Henderson's successor in the Chair was Professor George J. Romanes, Professor of Anatomy in Edinburgh University, who had been a Board member since 1956. His success and his popularity as Chairman are evident from the fact that he continued to be appointed to that office for 15 years until the Board of Management were disbanded under the Health Service re-organisation of 1974.

That account of the Board's four Chairmen has taken us a long way from the start of the National Health Service and to that point we must now return. On 5 July 1948 the newly-created Board of Management took over the management of the Royal Infirmary Group of hospitals on behalf of the South-Eastern Regional Hospital Board and the Secretary of State for Scotland. Mr. William F. Ferguson, Secretary and Treasurer of the Infirmary Board since 1942, continued in that post for the Group and Maj.-Gen. E. A. Sutton, late RAMC, who had been appointed in March 1948 as 'Superintendent' of the Infirmary became the Group's 'Medical Superintendent' a change of title which was not without significance as will be seen later. Within a few weeks, however, General Sutton's position as Group Medical Superintendent was slightly altered when the Department of Health suggested that the position of Dr. A. C. W. Hutchinson who had been Dean of the Dental Hospital since 1934 and, as such, that hospital's Chief Executive Officer should be 'clarified *vis-à-vis* the Medical Superintendent of the Group'. It was then agreed that Dr. Hutchinson should continue to be 'charged with the administrative responsibility of the Dental Hospital and be recognised as Superintendent of that Institution' particularly in view of the hospital's increasingly close association with the University. This relieved General Sutton, though not the Board of Management, of responsibility for the activities of the Dental Hospital.

All staff became employees of the Regional Hospital Board, but only certain senior appointments, chiefly those of specialists of the grade of registrar and above, were to be made by them. For all other staffs general powers of selection and appointment were delegated to the Board of Management and thus, for most everyday purposes, they became, in effect, employees of that Board.

When the new Board of Management met on 5 July 1948 to assume the task of administration, they were free from their predecessors' constant pre-occupation with the need to seek means of raising money from contributors and sympathetic donors. This did not mean freedom from all restraint on spending, as limits had necessarily to be imposed by higher authority; but it did mean that basic needs might be expected to be met, that reasonable improvements would usually be possible and that special requirements could be discussed on their merits. There were now, however, three things which had to be kept in mind and which were liable to cause some concern, especially to those who had formerly been Managers in full control.

The first point was that, although they were still able to make independent decisions about day-to-day running of the hospitals, any questions of broad policy, the introduction of a new service or the provision on any large scale of new buildings, extensions or equipment were now for the Regional Board to decide. Secondly, it had to be recognised that as the Regional Board had a duty to see that the needs of the whole region were effectively met it would be necessary for that Board to direct how resources should be deployed, thus sometimes increasing and sometimes reducing the Infirmary's activities.

Thirdly, as the new universal statutory service took over from the former charity, it was to be expected that the number of patients to be dealt with would increase and also that patients and their relatives might feel entitled to look for improved efficiency and greater comfort in non-medical fields—the excellence of the clinical and nursing attention in the Infirmary never having been in doubt. Strangely, in some instances the acceptance of out-dated arrangements lingered on far into the new era. To take a simple example—it had always been the practice for patients' visitors to be required, in fair weather or foul, to form a queue outside the hospital gates until these were opened a few minutes before visiting time. The attitude of those who allowed such a regulation to continue (and of those who accepted it uncomplainingly) must surely have belonged to the past. Yet it was not until 1958, ten years after the new regime had begun, that the Board gave instructions for the gates to be opened fifteen minutes before visiting hours and for visitors then to be admitted to wait in the lower corridors. Even so, this was to be done only for an experimental period of three months; and it was done at that time only because the recently appointed Secretary and Treasurer, a newcomer to Edinburgh, had been astonished to see a long queue of visitors patiently waiting outside the east gate during a snowstorm and had raised the matter with the Board. Not surprisingly, the 'experiment' became permanent and finally, as part of a general improvement of access roads in 1962, the gates were removed.

The responsibilities of the Regional Hospital Board in relation to the Infirmary included the appointment, grading and adjusting of contracts for senior medical staff and the fixing of an approved establishment for such staff and for others in the hospital, now all entitled to salaries on prescribed scales. The tasks of allotting each medical man or woman to the proper grade and determining a suitable establishment for each hospital could not be accomplished overnight. It occupied many months, during which most members of the Infirmary's former honorary medical staff continued to act as before, receiving payments to account of their salaries until their places in the new service were decided and their contracts were completed. The contracts provided in some cases for whole-time salaries and in others for payment for part-time services based on the number of 'notional half-days' of $3\frac{1}{2}$ hours each, normally worked by the person concerned. Those members of staff who were paid by the University as whole-time professors received honorary hospital appointments, carrying no salary.

As time went on changes introduced by the National Health Service (Scotland) Act had an effect on the arrangements for senior medical appointments in the Infirmary. It had formerly been the rule that members of the honorary medical staff with charge of wards would hold their appointments for a maximum of fifteen years (subject to an age limit of 65) after which they were usually invited to become honorary consulting physicians or surgeons so that their talents might not be entirely lost. It had also been a regular practice, on the resignation, retiral or death of a physician or surgeon, for the vacancy to be filled by promotion of the senior assistant on the Infirmary's own staff. Under the new statutory provisions, the 'fifteen years' rule was discontinued but the normal age of retiral remained 65. It also became a requirement that vacancies be advertised and that appointments be made after interview by appointments advisory committees in which representatives of Regional Board, Board of Management and University and members of a national panel of consultants would be included; the object being to ensure that selection of the successful candidate would be made on merit alone and that the way would be open for the possible introduction of new people of wide experience bringing with them new ideas. (Soon afterwards the rule was modified, enabling the most senior Assistant to be promoted in appropriate cases and only the consequential vacancy to be advertised.)

It had long been the practice for some members of the honorary medical staff of the Infirmary to attend from time to time at other voluntary hospitals, usually within the city and only occasionally further afield. Patients living outside Edinburgh were often referred by their own doctor, or by the local hospital, to the Royal Infirmary. While this would always be necessary for examinations requiring equipment beyond the resources of a small hospital, one of the aims of the new service was, so far as possible, to make the best advice readily available throughout the Region thus reducing the need for so many patients to travel to Edinburgh. Contracts of many of the consultants, therefore, provided for their making regular visits to outlying hospitals and clinics. The reputation of the Royal Infirmary, however, was such that not all the patients seen at these peripheral clinics were satisfied. One senior consultant used to tell the story of his visit to such a clinic soon after the new arrangements began. The response of a patient examined there (who was not suffering from any serious ailment) surprised him: 'Thank you doctor, but now I would like to go to the Infirmary and see a real specialist'. Without comment, the consultant made an appointment for his next out-patient session at the Infirmary. The surprise of the patient on recognising the 'real specialist' may be imagined. It was a minor incident but one that illustrates a major problem facing the Infirmary, because of its reputation, for years after the new service began. Although the holding of such peripheral clinics must have eased the situation to some extent, the difficulty of diverting a sufficient number of patients to them persisted.

Endowments Scheme—and the League Disbanded

Before taking further the story of the Royal Infirmary and its associated hospitals under their new Board of Management, it will be well to explain the distinction between the two kinds of property which came under the Board's care. First were the hospitals, clinics and related premises and equipment which had been transferred to the ownership of the Secretary of State and were now to be managed on his behalf by the Regional Hospital Board and the Board of Management within limits of expenditure and other rules to be prescribed by the Department of Health for Scotland. Secondly, there were the hospital endowment funds—properties, securities, investments and money which had accrued to the former Managers for the benefit of the hospitals from bequests and gifts over many years. The National Health Service (Scotland) Act did not neglect to make provision for the future use and management of these funds. Initially, they were to continue to be held by the Board in trust 'for the like uses and purposes' as those for which they were formerly held. Then, the Secretary of State was to constitute a Hospital Endowments Commission with a duty to ascertain the amount and value of all such endowments held on behalf of voluntary hospitals in Scotland and, after enquiry and consultation, to prepare a scheme for each Board of Management under which their endowments might be re-allocated, having regard to the intentions of founders or donors of particular funds and also to the extent to which the original purpose of a fund might since have been met by other means. The Commission were empowered to direct under such schemes that a proportion of the endowment funds be transferred to Regional Hospital Boards which, being new bodies, had no such resources at their disposal and to Boards of Management responsible for hospitals (including the former local authority hospitals) with no endowments. They were empowered, also, to allocate some part of the endowments to research purposes.

The Commission was formed in April 1949 with Sir Sydney Smith, Professor of Forensic Medicine at Edinburgh and a former Royal Infirmary Manager, as Chairman and with eight other members who had varied medical, legal and financial experience. They had been given a formidable task, involving much research and a great deal of legal and financial argument. It was therefore not surprising that the Endowments Scheme for the Royal Infirmary Board was not completed and approved until July 1954. When it finally appeared it contained much interesting information. It showed, for example, that at the 'appointed day' in 1948, while the total market value of the endowments held by all 400 hospitals in Scotland, with about 65,000 beds among them, was £13 million, the corresponding value of those held by the Royal Infirmary (stated by the Commission as having 1,157 beds at that time) was £1,283,900—say ten per cent of the total funds in respect of less than two per cent of the total beds. This, doubtless, partly reflects the immense reputation of the Infirmary and the affection in which it was held, almost world-wide, leading to large donations and bequests in its favour. It reflected also the care—some might say the excessive care—with which the hospital's funds had been managed and conserved over many years.

Totals of the endowments belonging to all the hospitals in the Royal Infirmary

Group, as at 5 July 1948, were shown by the Endowments Commission to have been as follows:

	Market Value (1948)
Royal Infirmary (1157 beds)	£1,283,923
Simpson Pavilion (169 beds)	14,063
Eye, Ear and Throat Infirmary (8 beds)	14,098
Convalescent House (80 beds)	11,930
Dental Hospital and School	114
Beechmount Hospital (46 beds)	Nil
	£1,324,128

In that statement, the sum of £1,283,923 shown for the Infirmary included £934,412 being the accumulated total of funds given over many years to endow named beds and cots.

Among such figures the Dental Hospital fund of £114 seems so insignificant as to call for an explanation. It was the remaining balance of a 'Painted Room Preservation Fund', initiated in 1939 to meet the cost of preserving mural paintings of classical landscapes which had survived in a room of the 17th-century house which still formed the nucleus of the Hospital's premises in Chambers Street. The old house had been the home for many years of a well-known Scottish Judge, Lord Glenlee, who had continued to live there until his death at the age of 90, in 1846, long after almost all his neighbours and colleagues had moved to the more fashionable New Town. He had clung to old fashions and customs even to the extent of walking daily to and from the Court in powdered wig, carrying his cocked hat and accompanied by a valet until, in his eighties, he had at last hired a sedan chair for the journey. His taste for the old had evidently extended to the interior adornment of his house, because one of its rooms contained five wall paintings of classical landscapes—a popular form of house decoration in early 18th century Edinburgh—said to have been painted by William Delacour, a French artist who had lived in Edinburgh and who died in 1768. In 1939, the part of the Dental Hospital which included the old 'painted room' was about to be demolished and the Hospital re-constructed. In order not to divert to the preservation of pictures money subscribed for reconstruction, the special fund was initiated to meet the cost, estimated at £250, of the delicate operation of transferring the pictures to another part of the Hospital. Delayed by the war and post-war restrictions, the demolition and reconstruction work were not completed until 1953. In course of the work, it was found possible to save three of the pictures and they may still be admired on the walls of a staff-room on the second floor of the Hospital.

The £114 listed by the Endowments Commission represented the amount of the preservation fund as it stood in 1948—the only Dental Hospital endowment available for transfer to the Board of Management. It seems that, before the National Health Service took over responsibility, the Dental Hospital was maintained almost entirely from dental students' fees and through the goodwill of those who worked there, as is narrated in an inscription on a pillar in the Hospital's reconstructed entrance hall which 'particularly recalls the period before 1948 when, at considerable cost to themselves, the staff kept the doors of the institution open to those in need of dental care and established a centre of dental education known throughout the world'.

It is time, however, to return from that digression to the Royal Infirmary of Edinburgh and Associated Hospitals Endowments Scheme of 1954. The Scheme showed that the Board of Management were then receiving from their endowments an annual income of £47,470 or approximately £32. 10s per bed, far above the figure of £2 per bed which the Endowments Commissioners considered to be the lowest level of endowment income any Board should have at their disposal. 'It therefore appeared' they wrote, 'that the Infirmary Board were in a good position to contribute to the needs of the Board of Management for the West Lothian (Bangour) Hospitals who are without funds; to the Board of Management for the Edinburgh Royal Victoria and Associated Hospitals, who have insufficient funds; to the South Eastern Regional Hospital Board; and to the Scottish Hospital Endowments Research Trust', a statutory trust which had been set up in 1953 in response to a suggestion by the Endowments Commission.

In accordance with these views the Scheme called upon the Royal Infirmary Board to transfer to the following bodies sufficient investments to bring in, as annual income, the amount shown opposite each:

	Annual Income
West Lothian (Bangour) Hospitals	£5,600
Edinburgh Royal Victoria and Associated Hospitals	640
South-Eastern Regional Hospital Board	250
Scottish Hospitals Endowments Research Trust	13,720
	£20,210

The Commission pointed out that the Royal Infirmary Board would then be left with an annual income from their endowment funds, drawn from properties, feu duties, heritable securities, trustee securities and other investments, of about £27,260 or £18.15 per bed.

This was the first of two occasions when funds which had belonged to the Infirmary were required to be transferred elsewhere. It was an early application of the principle which saw hospitals as no longer operating in isolation from one another but as parts of an integrated system. The second occasion was in 1972 when a Scottish Hospitals Trust was established to which the funds were transferred and a statutory scheme made to regulate distribution of the income from them. The Board of Management's reception of the transfer requirements, however, was less than enthusiastic and, on each occasion, assurances were obtained that future bequests and donations to the Infirmary would be immune from such encroachment, the object being to avoid possible discouragement of prospective donors.

The Endowments Scheme laid down certain general rules which the Board would have to follow in making use of their endowments, the most important being the requirement that expenditure exceeding £1,000 on any one building project or on the provision of any one piece of equipment other than as a replacement, must have the prior approval of the Regional Board. Subject to these restrictions, the Infirmary Board were enabled to use their endowment funds (and also their 'Board of Management Funds' consisting of bequests and gifts received after the transfer of the hospitals) for projects for which authority to incur expenditure out of central health service funds could not be obtained. As time went on many desirable improvements and new developments were financed wholly or partly by these means and were thus carried out sooner than would otherwise have been possible. Indeed, several might otherwise not have been undertaken at all.

Another aspect of the Infirmary's former financial arrangements which had to be considered as the old order gave way to the new was the position of the League of Subscribers. With hospital provision being financed nationally, would there be any place for such an organisation? The League members thought there should be and, at a special general meeting of the League in June 1948, the following resolution was passed:

> That this meeting is of the opinion that after the introduction of the
> National Health Service there will be room for an organisation which
> can provide comforts and amenities for patients supplementary to the
> benefits to be provided under the State Service and agrees that the
> organisation of the League of Subscribers should be retained and utilised
> under a system of modified contributions for an experimental period—not
> exceeding one year—in order to ascertain how and to what extent these
> additional benefits can usefully be provided.

The Managers of the Infirmary concurred in that view and, six months later, the new Board of Management recorded the same opinion. In January 1949, however, the Government made it clear that although unsolicited gifts and bequests would always be acceptable it would be against their policy for Boards to advertise or otherwise appeal for funds or to organise the collection of subscriptions in support of an essential public service, the cost of which all were now sharing through taxes and statutory contributions. The League of Subscribers were therefore formally disbanded at a special meeting in March 1949, described by one member as being 'in the nature of a funeral service'.

Ten months later a bronze plaque was placed in the main corridor of the surgical house. It bears, in bas-relief, a scene depicting against a background of the Infirmary 'roof-scape', a group of workers in various occupations. An inscription records that in its thirty years existence the League had contributed £851,539 to the Infirmary and that coal and shale workers had raised an additional £408,330 making a grand total of £1,259,869—'a thank-offering in recognition of the benefits bestowed on afflicted humanity by the Royal Infirmary of Edinburgh as a voluntary hospital'. The plaque was unveiled on 14 January 1950 by Edinburgh Councillor Mrs. Barbara Woodburn who was accompanied by her husband, the Rt. Hon. Arthur Woodburn, Secretary of State for Scotland.

Also present at the ceremony was Mr. Russell Paton, Organiser of the League for 24 of its 30 years. After his retiral in 1942 the work of organising had been continued by his former assistant, Mr. Charles Brown. With that work at an end Mr. Brown had been transferred to the secretariat of the Regional Hospital Board. Though his position there was a minor one, the deep concern for hospitals which had led him to his former post as well as his caring response to members of the public seeking advice at the Board's office, played a small but useful part in helping to demonstrate that the new service, even at its office level, remote from hospital wards, had a human face.

The King's Illness

Only eight months after assuming responsibility for their group of hospitals, the Infirmary Board of Management received an impressive reminder—if any such reminder had been necessary—of the high reputation of their principal hospital and the esteem in which the professional skills of those associated with it were held. Towards the end of 1948 the whole country had been deeply concerned to learn that the health of King George VI was causing The Queen and their medical advisers much anxiety. On 12 November Professor Learmonth was called into consultation. He diagnosed early arterio-sclerosis, as a result of which gangrene might possibly develop and amputation of the King's right leg might even become necessary. Regular attention and treatment over the next few months fortunately avoided the need for such drastic action. Then, in March 1949, there was a full consultation of doctors at Buckingham Palace, as a result of which it was decided that a lumbar sympathectomy operation should be undertaken to improve the flow of blood. Professor Learmonth had made an intensive study of that operation and of the condition it was designed to alleviate and had become a recognised authority on the subject. It was therefore decided that he should perform the operation and that it should take place on 12 March, not in a hospital or nursing-home, but in Buckingham Palace, where a bedroom would be converted into an operating theatre. So, to Buckingham Palace went Professor Learmonth with Mr. A. J. Slessor, assistant surgeon at the Western General Hospital, as his assistant; Dr. John Gillies as anaesthetist; and Sister Anna Gordon, the Professor's theatre sister from the Infirmary, to supervise the setting-up of the temporary theatre and to act as theatre sister during the operation along with a sister from St. Bartholomew's Hospital, London. They took with them boxes and laundry baskets containing equipment, instruments and dressings, already sterilised, so that everything in the temporary theatre might be in perfect order and as nearly as possible in the same condition as in the Professor's usual theatre in the Infirmary. The *Edinburgh Evening News* reported on 12 March 1949: 'Three of the nine medical men and one of the five nurses who were in attendance at Buckingham Palace to-day, during the King's operation are from Edinburgh'.

At 11.15 a.m. the following bulletin had been issued from the Palace: 'The operation of lumbar sympathectomy was performed on the King at 10 a.m. His Majesty's condition is entirely satisfactory'. It was signed by Sir Maurice Cassidy, Physician to the King; Sir John Weir, Physician in Ordinary to the King; Sir Thomas Dunhill, Sergeant Surgeon to the King; Dr. Horace Evans, Physician to

Queen Mary; Professor Paterson Ross of the Chair of Surgery at London University and his assistant, Dr. C. J. Longland; and by Professor Learmonth, Dr. Gillies and Mr. Slessor.

The King made a good recovery and on 25 March 1949, during a routine professional visit to the Palace, Professor Learmonth was formally received in audience and invested by His Majesty with the insignia of Knight Commander of the Royal Victorian Order, the personal order bestowed by the Sovereign for services to the Royal Family. The Board of Management, at their next meeting, were told that a few days after the operation the Secretary of the Regional Hospital Board had received the following letter from The King's Private Secretary:

> I am commanded by The King to ask you to be good enough to convey to your Board and to the Hospital authorities concerned, His Majesty's sincere thanks for their kindness in granting leave of absence to Professor J. R. Learmonth, Dr. John Gillies and Mr. A. D. Slessor and to Miss Gordon, Theatre Sister in the Royal Infirmary, Edinburgh, so that their services could be available to The King in his recent illness.
>
> His Majesty very deeply appreciates the skilful treatment and care which he has received and is grateful to the Board for making it possible.
>
> The Board also, as you know, provided and prepared equipment for the operating theatre at Buckingham Palace last week and for this, too, I am to ask you to express His Majesty's thanks. Yours truly,
>
> (sgd) A. Lascelles.

After the letter had been read to the Board, the Chairman referred to the Knighthood conferred on Professor Learmonth and to the Honours of Commander and Member of the Royal Victorian Order which, respectively, had been awarded to Dr. Gillies and Mr. Slessor. He reported, also, that Sister Anna Gordon had been presented with a memento in the form of a gold brooch bearing the Royal Cipher in diamonds. It was an occasion when the Board members, alongside their happiness in learning of the King's improvement in health, might justifiably feel pride in knowing that, at a crucial time, the Royal Family and their advisers in London had shown such clear confidence in the skills of surgeon, anaesthetist and sister from the Royal Infirmary of Edinburgh.

Surgical Neurology

In the early months of the National Health Service several special branches of surgery and medicine were subjects of much thought and discussion by both Regional Hospital Board and Board of Management. Among the first to be considered was surgical neurology.

Professor Dott had already drawn attention to the need for improvements in his accommodation and facilities both at the Infirmary and at Bangour Hospital; for conditions which had satisfied him during the stress of wartime were unlikely to satisfy him for long in more normal times. Post-war restrictions and limitations on expenditure meant that little could be done immediately. However, it was soon found possible to extend the 'Ward 20' accommodation into adjoining vacant premises formerly used as dormitories. Additional items of X-ray and other equipment were installed and paid for by the University Grants Committee because of their contribution to teaching.

During the decade of the 1950s increases in the volume and speed of traffic on the roads led to increases in the number and severity of road accidents in which head and spinal injuries so tragically figure. This brought steadily growing demands on the department of surgical neurology, the resources of which might be called upon at any time of the day or night. From time to time emergency operations were carried out in other hospitals by members of the Ward 20 team through their 'flying squad' service which was introduced in 1952. In the same year a telephone consultation service was introduced which was of value to doctors in outlying parts of the region seeking urgent specialist guidance on the treatment of patients, either before sending them by ambulance to Ward 20 or while awaiting arrival of the flying squad.

In addition to increasing emergency work there were important extensions in the types of patient who could be helped by the surgical neurologist. Progress was made in the surgical treatment of infantile hydrocephalus; it was found that some cases of sciatica and brachial neuritis could be cured by surgical intervention; apoplexies were sometimes due to rupture of arteries of the brain which could be located by X-ray angiography and repaired. In 1955 the Ward 20 team became pioneers in Great Britain in the surgical treatment of Parkinsonism, a development which was much helped two years later by the purchase through the Scottish Hospitals Endowments Research Trust of an image-intensifier, an item of equipment which opened up the whole field of stereotaxic intra-cranial surgery, including means of treating selected psychiatric disorders. The department also undertook the study and recording of electrical 'brain waves', the retraining of lost speech capacities and the relief of pain by surgical means. In addition to the department's work as the surgical neurology centre for the South-eastern Scottish Region, its reputation was such that it received many patients from other parts of the United Kingdom and from overseas. Thanks to co-operation with the large rehabilitation section at Bangour Hospital and a paraplegic unit at Edenhall Hospital, Musselburgh, Ward 20—still with only 20 beds—was able, in 1958/59 to deal with 1,100 patients.

Advances in techniques and the growing pressure of work made expansion essential. There was, however, no room for the department to expand in the Infirmary and the Department of Health had therefore been persuaded to buy land on which to extend the Western General Hospital by building, at a cost of £500,000, a fully equipped surgical neurology block which was opened by the Secretary of State for Scotland, the Rt. Hon. J. S. McLay (later Viscount Muirshiel) on 1 July 1960. It had been designed by the Regional Hospital Board Architect, Mr. John Holt and his staff to meet the exacting requirements of Professor Dott and his colleagues. A six-storey building, with twin operating theatres in a three storey wing, it had 60 beds with the most modern and comfortable ancillary accommodation, including physiotherapy and occupational therapy rooms. The operating theatres, 'of egg-shaped design to afford smooth air-flow', the anaesthesia rooms and the sterilising rooms were provided with sophisticated lighting and air-conditioning equipment of the latest design. Professor Dott wrote at the time;

'Surgical Neurology is challenging, exacting, inspiring—and at times arduous work . . . Such service should be facilitated by all that modern architecture, art and technology can provide.' In the new building everyone concerned had collaborated in their efforts to bring that about.

The new unit at the Western General Hospital was used mainly for elective (i.e.—pre-arranged) surgery, Ward 20 continuing as the acute head and spinal injuries part of the Infirmary's central accident service and also for out-patient consultations. This division of the surgical neurology department into two sections, some two miles apart, and in hospitals under different Boards of Management might be thought to be unsatisfactory, but a similar kind of sharing with Bangour Hospital had worked well enough during and since the war years. Thanks to goodwill on the part of the Edinburgh Northern Hospitals Board of Management who were responsible for the Western General, the new arrangement also worked well, especially after the installation two years later of a direct television link between the two sections had provided means of instant communication visual as well as oral.

Even with the help of the second-line beds at Bangour and Edenhall Hospitals, the opening of the new unit had come only just in time. Otherwise the expansion of the work into new fields and the ever-increasing number of road accident patients with severe head injuries would soon have made it impossible for Ward 20 to cope with the total load of work. In 1938 there had been 350 in-patients; in the year 1959/60 the number dealt with was 1,100 involving 900 operations and there were also 6,000 out-patients.

In 1962 Professor Dott retired from his University Chair and from the Infirmary. On 6 July in that year, at a civic ceremony in the Usher Hall, he was made an Honorary Freeman of the City, receiving his 'Burgess Ticket' from the Lord Provost, Sir John Greig Dunbar, 'in recognition of the honour and distinction he has brought to the City by virtue of his career as a surgeon'. He was the first surgeon to be so honoured since Sir William Turner, Principal and Vice-Chancellor of the University in 1909 and the first to receive the honour specifically in recognition of his surgical work since Lord Lister in 1898. In returning thanks at the ceremony, Professor Dott acknowledged the debt he owed to his medical and surgical colleagues and the nurses and technicians who had worked with him and he concluded by paying tribute to a group who might easily have been forgotten—his patients—whom he described as 'the great, courageous, pioneer patients who have adventured with me into the unknown . . . *they* should be standing here rather than their surgeon'.

Orthopaedics

To return to the first years of the National Health Service, the next specialty considered by the Board was Orthopaedics. By the middle of 1949—some eight months after taking up his appointments to the Chair of Orthopaedics and as Regional Adviser on Orthopaedics—Professor Walter Mercer had worked out proposals for organising the regional orthopaedic scheme which had been dear to his heart for so long and the coming of which had been prophesied more than twelve years earlier, when Sir Thomas Whitson opened Ward 2, at the south-east end of the surgical house, as the first ward specifically allocated to orthopaedics. In 1949 it was still in use for that specialty, in the care of Mr. R. I. Stirling, Mr. W. V. Anderson and Mr. Ewan Jack. Professor Mercer had been chief in general surgical wards 11 and 12 on the first floor at the west end of the surgical house but had just relinquished that charge to concentrate on orthopaedics.

At the Board of Management's Medical Committee meeting in June, Professor Mercer outlined his proposals for an 'Orthopaedic Scheme for the South Eastern Region of Scotland'. Its object, he said, was to improve, expand and co-ordinate. He was not in favour of providing a hospital for orthopaedics alone, not just because of the impossibility of building any new hospital at that time, but because so many fracture cases resulting from accidents required the skill of other specialists as well as the orthopaedic surgeon; and also because it was important for a teaching hospital to deal with a wide range of cases. Every hospital in the Region, he believed, should be included in the Orthopaedic Scheme and should have ready access to advice from orthopaedic specialists, because all hospitals had to deal from time to time with orthopaedic cases, but the relationship of the hospitals to the Scheme would vary according to local circumstances.

At the centre, under his plan, would be the Royal Infirmary, dealing largely with the early treatment of emergency and accident cases, and the Princess Margaret Rose Hospital to which adult patients (as well as children, who had always been sent there) could be transferred after early attention in the Infirmary if further treatment in bed was required, so facilitating a more rapid 'turnover' of the Infirmary beds. The Princess Margaret Rose Hospital, with its fine situation, was ideal for accommodating longer-stay patients and, unlike the Royal Infirmary, it had ample open space on which new buildings with clinical facilities and for research purposes could be built as the scheme developed.

Professor Mercer's plan involved some reduction in the number of beds available for general surgery in the Infirmary and against this a full meeting of the surgical staff lodged strong objection. The Regional Hospital Board, however, considered that the urgent need for increased orthopaedic facilities was such that the consequential loss of general surgery beds must be accepted, especially as they were hopeful that the policy on which they were embarking, of augmenting surgical facilities in outlying hospitals would, in the future, reduce pressure on the Infirmary. So Professor Mercer's proposals were approved. Wards 5 and 6 at the west end of the surgical house became the orthopaedic wards with their own operating-theatre and with an out-patient department in the disused Ward 5A and its hutted annexe beside the west entrance roadway which was later replaced by a permanent building for the out-patient department.

Professor Mercer retired in April 1958. In January of that year Wards 5 and 6 were turned over entirely to the treatment of acute trauma and the in-patient work of the unit came to be devoted wholly to accident work, all non-traumatic and reconstructive orthopaedic surgery being concentrated at the Princess Margaret Rose Hospital. Steadily the accident work had been increasing as had the proportion of elderly patients arriving at the unit with fractured limbs, especially during winter months. The Infirmary's annual report for 1958-59 recorded that the elderly woman patient with a fractured femur was presenting a difficult problem, Ward 5 being continually overcrowded and the youngest patient being sometimes more than 80 years old. In an ageing population it was a problem likely to continue and it still continues.

Professor Mercer's successor was Professor J. I. P. James, under whose dynamic leadership the capacity of the Infirmary's orthopaedic service steadily increased in a constant effort to keep pace with a growing influx of patients. In 1958 the Professors, working with two consultants, were responsible for 800 orthopaedic operations in the Infirmary. By 1978, the year before Professor James' retiral, the number of such operations was 3,200. By then he was assisted by a team of eight consultants who, however, had responsibilities also in other hospitals. But there was still only one operating theatre for the unit and it, of necessity, was used seven days a week and at all hours of day and night.

Cardiology

Following hard upon Professor Mercer's regional orthopaedic scheme came a memorandum by Dr. A. Rae Gilchrist which was submitted to the Regional Hospital Board in June 1950, with proposals for establishing a cardiac department in the Royal Infirmary. The importance of the proposals in his memorandum can best be appreciated against the background of developments over the previous twenty years or so, during which, following earlier work in the Infirmary by G. A. Gibson, A. Rainy and W. T. Ritchie, he had interested himself as a clinical tutor, assistant physician and physician-in-ordinary, in the problems of heart disease. During that time not only methods of diagnosis and treatment, but the incidence of heart disease itself had changed. In 1929, rheumatic fever was common and rheumatic heart disease accounted for one in eight of the admissions to the medical wards; by 1950 the number of such cases had diminished and by 1979 rheumatic valvular heart disease was seldom seen except in the elderly.

On the other hand, ischaemic heart disease, resulting from a deficient blood supply to the heart, was little recognised in 1929, myocardial infarction (destruction of a heart tissue through lack of blood supply) having been recognised clinically for the first time in the Royal Infirmary by Dr. Gilchrist in 1928. By the year 1978 the annual number of such cases admitted to the Infirmary had risen to 534.

Working with Mr. R. Danskin, who in 1919 had been appointed as the sole cardiac technician, Dr. Gilchrist saw the advance from primitive electro-cardiography to detailed intra-cardiac investigation. It is told of him that, as a clinical tutor in 1928, he showed one of the long glass ECG plates of that time to a ward chief and pointed out on it that the patient had suffered a coronary thrombosis, only to find that the chief had never heard of such a thing. This was perhaps not altogether surprising as the chief in question had been known to say that he did not approve of 'electro-cardiograms and such new-fangled things'; but it does illustrate the change in understanding of heart disease in modern times.

Dr. Gilchrist found a more responsive ear when he sought to interest Sir John Fraser in the idea of the surgical ligation (or 'tying-off') of a blood vessel, the ductus arteriosus, in a young child. As a result, Sir John became in 1940 the

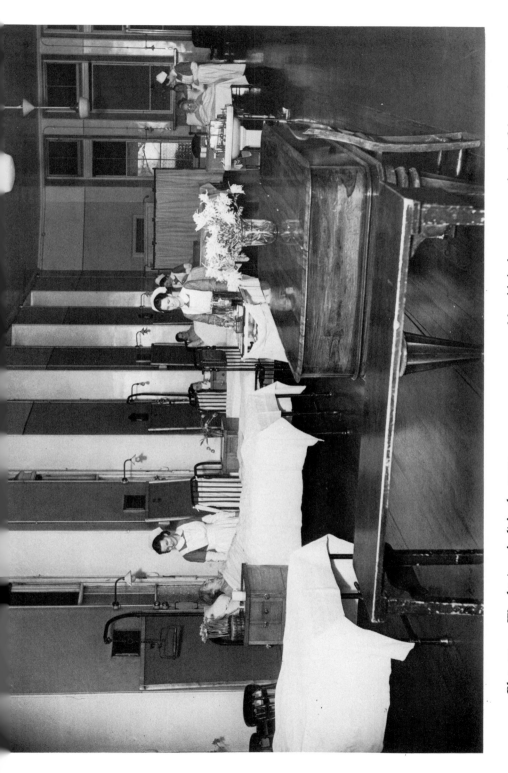

Plate 12   Ward 9 (surgical) in the 1940s

Movable bed-screens are at the end of the ward

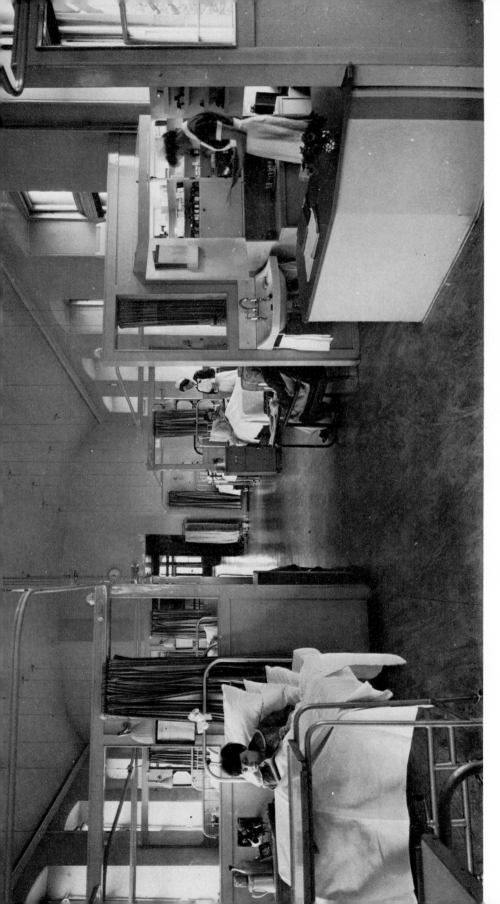

Plate 13   A renovated medical ward in 1965

Picture shows one end of a ward in which partitions have been provided to give privacy. The nurses' station, on right, is centrally situated with views towards both ends of the ward first surgeon in Britain to ligate an uninfected ductus, thus initiating cardiac surgery in the Royal Infirmary. In 1948 Mr. Walter Mercer, on the eve of leaving general surgery to concentrate on orthopaedics, was the first in the Infirmary to undertake a 'Blalock-Taussig' operation—connecting a branch of the aorta to a pulmonary artery—in a patient from the Royal Hospital for Sick Children referred to him by Dr. R. M. Marquis who was then working in that hospital on the assessment of patients for cardiac surgery.

These developments led to ever-increasing demands for cardiological out-patient consultations and, from 1945 onwards, on two mornings each week, such out-patients crowded into the corridor of Dr. Rae Gilchrist's Ward 25. The Scheme which he put forward in 1950 had been prepared in the light of that demand and of his years of investigation and practice in the field of cardiology. It specified four main objectives to be aimed at in a cardiac department in the Infirmary:

(a) In a consultative capacity, to diagnose, care for and supervise cardiac patients by modern methods, 'the expeditious and efficient handling of the cardiac out-patient being a crying need at the present time'; in pursuance of this aim the department should become a regional centre with associated clinics elsewhere in Edinburgh and in Fife, West Lothian and the Borders.

(b) to treat a selected number of patients with cardio-vascular disease and make provision for clinical teaching.

(c) to undertake research on cardio-vascular problems, all staff in the centre and at the peripheral clinics being expected to prosecute original work on such problems (an aim vigorously pursued in the following years by the staff and by research fellows attached to the department).

(d) to provide training for a limited number of senior post-graduates in the clinical and technical aspects of cardiology.

The Scheme called for the erection of a new building in which cardiac patients could be seen and examined on the ground floor, not far from transport and within easy reach of the radiology department. It also envisaged increased and modernised facilities for electro-cardiography and other forms of testing. All these requirements were approved by the Regional Board—but in principle only, with little hope of early fulfilment. However, Dr. Gilchrist had been realist enough to submit also, an interim scheme under which, in 1953, the Department of Cardiology was opened, not in a new building, but in a limited area beside the electro-cardiography department on the ground floor of the clinical medicine laboratory at the east end of the medical house. Deliberately, cardiology patients were not concentrated in one area but were distributed among several wards. This, it was claimed, ensured flexibility, increased the availability of beds and enabled a wider group of physicians and a larger body of students to become familiar with the range of cardiac disease, and with changing methods of their management. It also had the benefit of helping cardiologists to keep in close touch with several other branches of medicine.

Figures contained in a Board of Management Report issued in 1958 give a convenient picture, from the technician's viewpoint, of the extent to which the department developed in the years following on the adoption of Dr. Gilchrist's

H

interim scheme. In 1952, still using the single instrument which had been installed in 1927, 5,121 electro-cardiograms were recorded for the whole hospital. Three portable machines were then obtained, providing an improved service for patients confined to bed and in 1953 the number of electro-cardiograms increased by 25% to 6,489, the numbers for the next four years being 1954—8,129; 1955—8,330; 1956—10,040; 1957—11,509. By 1957 the importance of electro-cardiograms in the diagnosis of acute myocardial infarction was recognised as being so great that the services of technicians to undertake such tests were extended to Saturdays and Sundays. In 1953, also, new X-ray equipment was installed for angio-cardiograms (enabling the functioning of heart and coronary artery to be seen by the injection of opaque substances) and cardiac catheterisation was introduced. These techniques, requiring the co-operation of a closely-knit team of physician, radiologist, anaesthetist, nurse, radiographer and technician became ever more elaborate and time-consuming during the next few years as improved methods were developed. Over that period (1952 to 1957) the number of out-patient attendances increased by over 160% from 1,079 to 2,881.

In 1955 Dr. R. M. Marquis, following his experience in dealing with heart disorders in the Royal Hospital for Sick Children, was appointed second physician in the cardiology department of the Infirmary. It was the first of a series of appointments in the cardiology department which bore much fruit in the 1960s and 1970s.

In response to increasing pressure on the department and the growing need for cardiac operations, arrangements were made in 1959 for Mr. Andrew Logan, hitherto based at the Eastern General Hospital and already internationally known as a thoracic surgeon, to undertake cardiac surgery in the operating theatre attached to professorial Wards 7 and 8. His results there from the operation of mitral valvotomy (cutting into a valve of the heart) were outstanding. The success of his work was followed in April 1961 by an interchange whereby a general surgical unit, led by Mr. J. A. Ross, moved from Infirmary wards 17 and 18 to the Eastern General Hospital and Mr. Logan's thoracic unit at that hospital was transferred to the wards at the Infirmary. As a by-product of this move it became possible for the Eastern General Hospital to deal with a large number of general surgical cases and to act as a 'waiting hospital' for surgical emergencies on one day each week, thereby helping to ease pressure on the Infirmary.

The Regional Hospital Board were thus able to inform doctors that facilities for open heart surgery were available at the Infirmary. This was an important step forward in the efforts of cardiologist and cardiac surgeon to work together and with others to bring their special skills to the aid of patients with heart disease. It prepared the way for outstanding advances in the years ahead.

Haematology

Haematology—the study of the nature and functions of the blood and the diagnosis and treatment of its diseases—is a science with a long history in the Edinburgh Medical School, the first description of one such disease, pernicious anaemia, having been given by an Edinburgh physician, J. S. Combe, as long ago as 1822.

A century later two distinguished physicians, Professor Lovell Gulland and Dr. Alexander Goodall wrote a standard textbook on the blood and its diseases, based on their experience in the Royal Infirmary. But the organised practice of haematology there dates only from 1938 or, if one counts only the period within which a laboratory has been officially allocated for the purpose, from 1947.

In 1938 Professor Stanley Davidson returned from Aberdeen where the study of haematology had been one of his special interests. The position then remained exactly as he had known it as an Assistant Physician eight years earlier, the diagnosis of blood diseases still depending on microscopic examination of specimens in ward side-rooms.

By arrangement with Professor Dunlop, the use of three rooms was obtained for this purpose in the clinical medicine laboratory. There the embryo department began and there it remained for nine years.

In 1947 the Managers agreed to convert former domestic staff bedrooms above Ward 27 to provide facilities for blood testing and patient examination and thus the first official department of haematology in the Infirmary was begun. Its services, however, were limited to the investigation of patients referred to the Infirmary medical unit. Writing in the Edinburgh Medical Journal in 1952, Professor Davidson said:

> In the division of haematology I have a medical staff of one full-time and two part-time lecturers, two assistants and one haematological Registrar, while the non-medical staff consists of four technicians trained in haematological methods. In addition to accommodation located in the University and in the clinical research laboratory in the Royal Infirmary, the Board of Management of the hospital has provided me with consulting rooms, waiting rooms, offices for secretaries and for filing records and haematological laboratories for servicing the special clinics for the investigation and treatment of diseases of the blood. It would indeed be extraordinary, therefore, if the services available in Edinburgh at the present time were not incomparably superior both in quantity and quality to those in operation twenty-five years ago, when a part-time Professor of Medicine who was fully occupied by a vast consulting practice, was provided with one part-time assistant and no laboratory accommodation in hospital.

The medical staff, other than the Registrar referred to in that description of the establishment as it was in 1952, would be University staff concerned largely with research, although in this as in other medical fields the dividing line between research on the one hand and diagnosis or treatment on the other hand can often be difficult to draw and, indeed, neither could progress far without the other. In the late nineteen-fifties regret was expressed that the staff directly employed in the haematology department was still a technical one, medical direction and supervision being provided by the Department of Medicine assisted by University research fellows studying diseases of the blood.

The work steadily expanded. In 1956 the service was extended to enable general practitioners in the south-eastern region to send blood samples for examination; and a year later it was arranged that the laboratory would undertake work for the radio-therapy department. To meet the growing demands it was found possible to enlarge the laboratory accommodation, though not sufficiently to keep pace with all its requirements. In the following year, however, some relief was gained by the installation of an electric blood cell counter, said to be the first of its kind in the country outside London. With its 'electric eye' focussed on blood cells as they flowed past it could do in less than two minutes work which otherwise would occupy a technician for twenty minutes. Still the work increased and new techniques were introduced—among them, micro-biological assays as a means of investigating coagulation disorders and the use of radio-isotopes for such estimations as blood volume, red-cell survival and the measurement of iron absorption. By 1960 nearly 26,000 blood samples were being received by the laboratory annually, involving some 75,000 tests.

With so many advances into new and highly sophisticated methods of assessment and analysis, the need for a full-time medical consultant to direct the work became apparent and, in 1961, Dr. S. H. Davies who, as a Research Fellow attached to the Department, had made the study of haemophilia his special interest, was appointed Consultant Haematologist to take charge of the Department. Under his direction the Department continued its steady growth in the scope and volume of work. Its responsibilities now extended from the laboratory to the wards, from the routine screening of blood to the intensive care of leukaemic and haemophiliac patients and with important responsibilities, also, in the teaching of medical students and laboratory technicians.

Anaesthetics

In the years leading up to the introduction of the Health Service, as the specialties already described were rapidly developing, important advances were being made in the science and practice of anaesthetics. As described by Dr. John Gillies in 1948 in an article in *The Pelican* magazine, highly mechanised methods had by then been introduced. These involved 'the use of apparatus which looks impressive and complicated but which in reality makes the administration of inhalational anaes-thetics simple, very safe and highly efficient'. He continued: 'Modern techniques of controlled respiration, absorption of carbon dioxide and endotracheal anaes-thesia have made possible the more extensive and elaborate operations which are performed today . . . But the advance has not been in the sphere of inhalational anaesthesia alone. Improvements in the techniques of local and regional analgesia and the rapid development of intravenous anaesthesia have all played important supporting parts in increasing the scope of the anaesthetist and widening the horizons of surgery.'

By the early 1950s, Dr. Gillies, as Director of Anaesthetics in the Infirmary, had been provided with departmental accommodation on the top floor of the surgical house and thus the recognition of anaesthesia as a distinct specialty was carried one stage further although, academically, it was still within the Department of Clinical Surgery. The practice of anaesthesia was becoming rapidly more refined and at the same time more diverse and more complicated in its procedures.

By 1960 it was reported that of 16,300 general anaesthetics administered during the year, 13,500 were induced with an intravenous agent and 9,200 of the patients were given specific relaxant drugs. In addition to giving anaesthetics to patients undergoing operations, members of the department increasingly were being called upon to bring their knowledge and skill to the care of patients suffering from respiratory inadequacy from medical causes or as a result of chest injuries. Help of this kind was given by the Royal Infirmary anaesthetists both in the Infirmary and at the City and other hospitals.

Less than twenty years before, the anaesthetist had been thought of as the medical assistant who kept the patient unconscious while the surgeon operated. Then, as we saw earlier, the highest praise of him might be that 'the surgeon forgot he was there'. By 1960 the anaesthetist had become a highly-skilled partner in the surgical team, co-operating in meeting the special requirements of each operation and the specific needs of every individual patient.

In 1960, Dr. John Gillies, under whose guidance these advances had taken place in the Infirmary and who had become known far beyond its walls as a leading exponent of modern techniques in his field, retired from his appointments as Director of Anaesthetics in the Infirmary, Adviser on Anaesthetics to the Regional Hospital Board and Reader in Anaesthetics to which he had been promoted by the University in 1946. The member of his department who succeeded him, Dr. J. D. Robertson, received a joint National Health Service/University appointment. He continued to introduce to his Infirmary Department improved techniques and new methods. Soon, his University Department, from being a branch of the Department of Clinical Surgery became an independent Department of Anaesthesia within the Medical Faculty. In 1964 Dr. Robertson became a Reader and in 1969 he was appointed to a Personal Chair as Professor of Anaesthesia. Thus was brought to full fruition the academic standing of his specialty, the seeds of which had been sown by Dr. Gillies about thirty years earlier when he sought to introduce more systematic training in the practice of anaesthetics to the operating theatres and wards of the Royal Infirmary.

An assisted ventilation unit, established in Ward 19 in 1960, had four beds. By 1965 the Ward had been reconstructed and fully equipped for its special purpose. The new service soon demonstrated its value as is evident from the Report for 1964-65 which showed that 62 patients had been treated during the year. Of these, 21 had received crushing injuries to the chest, 20 were post-operative cases and others had neuro-muscular disorders or ventilatory failure following resuscitation from cardiac arrest. No doubt all would in any case have received the skilled attention of anaesthetists; the provision of this fully-equipped modern unit meant that those skills were given the greatest possible chance of success. The change of use ended Ward 19's seventy years of service as the "students' ward" reserved for any who became ill during their course of study.

Building in the Fifties

During the 1950s, while clinical and scientific advances were being made, some of which have been described, the staff of the Works Department of the Infirmary group of hospitals were kept busy about the buildings, adapting, improving and adding to them. The aim was to keep pace, if that were possible, with demands for more accommodation, for space in which to house new equipment and new processes and for improvement of living conditions and amenities for patients. The problem at the Infirmary was to find ways of doing these things on the congested site and within the crowded buildings. The ideal of siting each new department or service in the position best suited to its work and most convenient in relation to other departments had often to take second place to the practicality of fitting it in at all.

Despite such difficulties much was achieved. This was helped by the fact that, until his retiral in 1956, Thomas Turnbull, the Infirmary's Architect, was still available to plan, to advise and to supervise. After 1956, he continued to be employed as Architect for certain projects. His intimate knowledge, gained over some 30 years, of the Infirmary layout, of the intricacies of its miles of piping and electric wiring and of its wide variety of machinery and equipment proved invaluable to the works staff and also to outside architects and contractors to whom major projects were entrusted.

Thomas Turnbull's retiral, in fact, created some difficulty and involved much discussion with the Regional Hospital Board and the Department of Health for Scotland. His knowledge of hospital building and engineering requirements and techniques had been wide in range and comprehensive in detail. But the technicalities of hospital engineering were becoming even more complex and a qualified architect who also had the requisite breadth of engineering qualifications and experience would have been difficult or perhaps impossible to find. The Board of Management were disposed to seek such a person by advertisement but neither the Regional Board nor the Department of Health would agree, believing that the range of expertise required was too wide to be effectively provided by one person. Eventually, by way of compromise, a senior member of the Regional Board's architectural staff was seconded to the Royal Infirmary Board to be their Architect, initially as a temporary measure. He was Mr. A. A. Dixon, an Associate of the Royal Institute of British Architects and also an Associate Member of the Institute of Structural Engineers. He remained at the Infirmary serving the Board of Management to everyone's satisfaction for twenty years until his retiral in 1976, taking charge of the planning and execution of building work and adaptations and co-operating in those major schemes for which outside architects were engaged. A Superintendent Engineer was appointed to the Works Department staff and, when necessary, advice and supervision were provided by the Regional Board's Engineer, then Mr. William Russell, and by engineering consultants.

Dental Hospital and School

Of the larger building projects within the ambit of the Board of Management, the earliest to be completed was the reconstruction and extension of the Edinburgh Dental Hospital and School in Chambers Street. This was a modified version of an ambitious scheme for which the former Dental Hospital Governors had issued a public appeal for funds in 1937 but the start of which had been delayed by the war and by post-war building restrictions. Work had at last begun in 1948 and the formal re-opening of the reconstructed hospital by the Rt. Hon. James Stuart,

Secretary of State for Scotland, took place on 17 July 1953. As befitted such an important occasion for the city, the Lord Provost, Sir James Miller attended. The University of Edinburgh was represented by Sir Edward Appleton, Principal and Vice-Chancellor and Sir Sydney Smith, Dean of the Faculty of Medicine and the Hospital Service by Lord Mathers, Chairman of the Regional Hospital Board and Mr. Wallace Cowan, Chairman of the Board of Management. Both health service and academic interests were represented in the person of Professor A. C. W. Hutchinson, Dean of the Dental Hospital who, in 1951, had been appointed to the newly-created University Chair of Dental Surgery.

Although this was described as its 're-opening' the Dental Hospital had, in fact, never closed, treatment and teaching having continued, despite difficulties, throughout the reconstruction. The extended building was on five floors, a lower ground floor and a basement. It provided for an annual intake of 60 dental students and catered annually, in the 1950s, for some 17,000 new patients and 50,000 patient attendances. According to an account written at the time by Professor Hutchinson, 'an innovation so far as dental hospitals in this country are concerned is that the dental chairs and units are separated from each other by screens. This gives patients a privacy which they appreciate and also provides students with what amounts to individual surgeries although still keeping them under supervision'.

The architects for the reconstruction were Messrs. Rowand Anderson, Kininmonth and Paul of Edinburgh and the total cost was £500,000 shared equally by the University and the Health Service. At the time, the building and its equipment were accepted as providing the very best in dental treatment and teaching facilities. New developments and demands in that field, however, followed so rapidly that by 1960 proposals for building a new Dental Hospital were already being discussed and in 1970 a special Committee, appointed to examine the problems of the hospital, began their report with the words: 'The physical conditions under which the Hospital and School are now run are deplorable and are rapidly approaching a stage inconsistent with the effective continuance of dental education'.

So inadequate had the building become for the growing numbers of patients and for the needs of an increasingly detailed and scientific curriculum that sections of the work had to be carried on in six separate adapted premises elsewhere. Later the dental curriculum continued to develop to the extent that, instead of one Professor of Dental Surgery, there came to be five Professors—of Conservative Dentistry, Oral Medicine and Pathology, Oral Surgery, Preventive Dentistry and Restorative Dentistry. Treatment, too, was changing with a trend away from extraction of teeth towards their repair and retention wherever possible. This resulted in a greater use of crowns, bridges and orthodontic appliances for the production of which more laboratory and workroom space was needed. Meanwhile, the increasing use of fully-reclining dental chairs, with both dentist and dental surgery assistant working beside the patient, required more space around each chair.

In 1979 the 'outhousing' problem was eased by the allocation to dentistry of accommodation in the old College of Surgeons at High School Yards, belonging to the University. At last, in 1980, authority was granted for the building of a new dental hospital and school to form part of the University complex in Bristo Square, not far from the present Dental Hospital to be begun when financial resources become available.

Oral Surgery

From the Dental Hospital, a logical point at which to resume the subject of developments in the Infirmary is the Department of Oral Surgery for which specially equipped accommodation was provided in June 1957. Since 1863 the Infirmary had had a dental surgeon or surgeons among its honorary staff, except between 1889 and 1893 when, as noted earlier, dental services were provided by the Edinburgh Dental Hospital, then occupying Infirmary premises in Lauriston Lane. During the war years, 1939-45, a special unit dealing with injuries to the mouth and jaw, tumours of the mouth and major tooth troubles had been allotted a small number of beds in Ward 2. There the oral surgery department had its origin under the charge of Dr. D. Skene Middleton and Dr. F. G. Gibbs, both of whom had been members of the Infirmary's honorary surgical staff since 1927.

By 1955 the number of operations carried out annually by the unit had reached 840 and was steadily increasing. The need for the unit to have a separate department had been recognised for some time but the problem, as with all such developments, was to find the necessary space. Eventually, with much ingenuity, the unit was fitted into part of the basement area of the Jubilee Pavilion beneath Ward 34 where its requirements could be met, though only with difficulty. Part of the corridor leading to the unit had to serve as the waiting-room for out-patients and there was no space in which to provide an adequate dental workshop.

In the new department twelve beds were provided, along with consulting rooms, a specially-equipped operating theatre and an X-ray room. The conversion planned by Thomas Turnbull and undertaken partly by contract and partly by the Board's Works Department, incorporated some intricate electrical devices designed by Richard Longden, the chief electrical engineer in that department, which greatly impressed a *Scotsman* correspondent who was conducted through the new oral surgery department a few days before its opening. They included tell-tale devices enabling faults in the operating theatre equipment to be located and remedied rapidly. The same writer, describing the work of the oral surgery unit immediately before its transfer to the new premises, pointed out that 'whereas it was a common thing to extract 32 teeth from a patient's mouth at the Dental Hospital and send the patient out to find his way, rather shakily, home immediately afterwards, such a total extraction is nowadays compassionately regarded as a major operation; many such extractions are done in the oral surgery department, where the patient is kept in bed to recover.'

Within a year of the opening of the department, Dr. F. G. Gibbs retired on reaching the age limit. The vacancy was filled by the recently appointed Professor of Dental Surgery, Professor John Boyes, but on the understanding that Dr. D. Skene Middleton, by virtue of his long service to dentistry in the Royal Infirmary, would continue to be the department's senior consultant. The appointment, as his colleague, of the new Professor who was already Dean of the Dental School had the advantage of strengthening collaboration between the Dental Hospital and the Infirmary department; and there was also close co-operation with the facio-maxillary unit at Bangour Hospital which, like the Infirmary oral surgery unit, had been established during the war.

The Board of Management's Report for 1958 recorded that, during the department's first year in the new accommodation, 1,338 new patients had been examined, 232 of them from inside the Infirmary. The report continued: 'There are three regular operating sessions—Monday, Wednesday and Friday. A wide variety of work is undertaken, from simple extractions to major surgical procedures in the mouth . . . The department works in close co-operation with the medical wards in the dental treatment of diabetics, haemophiliacs and cardiac conditions and with the surgical wards and other specialties. In February 1958 a dental service for the nursing staff was instituted and the work is being undertaken in the department.'

At the time of its opening, the oral surgery department was said to be the only one of its kind in a hospital in Britain. Since then, despite the limitations imposed by its restricted accommodation, it has continued to maintain a position in the forefront of its special branch of surgery and to play a prominent part in the teaching of both medical and dental students.

Dual-Purpose Project

After the Dental Hospital reconstruction, the next large building project—though not on so great a scale—was a dual one, involving the construction at the Infirmary of a gynaecology out-patient department and a suite of classrooms for nurses in training. Both were much needed. They were combined in a single building sited in the open space between medical ward 31 and gynaecology ward 34 in the Jubilee Pavilion. The new building had been planned by Thomas Turnbull as almost his last task before retiring and after his retirement he continued on behalf of the Board to supervise its construction by the contractors. It was one of the first buildings to encroach seriously on the much-prized open areas between the wards of the medical house.

The need for the out-patient department had been increasingly felt since the 1930s when, as described earlier, a proposal to build a new gynaecology department along with the Simpson Memorial Maternity Pavilion had to be abandoned. Since then, gynaecology out-patients had continued to be seen within the ward area in accommodation which, in 1949, Professor Johnstone, then Chairman, described as having been 'lamentably inadequate for many years'. Besides providing more comfort for the patients, the new accommodation, by its greater space and efficient lay-out and equipment, seems also to have contributed to a reduction in patients' waiting-times; and, apart from the time factor, the greater comfort and privacy benefited everyone concerned.

The new teaching unit for nurses was an equally necessary and important addition. Since the establishment of the first nurse-training arrangements in 1872, the Infirmary had had an enviable reputation for the quality of its nursing instruction but the accommodation available for teaching had long been insufficient.

So far as preliminary training was concerned, there had been an improvement in 1951 when a former hotel in Melville Crescent (about one mile from the Infirmary) was acquired from endowment funds at a cost of about £50,000 and converted for that purpose but the more advanced teaching had still to be carried on in cramped and scattered accommodation in the Infirmary. The main class-rooms, since 1929, had been in the small detached red-brick building near the foot of the west entrance roadway, which is now a cafeteria. It had been built in the 1880s as an isolation block for suspected infectious patients and had later become a laboratory. For 27 years it served as the main nurse-teaching unit, while other aspects of teaching took place, inconveniently, in rooms above Gynaecology Ward 33 and below Ward 34 and in a small teaching kitchen above Ward 24, at the opposite end of the medical house. The up-to-date nurse-teaching unit incorporated in the new building in 1956 was clearly long overdue. The new building was formally opened on 7 November 1956 by the Countess of Wemyss who, having been a patient in the Infirmary less than a year before, was able to pay a graceful tribute to the excellence of the nursing she had received—'I have never been better looked after than I was here'.

The new teaching unit included a large lecture-room which could seat 200 people, but was partitioned to form a lecture-room for 64 people and two study rooms seating 20. There were also two smaller study-rooms, tutors' offices and a kitchen. Upstairs there was a practical room and a library. At the time, there was much appreciative comment on the bright colour scheme adopted, 'the main colour being yellow, with red-topped cupboards, red curtains and red mesh screens on the radiators'. Even 'Jimmy' the demonstration skeleton, regarded almost as a mascot of the training school, who had been brought from the former premises, now stood in a bright yellow box.

The cost of the combined building was £40,000. It might have been expected that two additions so necessary and so urgently required as the gynaecology out-patient department and the nurse-teaching unit would have been paid for from exchequer funds. But in the 1950s the allocation from national resources available to the Regional Hospital Board was limited and so many essential projects through-out the South-Eastern Region had to be financed that this project did not receive high priority in the queue for funds. As the Board of Management Chairman, Sir George Henderson, explained at the opening ceremony, it had been financed from a legacy of the late Mr. Robert Irvine of Granton, a gift which, he said 'illustrates the great value to the Board of Management of having available funds which do not depend on national resources'.

Behind the Chairman's reference to that legacy lies an interesting story, taking us from Edinburgh to an island in the Indian Ocean and back. It is, no doubt, only one of many stories that could be told of circumstances otherwise unconnected with the Infirmary which have come together to bring much benefit to it. This story begins towards the end of the 19th century. At that time, Robert Irvine, chemical director of A. B. Fleming & Co. Ltd., printing ink manufacturers, lived in the 17th-century Caroline Park House near his company's works at Granton. Less than a mile away at Challenger Lodge, Boswall Road (now St. Columba's Hospice), lived his friend Sir John Murray, a distinguished marine zoologist who had taken part in the *Challenger* oceanic expedition in the 1870s and then, for many years, was assistant editor and later, editor of the expedition's reports. Among that expedition's discoveries which interested both these men was the massive deposit of phosphate of lime, a substance of great commercial potential, on Christmas Island in the Indian Ocean, some 200 miles south of Java. The island, which had been discovered on Christmas Day in 1643, was annexed by Britain in 1888 (it became Australian territory in 1958). In 1897, the Christmas Island Phosphate Co. Ltd., was formed and Robert Irvine became a shareholder. He died in 1902, having been pre-deceased by his wife who had been a victim of cancer. In his will he directed that the proceeds from his shares in the company should be allowed to accumulate until enough money was available to found a Chair of Bacteriology at Edinburgh University. Thereafter, the shares were to be sold by his Trustees and the proceeds divided equally among the Longmore Hospital for Incurables, Edinburgh (now a general hospital within the South Lothian District), the Royal Infirmary of Edinburgh and the Dunlop Cancer Fund.

In Irvine's lifetime his shares produced no dividends but soon after his death the Phosphate Company began to prosper greatly. In 1911 the Trustees were able to pay £30,000 to the University, thereby enabling the Robert Irvine Chair of Bacteriology to be instituted in 1913; and from that part of the bequest the Infirmary has also benefited through the work of the five successive incumbents of that Chair.

During the 1914-18 war the shares lost their value but the three named charities asked the Trustees to continue to hold them; between the wars the Company again prospered but during the second world war Christmas Island was taken over by the Japanese and the shares once more became worthless. Then in 1948, the Company was bought out by the Australian and New Zealand Governments and a sum of £99,000 was received by the Trustees for the shares left by Robert Irvine. That sum was divided equally among the three beneficiaries. By 1956, the Royal Infirmary's portion had increased to £40,000.

Meanwhile in 1949 the Trustees (who at that time included Mr. Wallace Cowan, later Royal Infirmary Board Chairman) had agreed that Robert Irvine's concern would have been to help any aspect of research into cancer. Since such research was well supported from other funds and among the patients attending the gynaecology clinic some were sufferers or potential sufferers from cancer, they decided that it would not be inappropriate to devote part of the bequest to the provision of up-to-date facilities there. So, sixty years after the Phosphate Company began its work on far-off Christmas Island, some of that Company's profits took permanent form in two new departments of the Royal Infirmary, thanks to Robert Irvine's bequest.

Queen Mary Maternity Home

The building project next completed was a relatively small one, planned by Thomas Turnbull and undertaken by the Infirmary's own works staff. This was the adaptation of the former Queen Mary Nursing Home at Nos. 27 to 35

Chalmers Street, immediately to the west of the Simpson Pavilion, to form a general practice maternity unit of twelve beds and to provide living accommodation for nurses. Although the maternity unit had a life of only eighteen years, it served a useful purpose during that time.

The Queen Mary Nursing Home had consisted originally of two terraced houses which had been bought in 1911 by a benevolent committee and converted to form a nursing home which would charge moderate fees and was described at the time as being 'of a new type . . . an institution for patients of limited means, equipped and staffed so as to provide the most effective treatment for medical and surgical patients who, unable to meet the high charges of private Homes, have to remain in their residences or accept the charity of the free institutions'. Later, it was extended to incorporate three adjoining houses.

Opened in 1913, the Home, for 35 pre-National Health Service years, provided a service much appreciated by its patients. After 1948, however, rising running costs resulted in an annual deficit which could have been avoided only by unacceptable increases in the charges made to patients. In 1953, therefore, its Governors offered to transfer their Nursing Home to the Health Service. The offer was accepted and the Nursing Home, by then containing 61 beds (of which 24 were in single rooms) two operating theatres and a labour room was allocated to the Edinburgh Southern Hospitals Board of Management.

Two years later the Southern Board reported that they could no longer use the accommodation economically, partly because of the difficulty of continuing to satisfy rising health and safety standards for such premises. It was agreed, therefore, that the building should be transferred to the Management of the Royal Infirmary Board and should be adapted and upgraded to provide twelve maternity beds on the ground floor in which patients, on payment of a charge fixed in accordance with National Health Service regulations, could be attended by their own doctors; specialist attention, operating theatre, X-ray and other facilities being provided, when required, by the Simpson Memorial Maternity Pavilion to which the Home (to be known as the Queen Mary Maternity Home) was connected by a covered way. The upper floors were adapted to form living accommodation for nurses.

The conversion was completed in the spring of 1958. The Board of Management decided to mark the opening of the Home in its new form by giving a silver mug to the first baby born there and the presentation was made by Miss Agnes K. Shaw who had been matron of the Home in its original form for the first 26 years of its existence, from 1913 until 1939.

Under the new arrangement the midwives in the Home were supervised by the Matron of the Simpson Pavilion. Specialists from 'the Simpson' were available at a moment's notice and anaesthetists were provided by the Infirmary department of anaesthetics. It was an arrangement which combined the almost domestic atmosphere of a small home with all the highly developed skills and facilities of the Infirmary of which the Queen Mary Maternity Home became, in effect, an annexe. In the third year of its operation the Board reported that, during the year, it had accommodated 378 mothers of whom only 18 (less than 5%) had had to be transferred to the Simpson Pavilion to receive special attention. The report continued: 'There were two still-births and no neo-natal deaths and a perinatal mortality of 5 per thousand—most creditable. This is an important experiment in the provision of adequate modern obstetrical facilities for the care and delivery of patients by their family doctor. The unit is attractively appointed and the results are satisfactory. Requests by general practitioners and patients for the limited number of beds greatly exceed the supply and indicate the desire for an extension of these facilities.'

That was in 1961. In the same year the nurses' accommodation on the upper floors for which the demand was diminishing as the practice of nurses 'living out' grew, was adapted to accommodate the preliminary training school which was transferred from Melville Crescent. Comfortable study-bedrooms were provided and the move enabled the preliminary and more advanced teaching of nurses to be more closely integrated.

The Queen Mary Maternity Home continued to occupy the ground floor. From about 1965, however, the number of patients annually transferred from the Home to the Simpson Pavilion tended to grow. This may have been due partly to changing attitudes causing the simpler provision in the Home to appear less adequate than it seemed before and partly to a growing desire among doctors to enable their patients to benefit, in any but the most straight-forward cases, from the increasingly high standard of facilities in the Simpson Pavilion. Whatever the reason, by 1973 when 493 patients were admitted, the number transferred was 178, or 36%. In that year, also, arrangements were made for a number of general practitioners to have the use of beds within the Simpson Pavilion—a move welcomed as a means of strengthening further the collaboration between the hospital and general practitioner branches of the Health Service. Meanwhile, as staffing and other costs increased, the operation of so small a unit as the 'Queen Mary' was becoming more difficult to justify. All things considered, therefore, it is not surprising that in 1976 the Maternity Home was closed. The vacated accommodation was again adapted and became part of the Health Board's newly-created South Lothian College of Nursing and Midwifery.

Convalescent House becomes Corstorphine Hospital

A more ambitious project for which Thomas Turnbull was responsible as architect after his retiral from the Infirmary Board staff was the extension and modernisation of Convalescent House near Corstorphine, a little more than three miles west of the Infirmary. It had been designed by Edinburgh Architects, Kinnear and Peddie, built at a cost of £12,000 and given to the Infirmary along with five acres of ground in 1867 by Mr. William Seton Brown, a business man with interests in Bombay and Shanghai. The building's fine situation on the southern slope of Corstorphine Hill made it ideal as a home to which patients could be transferred to recuperate after the acute stage of their illness had passed, thereby providing valuable relief of the pressure on Infirmary beds. It at first accommodated fifty patients. In 1893 it was extended, by the addition of two wings, to provide beds for forty more patients. The cost on that occasion was met from a bequest by James Nasmyth, the Edinburgh-born engineer renowned for his invention of the steam hammer.

Convalescent House gave valuable service for its initial purpose and accommodated also some longer term patients. As we saw earlier, it served as an auxiliary hospital during the 1939-45 war. However, it had been built and equipped to meet 19th-century standards and, despite several internal improvements, it was described by a Committee of the Board of Management who inspected it in 1955 as 'resembling a poor law institution of the earlier part of the century'. It would have been difficult for the Committee to find a more damning description than that and the Board realised that the time had come for complete renovation.

At first renovation was all they contemplated but in 1957, after consultation with the Regional Board, it was decided to enlarge the building so as to provide an up-to-date hospital of 112 beds and also to build a home in the grounds for the nurses who, until then, were housed on an upper floor of the main building. From a modernisation scheme estimated to cost £58,000 this became a major scheme of renovation and new building. The final cost was £250,000 paid for from the Board of Management's own funds.

For about two years as the work progressed the hospital was closed, or partly closed. Wards at the improved and extended hospital were then pressed into use for some time for patients from wards in the Royal Infirmary which were being modernised, one ward continuing in use for this purpose for several years while the programme of modernisation continued at the Infirmary.

On 25 May 1962 Convalescent House was formally re-opened by the Earl of Mansfield, then Lord High Commissioner to the General Assembly of the Church of Scotland and, at the same time, the hospital had bestowed on it the new name 'Corstorphine Hospital' by which it has since been known. Much improved kitchen facilities were brought into use with guidance from the Scottish Home and Health Department's Catering Adviser and enabled a choice of menu to be offered to patients and staff. This was then something of a novelty in hospital life and its introduction was greatly appreciated. A year later the reconditioned hospital, with the approval of the General Nursing Council, took its place in the Royal Infirmary of Edinburgh training scheme for state-enrolled nurses, a status it could not previously have achieved.

In its new form Corstorphine Hospital continued to serve as an annexe of the Infirmary until the re-organisation of the National Health Service in 1974. Since then, along with its near neighbour, Beechmount Hospital, it has been administered separately through the North Lothian District organisation of the Lothian Health Board. They now provide geriatric, convalescent and rehabilitation facilities for patients who may be admitted direct or from the Infirmary or some other hospital according to need.

Improvements and Amenities

The ward improvements at the Infirmary, towards which Corstorphine Hospital contributed by acting as a temporary refuge for patients, had had their beginning about twelve years earlier, in 1950, when it was reported that many wards urgently required attention, some not having been painted for more than 25 years and all of them suffering from the drab colours, or lack of colour, that used to be a normal feature of institutional accommodation. It was then agreed that something must be done and the plan eventually adopted was that all 54 wards in the Infirmary and the Simpson Pavilion should be renovated in turn by the works department staff with some help from contractors. The cost was estimated at £2,700 for each ward and it was agreed with the Regional Board that for every ward paid for out of State funds, two would be paid for from endowment funds. It was expected that completion of the full programme would occupy eighteen years.

In 1952 another important aspect of amenity came under discussion—the question of installing curtains, hung from rails fixed above each bed, which could be drawn around the bed when desired. At that time, and for many years before, each ward was equipped with a number of folding screens which the hard-working nurses had to manhandle and hastily arrange round the bed of any patient temporarily requiring such privacy as the screens could provide. Surprising though it may now seem, the proposal to instal individual bed curtains met opposition from some members of the surgical and medical staffs who feared that fixed curtains, especially in the surgical wards, would be more likely to harbour harmful germs than the movable screens to which they were accustomed. Other objections were on grounds of expense and the limitation which fixed curtain-rails would place on the positioning of beds. In December 1952, the proposal was firmly rejected by the Board of Management.

However, Miss Marshall, the highly-respected Lady Superintendent of Nurses, was not disposed to accept that decision without comment. She protested and sought permission to bring a deputation to a meeting of the Medical Committee of the Board, for neither Lady Superintendent nor any member of her staff then attended such meetings as a matter of course. Permission having been given, she and two ward sisters were received by the Committee in February 1953. Their concern was primarily for the feelings of women patients. They told the Committee that their nurses had 'for long been shocked by the way female patients are attended to in public view and the lack of privacy at certain times is very distressing to the patients'. Miss Marshall said that the supply of movable screens was inadequate and that their use added greatly to the nurses' work. As for the danger of infection from fixed curtains, she pointed out that these would be made of washable materials and added that she did not know of any matron or sister in any hospital where such curtains were in use who would wish to revert to the use of screens. Her plea was only partly successful. The Committee agreed to recommend the use of bed curtains on rails but only as an experiment in one gynaecology ward. A year later, following requests from medical staff, it was decided to equip all the medical wards with bed curtains. On the suggestion of Miss Marshall it was agreed that the curtains should be made of brightly coloured materials thus adding to the cheerful atmosphere in the re-decorated medical wards. Yet in July 1957, the wisdom or unwisdom of installing curtains in the surgical wards was still being debated.

By 1957, nine wards—three gynaecological and six medical—had been renovated, and according to a press report were 'sparkling new and up-to-date'. Side rooms were also being improved and cork matting was being laid over the stone floors of ward corridors. Until then, all corridors still had the original bare stone-flagged floors except the main surgical corridor for which rubber covering had been provided, years before, by rubber planters of the Federated Malay States.

Referring to the improvements, Dr. Francis said that many of the ideas adopted had been suggested by ward sisters, nurses and other staff, each sister having been invited to collect and submit ideas, all of which had been discussed at meetings of Medical Superintendent, Architect, Lady Superintendent and Sisters. He added that one result of this series of consultations was that each completed ward showed some improvement on the previous one, proving the wisdom of accepting advice from those with practical working knowledge of the needs.

While the work of renovation was going on, improving the comfort and the general atmosphere of the wards, the Clinical Medicine Board (members of the medical staff responsible for clinical teaching arrangements) drew attention to the need for more extensive improvements if the Infirmary was to maintain its high reputation. In March 1955 they wrote:

> We have no desire for a radical re-building of the medical pavilions.
> We consider that the wards are excellent for their purpose, large, well ventilated, spacious and light and that they only require certain modifications and additions to make them entirely suitable for their purpose

but the modifications which they suggested were quite extensive. They recommended the conversion of accommodation at the north, or corridor, end of each medical ward to form single rooms in which critically ill or disturbed patients could be looked after, the improvement of lavatory and bathroom accommodation and the construction of a day-room and sun-parlour at the south end of each ward, overlooking the Meadows. 'The present arrangements', their letter added, 'by which convalescent patients sit on a hard chair by their beds or at the end of the ward before a single-bar radiator is antiquated and inhuman.' These improvements, they explained, were becoming more important as the practice of encouraging patients to spend more time out of bed was being increasingly adopted.

The suggestions were commended by the Medical Committee of the Board of Management and a scheme incorporating them was submitted to the Regional Hospital Board for approval. The scheme envisaged that during the next few years, the twelve medical Wards (22 to 33 in the pavilions facing the Meadows) would be adapted, in sequence, in the way proposed; but four years later, the Regional Board had still been unable to sanction the expenditure involved.

In 1958 a comparable scheme for one surgical ward (Ward 18 in the west-most surgical pavilion) was undertaken. Like the scheme proposed earlier it included the formation of small rooms at the inner end of the ward and the improvement of toilet facilities and construction of a day room at the outer end of the ward. The surgical wards had always had narrow open balconies there. Now, an enclosed glass-fronted lounge, comfortably furnished, was provided at the end of Ward 18, constructed partly in the former balcony space.

This was the first stage of a new programme which envisaged two surgical

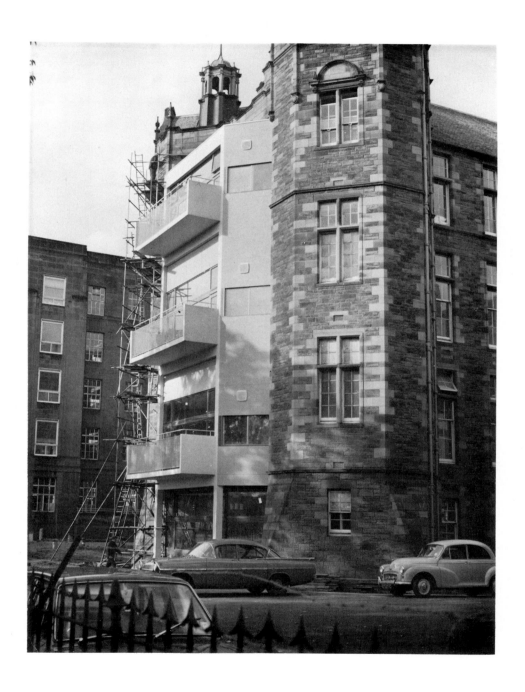

Plate 14   Formation of ward day-rooms

These were built outwards between turrets. This extension is to the Jubilee Pavilion

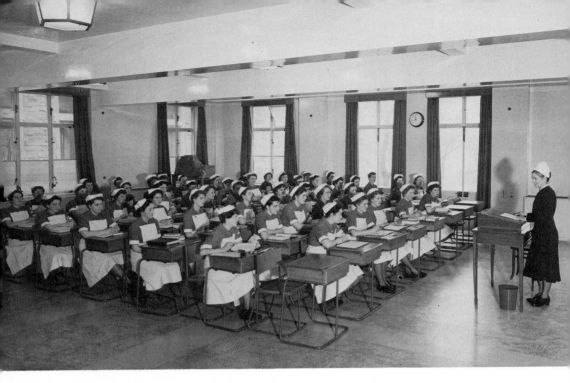

Plate 15   Student nurses in their new class-room — 1956

The lecturer is Miss Barbara Renton, Lady Superintendent of Nurses 1955-59

Plate 16   Night nurses' bus

These nurses, coming off duty in 1950, are boarding their special bus which took them daily to and from Woodburn House, Canaan Lane, Morningside, used as a night nurses' home from 1922 until 1966.

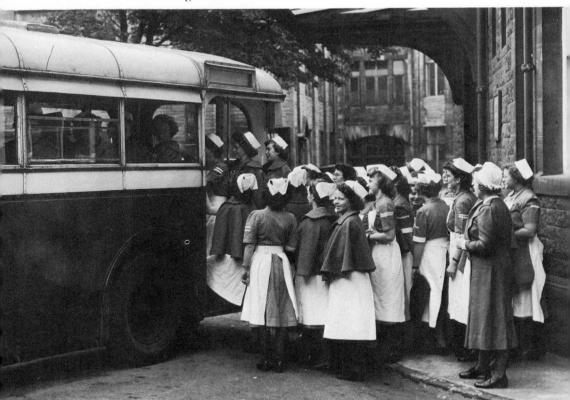

wards being reconstructed each year until all had been adapted to meet the most up-to-date requirements. For this first stage, two-thirds of the cost was to be met from endowment funds. The allocation of costs of further stages was left for later discussion.

When reconstruction of surgical Ward 18 was completed in January 1959 the physicians understandably were curious to know what had become of their proposals for the medical wards. Their concern was noted and it was soon agreed that a comprehensive programme should be adopted under which two major ward reconstructions would be undertaken each year until all wards in the main building had been brought up to date on roughly similar lines, the cost to be shared between exchequer and endowment funds in proportions to be agreed.

By March 1963 six medical Wards had been reconstructed—22, 23 and 24 in the eastmost medical pavilion and 25, 26 and 27 in the next pavilion. In each case the suggested day-room and sun-parlour had been formed out of part of the south end of each ward and by building outwards between the turrets, as had been done in surgical Ward 18, but with two minor differences. Planning restrictions had required the sun-parlour facing on to Lauriston Place to be kept within the outer limit of the turret walls, but those facing the Meadows were allowed to project slightly beyond that line, giving some extra interior space; and while the extensions of the medical wards were supported by stanchions from ground level, those of the surgical wards were cantilevered out from the ward floors so as not to impede essential traffic using the narrow roadway below.

The results of the reconstruction of the first six medical wards were described in 1963 as follows:

> A feature of the reconstructed wards is the degree of privacy provided to the patients by the bay partitioning and bed lay-out which combats the institutional atmosphere of the older type of ward whilst still retaining ready access to every patient for nursing care and observation. Each bed position is wired for radio, individual bed-head lighting and nurses call-system. Plug-in points have been provided, allowing the use of a mobile telephone at every bed. Bathing and toilet facilities and nurses work-room space, previously very limited . . . are more generously provided for. The reconstructed wards also provide comfortable sitting-rooms for patients able to get up and much improved facilities for the medical staff and for teaching.

At that time, planning for complete rebuilding of the Infirmary was under way and it would have been easy for the Board of Management to regard that as a good reason for going no further with their upgrading schemes. They decided, however, that it would be unfair to patients and staff alike to allow the promise of future perfection to be used as an excuse for tolerating, longer than absolutely necessary, conditions which were unsatisfactory. Timing of the upgrading of the wards in the main building was dictated not just by financial considerations but also by the availability of alternative accommodation, sometimes as far afield as the City Hospital, to which patients could be transferred while the work progressed. At last, in 1971, all wards in the main building had been upgraded and provided with day-rooms.

I

Two Senior Officers

Under the National Health Service, the Board of Management carried on their functions, as the former Managers had done, through a series of committees appointed from among their own members, chief among these being the General Purposes, Finance and Law, Establishment, Medical, Nursing and Works and Buildings Committees; and they encouraged to a greater degree than before, the giving of advice and submission of representations from formally constituted Committees of the medical and surgical staffs.

The two chief officers of the Board of Management—both of whom were now appointed by the Regional Hospital Board after consideration jointly by representatives of both Boards—were the Secretary and Treasurer and the Medical Superintendent. In July 1948 these posts were occupied respectively by Mr. William F. Ferguson, FHA, Solicitor, who had held the corresponding post under the former Managers since 1942 and Maj.-Gen. E. A. Sutton, CB, CBE, MC, (late RAMC) who had been appointed as 'Superintendent' by the former Managers in November 1947, with effect on 1st March 1948, only about four months before the change-over. The post of Secretary and Treasurer had been so designated since 1929 when Mr. Henry Maw had been appointed on the retiral of Mr. William S. Caw (after 49 years service in the Infirmary) who had been 'Treasurer and Clerk' since 1893. The change of designation in 1929 had been seen by some as subtly implying an upward trend in the holder's position in the hierarchy of administration and Henry Maw, during his 13 years in office, acted in some sense as a 'lay administrator' directing some aspects of the hospital's affairs beyond the strictly secretarial and financial responsibilities to which his immediate successor was more inclined to adhere. In 1948, the prefixing in hospitals throughout Scotland of the word 'Medical' to the title of 'Superintendent' seemed to imply a limitation of the span of control of that post to matters which had a medical bearing.

Major-General Sutton resigned in October 1952. Before advertising the vacancy, the Regional Board and the Board of Management were at pains to adjust the pre-1948 regulations under which the two officers had hitherto worked. These regulations began with a general statement that the Superintendent was to have the chief authority within the hospital but went on, in a later section, to say that he was to be responsible for all officials and their work 'with the exception of the Secretary and Treasurer and the business falling to be done by him'. The Board of Management now proposed to omit from the revised document the words within these quotation marks. The Secretary and Treasurer objected that to do so would, in effect, curtail his authority and be contrary to the terms of the contract under which he had been employed since 1942. Not only so, but the Regional Board also pointed out that the proposed omission, by giving the Medical Superintendent full control over the Secretary and Treasurer, would be inconsistent with a directive issued by the Department of Health for Scotland in 1948 that under the National Health Service 'the Medical Superintendent and the Secretary and Treasurer should be two senior officers of equal status working together'. So the Board of Management agreed that 'a more general statement of duties' should be adopted which would not contravene the intention of the Department's directive but they added that they did so 'on the understanding that this did not indicate any weakening of their opposition' to the terms of the directive.

The difficulty really stemmed from the long-standing belief in Scotland that a hospital superintendent must be ultimately responsible for every aspect of administration because everything done in a hospital, whether connected with medical matters or not, might affect in one way or another the welfare of the patients which was his prime concern. The other point of view, more prevalent in England, was that there were many matters important to the patients' well-being which could be effectively directed by a lay administrator, thereby leaving his medically-qualified colleague free to devote more time to aspects of administration which have a direct bearing on the treatment and medical condition of the patients. That seems to have been the view on which the Department of Health had based their directive.

In April 1953, after the necessary consultation, the Regional Hospital Board appointed as General Sutton's successor in the office of Group Medical Superintendent, Dr. S. G. M. Francis, TD, MB, ChB, who had been Deputy Medical Superintendent since 1951. His was the eighth appointment since the post of Superintendent was created in 1871. All seven of his predecessors in office had been high-ranking military medical men, four having had careers in the Army Medical Service and three in the Indian Medical Service, before coming to the Infirmary. In former more authoritarian days, a background of military-style discipline may well have been a valuable asset for anyone given the task of governing a large charitable institution such as the Infirmary and certainly the later Superintendents—Colonel G. D. St. Clair Thom, CB, AMS (1924 to 1935), Lt.-Col. A. D. Stewart, CIE, IMS (1935 to 1948) and Maj.-Gen. E. A. Sutton—each enjoyed an outstanding reputation for the firmness, combined with tact, sympathy and understanding with which they had exercised their authority. Now, however, as the administrative organisation of the health service was developing, the time seemed right for a medical superintendent with a different background to be appointed.

Dr. Francis had graduated in Edinburgh in 1936. Though holding the rank of Major, RAMC in the Territorial Army, his main experience had been in civilian hospital work, including periods as Resident Medical Officer in Birmingham Children's Hospital and as Assistant Paediatrician in the Simpson Memorial Maternity Pavilion. More recently, as Deputy Medical Superintendent, he had gained valuable knowledge of the intricate organisation of the Royal Infirmary and its special problems. He remained in office as Group Medical Superintendent for 21 years, until that post was discontinued under the National Health Service re-organisation of 1974. From then until his retiral in 1977 he was a Community Medicine Specialist, still retaining a special link with the Infirmary where he continued to have an office. As Medical Superintendent he played an important part in the formulation of long-term plans for re-building the hospital and in the shorter term arrangements for forming new departments and modernising others.

Within four years of Dr. Francis' appointment the question of the relationship of his post with that of the Secretary and Treasurer arose again, this time as a result of the retiral of Mr. W. F. Ferguson from that post in January 1957 owing to ill-health. With the need to adjust conditions of appointment for issue to candidates, the question of co-ordinating the functions of the two positions was again raised. This time the Board of Management had more definite guidance to refer to than the mere assertion that the two officers should be of equal status working together. Only a month earlier, in December 1956, the Secretary of State's advisory Scottish Health Services Council had adopted and published a report by one of their sub-committees whose terms of reference had included a remit 'to consider how medical participation in the control and management of hospitals can best be secured in Scottish conditions with special reference to (a) the employment of medical superintendents, their functions, recruitment and training . . .' That report was of special interest to the Board of Management because Sir George Henderson, their Chairman, had also been Chairman of the Health Services Council's Sub-Committee responsible for the Report. In March 1957 he drew the Board's attention to the fact that the Report had rejected the suggestion that *all* management duties in hospital should be the responsibility of the Medical Superintendent and had advised that a lay administrator should be responsible directly to the management board for matters in which the lay interest was predominant.

Bearing that advice in mind, the Board of Management, in April, approved of arrangements under which separate functions would be specifically allocated to each post. Accordingly the stage was set for the vacancy of Secretary and Treasurer to be advertised. But in seeking to state specifically the division of functions, the Board had attempted a very difficult task. Given the increasing volume and complexity of hospital work, questions of demarcation and emphasis were bound to arise and, in the following years they did arise from time to time, though it would now be pointless to narrate them. One is left with the thought that perhaps, after all, no detailed description of duties could have improved upon the Department of Health's initial dictum that the Medical Superintendent and the Secretary and Treasurer 'should be two senior officers of equal status working together'.

In July 1957 the Regional Board, in consultation with the Board of Management, appointed as the new Secretary and Treasurer of the Royal Infirmary of Edinburgh and Associated Hospitals, Tom Hurst. A Fellow of the Institute of Hospital Administrators and an Associate of the Chartered Institute of Secretaries, he had already had a successful career in hospital administration. Since 1948 he had been Group Secretary of the Wigan and Leigh Hospital Management Committee (English equivalent of 'Board of Management') within the area of the Manchester Regional Hospital Board.

Tom Hurst attended his first Board meeting as Secretary and Treasurer in November 1957. He remained at the Infirmary until 1971 when he resigned to take up an appointment with the National Health Service Advisory Service in London. During his fourteen years at the Infirmary the pace of developments there certainly accelerated. The up-grading of wards (as distinct from their renovation), the introduction of the pre-set tray system for issue to operating theatres of sterile sets of instruments and dressings, progress towards the centralisation of medical records—these and other advances were made during those years. All involved the initiative and effort of many people but progress on each of them owed something to Tom Hurst's enthusiasm.

Some of these developments will be described later but one action, taken soon after Hurst's arrival, deserves to be mentioned now. It is one for which every chronicler of events during the period must be grateful—the introduction of the Board of Management's Annual Report. The former Managers of the Royal Infirmary, in compliance with their Royal Charter, had issued a report every year, their last being the one for 1946, published late in 1947. By the time their 1947 Report would have appeared, they had demitted office and, under the National Health Service, the new Board of Management had taken charge. Perhaps because one of the main purposes of the Report had formerly been to encourage donations and subscriptions, the new Board, relieved of that concern and with so many other urgent responsibilities on their minds, saw no need to continue such a publication and for ten years no report appeared—a fact which astonished the new Secretary and Treasurer on his arrival. With the approval of the Chairman and of the Board of Management, he at once set about remedying the omission. In 1959 a summary report for the years 1948 to 1958 was issued and, for fourteen years thereafter, annual reports appeared. Together they form a valuable record of an important period in the story of the Infirmary and its associated hospitals. Unhappily, with the approach of the Health Service re-organisation of 1974, history repeated itself and, after the issue of the Report for 1972-73, the publication of annual reports again ceased.

Tom Hurst was succeeded at the Infirmary by George G. Savage who had previously occupied the corresponding post in the Edinburgh Northern Hospitals Group. In 1973, however, as re-organisation approached, Mr. Savage became Secretary of the newly-created Lanarkshire Health Board. In 1974, the posts of Medical Superintendent and Secretary and Treasurer were discontinued on the disbandment of the Board of Management.

Personnel Department

Among the duties undertaken by the Medical Superintendent and the Secretary and Treasurer, each in his own sphere, was the appointment of staff other than those on the most senior grades, who were appointed by the Regional Hospital Board and nurses, for whose appointment the Lady Superintendent was responsible. Even although recruitment to many sections within the hospitals in the Group was delegated to section heads, the increase in the total numbers employed put a growing strain on the senior officers; and the distribution of responsibility among departments meant that staff records were scattered and unco-ordinated.

In 1958 the Department of Health for Scotland suggested that as an experiment a Group personnel department should be set up in the Infirmary. In response to that suggestion a personnel officer was appointed and provided with a secretary. This was the first such department in a Scottish hospital, the only precedent in Britain having been the establishment of the personnel department of St. Thomas's

Hospital in London in 1947. Office accommodation was provided in one room of the central gate lodge which was no longer in use as the Chief Porter's house.

Progress at first was slow. There was initial resistance from some departmental and section heads. Although it would be the personnel officer's function to relieve them of much of the 'drudgery' of appointments procedures and although they would always be consulted and would normally make the final decisions on choice of candidate, they tended to see the new arrangement as an encroachment on their authority.

Reviews by the Department of Health in 1960 and by the Regional work-study team in 1965 helped to demonstrate the advantages to be gained by a fuller use of the Personnel Officer and to suggest ways in which his role might be expanded to include, in addition to recruitment, help in arranging transfers and promotions, the giving of advice on staff complements and gradings, the specification of conditions of service and—all important—the maintenance of staff records.

Though accommodation expanded within the restricted limits of the gate-lodge it continued to be insufficient until, in 1968, the department moved into part of the Red Home. By then their staff complement had increased to a total of four; despite that modest number, they were by then actively engaged in all stages of appointment of almost all staff except medical and nursing personnel. Under the 1974 re-organisation, District and Area Personnel Officers were appointed and their presence helped in the standardisation of practices and procedures. The mass of employment legislation and increasingly voluminous Whitley Council conditions introduced during the 1970s, combined with greater trade union activity among hospital staffs, made the presence of a department able to keep pace with all the complexities of these developments and to act in accordance with their requirements, an essential part of such a large organisation. By 1979 the Personnel Officer and his staff of six were providing a centralised service which covered about 2,500 staff in the Infirmary, the Simpson Pavilion, Chalmers Hospital, the Eye Pavilion and the Dental Hospital—i.e. all staff except nurses and senior medical officers; junior medical posts having been brought partly within the department's scope in 1978. It had become unlikely that any departmental head would now complain, as some had done twenty years before, of being relieved of a function which had become a complicated and time-consuming one requiring specialised knowledge.

4

Planning Ahead

Towards a New Infirmary

In anticipation of the Health Service, the Department of Health for Scotland published in 1946 a comprehensive Survey of Hospitals in Scotland which included a Report on those in the South-Eastern Region by Mr. J. W. Struthers (Surgeon-in-Ordinary in the Infirmary from 1925 until 1941 and thereafter Consulting Surgeon) and Dr. Henry E. Seiler (then Depute Medical Officer of Health and later MOH of Edinburgh). In sections of their report dealing with the Royal Infirmary they wrote: 'It is evident that if the hospital is to meet the increasing demands made on it radical alterations will be required, especially in the older parts of the buildings'; and 'the only hope of carrying out much-needed improvement appears to lie in replacing the original pavilions by new buildings'. They pointed out, also, that as the crowded site was already occupied by a collection of buildings of varying sizes and styles, 'future plans for re-building need not therefore be conditioned by any necessity to adhere to a uniform architectural style'. Right from the start, therefore, there was recognition that, sooner rather than later, the original Infirmary buildings would have to be replaced.

Before pursuing the idea of replacing them on the same site, with all the problems that was bound to cause, the Department of Health and the Regional Hospital Board seriously considered the possibility of building a new large teaching hospital on the outskirts of the city where construction would be straightforward and ample space could be reserved for future extension. In September 1950 the Regional Board asked the Department to acquire for that purpose an area of farmland on Mortonhall estate on the southern edge of the city, not far from the Princess Margaret Rose Hospital. A modern teaching hospital there, they argued, would relieve pressure on the Infirmary. It would also relieve other Edinburgh hospitals and would make a wide range of treatment easily accessible to some 100,000 people in the County of Midlothian without the need for them to travel to the centre of the city. In the City Development Plan published by the Town Council in 1953, a site of 30 acres at Fairmilehead was zoned for hospital building in the following '6 to 20 years' period, altered to the period 'beyond 20 years' in the Plan approved by the Secretary of State in 1957. There the proceedings relating to that site seem to have halted.

Not everyone, and least of all the University, had been convinced that the plan was a good one and, in the early 1950s, when the University decided to go ahead with their own developments in and near George Square close to the existing Medical School, the idea of replacing the Infirmary, wholly or partly, as a teaching

hospital, by one sited four miles away seemed quite unattractive. Nor did the demise of
that hospital plan cause much disappointment to the Infirmary Board of Management.

   Although slightly out of sequence this may be the best point at which to
record an attempt to plan for the building of a new and up-to-date Infirmary close
to its present site without having to face the problems inherent in any scheme for
demolition and replacement of buildings step by step while work in those awaiting
demolition continues amid noise and dust. Such problems are serious in any context; in a hospital, much more so. It is therefore not surprising that the suggestion
was made that all these problems could be avoided if a new Infirmary were to be
built on the eastern end of the Meadows, close to George Square and thus close to
the Medical School and if, after the new hospital was completed and occupied, the
existing Infirmary buildings could be demolished and their site, cleared and
attractively planted with grass and trees, could be handed over to the local
authority to be added to the Meadows in exchange for the section built upon. A
keen proponent of this idea was Professor Norman Dott. Officiating at a graduation
ceremony in the McEwan Hall in July 1958 he stressed the urgent need for a new
Infirmary to replace the old which, he said, was 'completely out-of-date and
unadaptable. No price is too high to keep Edinburgh medicine from dangerous
decline and there is danger today from the inadequacy of our facilities. Do you
think the City Fathers would refuse the site for this great purpose if assured that
the present site would be returned to meadowland in a few brief years? The city
founded and nurtured both the University and the Royal Infirmary through her
own illustrious children. How could her citizens refuse to carry them onwards
and upwards?'

   How could they, indeed—except that the open space of the Meadows (site of
the former Burgh or South Loch) had been cherished for 200 years or more as one
of the city's 'lungs' and was protected by Act of Parliament against the erection of
any buildings except bandstands and other minor public utility structures. Otherwise, the idea was an attractive one, in that a new hospital could be built there
without any disturbance to the existing hospital and much more quickly than by
building it piecemeal on the occupied site; and, in the long run, the public would
have been no worse, and perhaps better, served as regards recreational open space.

   The idea was mentioned several times in course of discussions about Infirmary
re-building plans but was never formally raised with the Town Council. To
adopt the scheme, not only the Town Council's consent, but legislation would
have been necessary and the barrage of objections that would have been raised by
amenity societies and others can readily be imagined. Even if authority had finally
been obtained, that could only have been after long delay during which the
uncertainty of the situation would doubtless have inhibited the making of improvements and additions to the old buildings. So the Regional Hospital Board and the
Board of Management were probably wise to accept as conclusive the advice given
by the Department of Health and conveyed to the Board of Management in
August 1958 (four weeks after Professor Dott had made his plea) that, after careful
consideration by their Planning and Hospitals Divisions, 'the Department see no
prospect whatever of the planning authorities giving consent to the use of a section
of the East Meadows for this purpose'.

Meanwhile much thought had been given to the need for re-building the hospital and to finding a practicable means of doing so. Such a major project, it was recognised, would be mainly the responsibility of the Regional Hospital Board and the Department of Health, but there was no reason why the initiative in working out a scheme should not be taken by the Board of Management. So a meeting of that Board's General Purposes Committee was held on 28 June 1955 which the Chairman, Sir George Henderson, described as 'a most important meeting'. He then invited the Medical Superintendent, Dr. Francis, to present a plan which had been evolved after discussion with many members of the clinical staff, with the Lady Superintendent of Nurses (Miss Marshall) and the Matron of the Simpson Pavilion (Miss Ferlie) and with the Architect (Mr. Turnbull). The plan was for adaptation and major re-building on the existing site. It was proposed to be carried out in four stages:

Stage one: to consist of internal adaptations and additions to give
               improved accommodation for departments and units in
               urgent need of expansion or upgrading.

Stage two: to be in three parts:
               (1) four houses in Chalmers Street to be acquired and demolished;
               (2) on the site so cleared a nurses' home to be built;
               (3) the Red Home to be demolished and a 'U-shaped'
                   building of six storeys to be built on the site. Three
                   floors would accommodate 'a first class polyclinic close to
                   the radiotherapy, gynaecology, ante-natal and dermatology
                   out-patient departments'.

Stage three: the three uppermost floors of the new building would house
               three surgical charges at a time, while the surgical house was
               being re-built to modern standards.

Stage four: this envisaged the purchase of neighbouring properties to
               provide a site for a Post-Graduate Institute, an idea which was
               not pursued in the consideration of later plans.

Such was the initial scheme for the re-development of the Royal Infirmary. In the years since then the concept has suffered many delays and has gone through many vicissitudes. Now, more than twenty-five years later, two major new buildings have been completed. They are the Princess Alexandra Eye Pavilion in Chalmers Street, opened in 1969, and the new 'Phase 1' block, completed in 1981, in Lauriston Place between Archibald Place and Chalmers Street. Both are outside the main hospital site but both are part of the complete reconstruction scheme. As will be explained later, that scheme is very different from the one suggested in 1955 and it is still liable to change.

No decision on the 1955 plan was sought at the time of its first presentation. Instead it was suggested that the opinion of a consultant architect should be obtained on the merits or demerits of the proposals. Ten days later the Regional Hospital Board, to whom the scheme had been submitted, pointed out that much more information would be needed before it could be considered against the whole building programme for major projects in the Region. They suggested that the Board of Management should appoint a consulting architect not just to comment on their scheme but 'to produce a master-plan for the co-ordination of all the proposed developments'.

The immediate outcome was that Professor (later Sir) Robert Matthew of the Chair of Architecture at Edinburgh University was engaged to examine the scheme and, after discussion with members of the clinical staff, to prepare a report on it. His report was presented in March 1956. Having suggested some modifications on *Stage 1* of the proposed scheme, he went on to suggest a complete re-shaping of *Stage 2*. On this his view was that a 'U-shaped' block would be difficult to plan economically and was not really suitable for high building. Instead, he suggested that the block to be built on the Red Home site should be a rectangular one, eight or ten storeys high; and in place of *Stages 3 and 4* he submitted his own preliminary outline plan and gave his opinion that 'it would be possible to re-plan the hospital on modern lines, in stages, provided that the heights of the new buildings proposed are allowed by the Authorities'—a significant proviso in the light of later events.

During the next three years much discussion took place and meetings of many committees and sub-committees were held to consider the hospital needs of the South-Eastern Region as a whole and of the Edinburgh area in particular and to seek decisions as to the extent to which and the means by which a reconstructed Royal Infirmary should be expected to meet such needs.

Towards the end of 1957 a Joint Planning Committee was established with members drawn from Regional Hospital Board, University, Department of Health for Scotland and Boards of Management of the Royal Infirmary and the Edinburgh Northern Hospitals (which included the Western General). The Chairman of the Regional Board (then Major Sir Humphrey Broun Lindsay, DSO, DL, JP) was Chairman of the Joint Committee. Their task was to consider the needs of the Region, how they should be met by hospitals in the Edinburgh area and the part the Royal Infirmary should play in doing so.

After two years study of reports from the University Faculty of Medicine and several sub-committees the Joint Committee recommended that:

 (*a*) each of the 'catchment areas' of Fife, West Lothian and the Borders should have a district hospital equipped to provide most forms of treatment (which, in fact, had been the policy since 1948);

 (*b*) the Edinburgh 'catchment area' should be chiefly served by the Royal Infirmary and the Western General Hospital, both of which should be re-built to modern standards;

 (*c*) these two hospitals should also provide, for the whole south-eastern region and even further afield, such highly specialised services as can be effectively provided only in large central hospitals—i.e. facilities for radiotherapy and for thoracic, neurological, urological and plastic surgery;

 (*d*) except for areas within the Region whose populations might warrant separate provision being made, these two hospitals should provide regional facilities for ophthalmology, dermatology, ear, nose and throat treatment and medical paediatrics.

The subject which gave the Joint Planning Committee most food for thought and, for a time, caused serious dissension among the Committee members was that of the number of beds to be provided in a re-built Royal Infirmary. The Department of Health representatives were adamant in their view that the maximum number of beds suitable for a major teaching hospital was 800. Other members were insistent that, to ensure a sufficient number and variety of patients to meet medical teaching needs, and also for economic reasons, the number should not be significantly less than the current complement of about 1,000 beds.

Eventually with some reluctance, the Joint Committee accepted the Department's view and in June 1959 they reported to the Regional Board their conclusions that the new Royal Infirmary should have 800 beds and that the Western General Hospital should have 700 beds. These recommendations were approved by the Regional Board, though not without vociferous protest by the Royal Infirmary Board of Management. It was, however, accepted that planning should proceed on the assumption that the bed complement of the re-built Infirmary (excluding the Simpson Pavilion) should be 800.

The Joint Planning Committee also stressed the importance to the future development and status of the Infirmary that highly specialised units should be included within medicine and surgery and should be represented in out-patient departments by the provision of appropriate diagnostic facilities; but that when a large number of beds were required for such units they should normally be found in other hospitals.

In January 1959 the Regional Board had resolved that the Infirmary should, 'if practicable, be reconstructed on its present site and that the Red Home be demolished as a first step'. They had been encouraged to make this pronouncement by a report that the Royal Victoria Hospital in Montreal, the original design of which in 1894 had been copied from that of the Edinburgh Royal Infirmary, had recently been completely reconstructed and had been able to function satisfactorily throughout the reconstruction. So, in July 1959, the Regional Board discussed the recommendations of the Joint Planning Committee in the light of comments by the University, the Boards of Management concerned and the Medical Staff Committee of the Infirmary. 'After detailed clarification of the issues' they accepted the recommendations as the basis of their forward planning.

An important statement on hospital building was made in Parliament by the Secretary of State for Scotland, Mr. J. S. Maclay on 17 November 1959. He said: 'Capital expenditure on hospital building in Scotland . . . will be £3.2 million in 1960-61 and £3.9 million in 1961-62. . . . I am asking the Regional Hospital Boards concerned to complete plans for the following major projects—(1) at the Royal Infirmary, Edinburgh, a new out-patient department and casualty accommodation. This will be the first stage of the reconstruction of the hospital and will probably also include some in-patient accommodation designed to facilitate the next stage of the reconstruction . . .'

That statement which went on also to refer to the Western General Hospital, was the cue for the Department of Health to ask the Regional Board to proceed with the planning of the first stages of reconstruction of the two hospitals; and the Board's response to that request, at their meeting on 30 November, was to confirm the appointments, already provisionally made, of Professor Robert Matthew as Architect and Mr. Llewellyn Davies (distinguished Architect of the King Edward's

Hospital Fund for London), as Consultant Architect for the Royal Infirmary project. Planning of the development of the Western General Hospital was entrusted to Mr. John Holt, the Regional Board's own Architect.

There now began to come into being a plethora of committees, sub-committees and working groups charged with assessing in all possible detail the requirements of specialties and departments and how these should be met and related to one another in the two hospitals. For the Royal Infirmary a Joint Planning Committee was appointed, representative of Regional Board, Board of Management, University and Department of Health under the chairmanship (as Vice-chairman of the Regional Board) of Mr. T. McWalter Millar, Honorary Consulting Surgeon who had recently retired after thirty years service as Assistant Surgeon and Surgeon in the Infirmary. The terms of reference of this Committee were: 'On the basis of the recommendations of the Regional Joint Planning Committee as accepted by the Regional Board, to report on an overall develop-ment plan for the Royal Infirmary; and, having regard for necessary priorities, to advise on the phased reconstruction of the hospital and the planning of each phase'. At their first meeting in January 1960 the Committee set about appointing more than a dozen working groups and technical sub-committees to study and eventually report on many aspects of the hospital's needs. At the close of that first meeting, the Chairman (showing, as it now seems, incredible optimism) pointed out that 'if building is to commence, as it is hoped, in 1961/62, it is essential that the Committee should go forward as quickly as possible . . .'.

At that point let us leave the Infirmary Joint Planning Committee facing their daunting task and return to the Architect and Consulting Architect. Their immediate objective, pending receipt of a fully detailed brief from the Committee, was to demonstrate in outline how a hospital of the size and with the range of services contemplated could be built on the site in stages so as to replace, eventually, the whole complex of buildings except the Simpson Pavilion and the Florence Nightingale Nurses Home. Little more than a year later, in January 1961, Professor Matthew with the help of a large-scale architectural model described their proposals, which had already been seen by the Board of Management, to an important group including the Secretary of State for Scotland (Mr. J. S. McLay), the Lord Provost of the City (The Rt. Hon., later Sir, John G. Dunbar), the Principal of the University (Sir Edward Appleton) and the Chairman of the Regional Hospital Board (Mr. Charles S. Gumley, W.S.). They are seen examining the model in Plate 19.

Professor Matthew explained that the first steps would involve the replace-ment, at the north-west corner of the site, of the boilerhouse, laundry and certain other buildings, and the provision of some new accommodation for nurses. This would be followed by the demolition of the Red Home and removal of the ear, nose and throat, the ophthalmology and the dermatology and venereal diseases pavilions, their occupants to be temporarily accommodated elsewhere. On the site so cleared, the main new building would be constructed. This would be a T-shaped structure with the 'leg' of the T reaching northward almost to Lauriston Place. It was to be a massive 17-storey block and would provide a large proportion of the required in-patient and out-patient accommodation and yet would not encroach on either the surgical house or the medical house and Jubilee pavilion which would therefore be able to function normally while the new block was being built. At a later stage they would be demolished and their sites partly used for lesser buildings and partly left as open space.

In this scheme there was an important difficulty, the possibility of which had been hinted at by Professor Matthew five years earlier, namely the great height of the main block which would have towered 52 metres above Lauriston Place and from several viewpoints would have obtruded itself on the skyline of Edinburgh Castle. This raised doubts, criticisms and arguments and later in the year the scheme was submitted to the Royal Fine Art Commission for Scotland. The Commission, though an advisory body with no powers of veto themselves, are nevertheless listened to with respect and their opinions are not lightly disregarded by planning and other authorities. According to the Commission this was the first time since their inception in 1927 that the design of a hospital had been submitted for their consideration. Their views on the submission were conveniently summarised in their official report for 1962-63:

> The beauty and unique character of the Capital City is so finely balanced
> that the intrusion of even one inharmonious building on an important
> site can have a disastrous effect. . . . We felt bound to express our regret
> that so massive a building should be erected on this particular site and our
> hope that it might be possible to reduce its dominance by re-building on
> lower ground adjacent to the Meadows. We recognised, however, that if
> for sound technical or functional reasons the upper part of the site had to
> be used, it would be difficult to evolve any more sympathetic lay-out
> or massing than those submitted to us.

The lower part of the Infirmary site, of course, could not be used because that would have made it necessary to demolish the Jubilee Pavilion and all, or a large part, of the Medical House before rebuilding began which would have defeated the main aim of the phased programme, as then envisaged.

The Fine Art Commission were not alone in criticising the height and mass of the proposed main hospital block. There were a good many others who disliked it. Because of these criticisms and after a tentative attempt to modify the design, the Architects were asked to produce a new outline scheme which would bring the overall height down to an acceptable level. That, however, re-introduced the old problem. The high block would have occupied a relatively small ground area and, as we have seen, could have been completed without encroaching upon the main buildings of the existing hospital. A more expansive layout, even for quite early stages of construction, would require the demolition of parts of these, thus increasing the need for preliminary 'decanting' of patients and departments and increasing the disturbance from building operations.

When a provisional development plan for the project was discussed by the Regional Board in March 1963 much concern was expressed about the disturbance problem. 'For ten years', one Board member complained, 'the Royal Infirmary will be working in the midst of a builder's yard'. However, Sir Robert Matthew (he had been knighted in 1962) assured the Board that techniques for minimising disturbance from building works were by then well established and that a complete protection scheme had been drawn up which would allow the Infirmary's services to continue without excessive disturbance.

Meanwhile, Joint Planning Committee meetings and meetings of hospital and University working groups continued to be held and, in 1964, a conference of representatives from all of them attempted to 'marry' together clinical, academic and technical requirements in such a way that hospital and University facilities in the new building would be effectively integrated, with advantage to both. The number and variety of requirements to be met and the number of persons whose widely differing and sometimes conflicting interests had to be taken into account made this a singularly complicated exercise. The 'Functional Brief and Schedules of Accommodation (First Edition)' produced in December 1964 contained a total of more than 400 pages, in three volumes.

The Report's introductory paragraphs included an important statement of principle: 'While each of the three functions—teaching, research and hospital service—can be separately described and even although teaching and research are mainly a commitment of the University of Edinburgh, and hospital service and some research that of the South Eastern Regional Hospital Board, it is not intended that, in the design of the hospital, there will be distinct dividing lines between the functional areas; it is most important that the design should demonstrate clearly how the areas overlap in function and how staff can move from one area to another'. Thus it was clearly indicated to the Architects that their design for the new Royal Infirmary, while incorporating all the detailed requirements of the 400-page report should both grow out of and stimulate the essential inter-dependence of the hospital's three main concerns—the treatment of patients, the teaching of medicine and nursing, and the widening of knowledge for the benefit of future patients, doctors and nurses alike.

In October 1964, Sir Robert Matthew had demonstrated, with the help of a new architectural model, how the operation of building a more widely spread hospital on the old Infirmary site could be achieved. His new model, seen in Plate 20 showed the 'Phase 1' building beside Lauriston Place, between Archibald Place and Chalmers Street and thus outside the main hospital site, in the position now occupied by the modified Phase 1 building completed in 1981. The proposed main hospital building to which the Phase 1 building would eventually be linked was to be constructed, in a series of five phases, with its main frontage along Lauriston Place. Within the whole formation there were to be nine open quadrangles admitting light and air to the wards. The main entrance would be centrally situated in Lauriston Place.

While the building programme was being worked out, discussions were complicated by several issues. One of these was the question of the siting of a new Children's Hospital. The Scottish Home and Health Department (successors, from June 1962, of the Department of Health for Scotland) had agreed with the Regional Hospital Board that the Royal Edinburgh Hospital for Sick Children in Sciennes Road (directly across the Meadows from the Infirmary) which had been opened in 1895 was out-of-date and must be replaced and that the replacement must be sited within the curtilage of a large general hospital. The Royal Infirmary Board, believing it important that a modern teaching hospital should include a viable children's department, argued that the new children's hospital should be incorporated in their new building or, alternatively, should be built on the west side of Chalmers Street as part of a wider Infirmary complex. After much, and sometimes bitter, wrangling the Regional Board, supported by the Scottish Home and Health Department, in October 1965 gave their final ruling that the new Children's Hospital would be built beside the Western General Hospital where ample clear space was available. The Board of Management, however, still argued for the inclusion of a paediatric unit in the new Infirmary. Eighteen years later, in 1983, the Sick Children's Hospital in Sciennes Road continues to give good service although its replacement is still regarded, in the longer term, as a necessary step to improve patient and teaching facilities in Edinburgh.

When it became clear that, to make way for new building, the Moray Eye Pavilion and the Ear, Nose and Throat Pavilion, both opened in 1903, would be among the first blocks to be demolished it became necessary to consider plans for their replacement either on a temporary or permanent basis. For the ear, nose and throat department the problem was solved by arranging for in-patients to be transferred (in 1965) to the City Hospital where accommodation was specially adapted and up-graded for the purpose, out-patients continuing to be attended to at the Infirmary. For eye patients it was decided that a new department designed and equipped to take full advantage of the 20th-century's striking advances in the techniques of ophthalmology should be built close to the Infirmary and a site was found on the west side of Chalmers Street. In February 1963 the brief for the new eye department was completed. Building began in June 1965 and, as will be described later, The Princess Alexandra Eye Pavilion came into use in 1969.

That decision to make permanent separate provision for ophthalmology made it necessary to reconsider the allocation of the 800 beds which it had been decided in 1959 should be the total complement of the new Infirmary's main building. In the interval, also, the need to incorporate beds for geriatric medicine and psychological medicine had been recognised. In September 1964, the proposed total bed complement of the main building was increased to 860 beds, the allocations as decided in 1959 and 1964 being as follows:

Department	Allocation proposed	
	in 1959	in 1964
Clinical medicine	320	320
Geriatric Medicine	—	30
Psychological medicine	—	30
Clinical surgery (including accident and emergency provision)	360	360
Gynaecology	60	60
Ear, nose and throat	20	30
Dermatology	20	30
Ophthalmology	20	—
	800	860
Ophthalmology (in new Eye Pavilion)		72

It was noted also by the Boards, in approving of the increased allocation that there would be 215 beds in the Simpson Memorial Maternity Pavilion of which 187 would be for obstetrics and 28 for premature and sick babies, bringing the total number of beds in the whole Infirmary to 1,147.

About a year later—in October 1965—the preliminary plans for the new 860-bed hospital were ready for submission to the Scottish Home and Health Department and to the Town Council as planning authority. A press statement was issued by the Regional Board and on 5 October 1965 a report appeared in *The Scotsman* which included the following information:

> Edinburgh Royal Infirmary is to be rebuilt, over ten years, on the same site, at a provisional cost of £15-million. Work is due to start in 1968. . . . The [Regional Hospital] Board were told by Mr. J. Holt, their regional architect, that the architects, Robert Matthew, Johnson-Marshall and Partners, had produced 'really an ingenious plan'. The site was very congested and the placing of new buildings in such a way that the present hospital could continue to function was no mean achievement . . .
>
> After the plan had been considered by the Royal Infirmary Board of Management last night the Secretary, Mr. T. W. Hurst, said the number of beds would be less than at present—860 against 980. But he added, 'This new hospital is a viable unit and could be extended if necessary'.
>
> The Board were extremely happy with the plan.

Between being happy with the plan and seeing the plan begin to take shape on the ground there can be a long and distressing gap, as the Board of Management, the Regional Board and (after April 1974) the Lothian Health Board discovered. In this case the gap extended to 9½ years due, mainly, to the inability or unwillingness of successive governments to sanction capital expenditure on hospital building at a level that would have allowed the work to go ahead.

The story of eight of those frustrating years can be concisely traced from the Annual Reports of the Royal Infirmary Board:

> 1965-66: financial clearance awaited
>
> 1966-67: still in planning stage; provisional cost limit of £14,385,607 agreed for new Infirmary.
>
> 1967-68: major re-development postponed; first phase (£2/3 million) scheduled to start in 1971.
>
> 1968-69: after 1971-72, priority expected to be given for second phase (estimated cost between £6 million and £7 million).
>
> 1969-70: Secretary of State (Rt. Hon. William Ross) reported in House of Commons that Phase 1 was due to start in 1970-71.
>
> 1970-71: building of Phase 1 now expected to start in August 1973.
>
> 1971-72: Phase 1 now expected to start in late Autumn 1973.
>
> 1972-73: 'It has been a great disappointment to the Board that in the period under review demolition has not yet taken place to make way for Phase 1 . . . the Board of Management did not wish to demit office in 1974 without seeing a start to what it regarded as the culmination of its work—the re-building of the Royal Infirmary.'

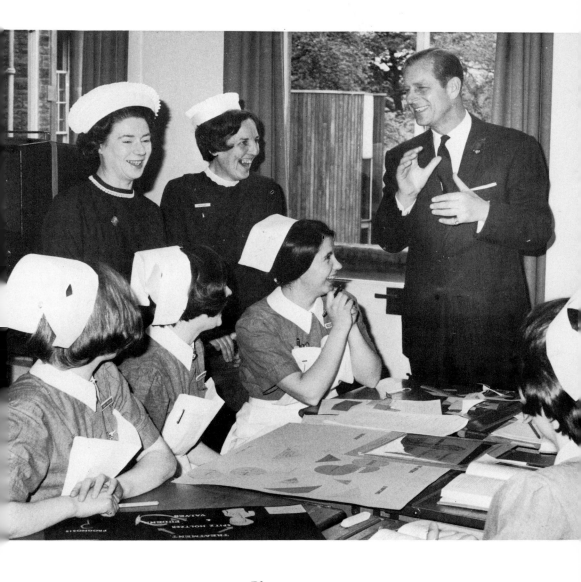

Plate 17

Royal Infirmary School of Nursing

H.R.H. Prince Philip, Duke of Edinburgh, shares a joke with tutors and students — May 1969

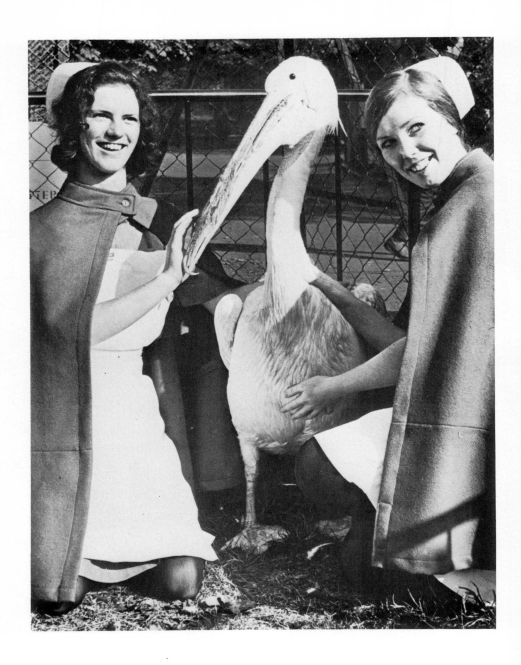

Plate 18   Peter the Pelican

With two friends at Edinburgh Zoo after being 'adopted' by the student nurses as part of the School's 100th Anniversary commemorative programme in 1972.

The Report for 1972-73 was the last Annual Report on the work of the Royal Infirmary Board of Management, disbanded on 31 March 1974 when their functions were absorbed in those of the Lothian Health Board. During the last year of the Board of Management's existence, further frustrating delay occurred. It was caused partly by financial stringency, partly by difficulties connected with the acquisition and demolition of properties in Lauriston Place and Chalmers Street and partly by the problem of the new boilerhouse chimney.

The financial difficulty was cleared in November 1973 when the Scottish Home and Health Department approved the final cost limit of Phase 1 (excluding equipment) at £4,965,437. The property acquisition and demolition difficulties were also disposed of in the autumn of 1973 when authority was finally given to demolish some 'listed' early nineteenth-century houses in Lauriston Place.

The chimney problem proved more difficult. To comply with clean air regulations a chimney height of 45 metres would have been appropriate, but the Secretary of State had given a ruling that to ensure complete dispersal of smoke and fumes, the design of new hospital chimneys must be subjected to rigorous wind-tunnel tests and be adjusted to conform to the findings of these tests even if that resulted in a higher chimney than would otherwise be necessary. Exhaustive tests were, therefore, carried out at the National Physical Laboratory at Teddington, Middlesex. These took into account the surrounding topography and the effect on wind currents of the proximity of Edinburgh Castle on its high ridge. Final approval of the Phase 1 plans, including the chimney designed on the basis of those tests, was given in April 1974. As built, the chimney rises 38 metres above the roof of the Phase 1 building, and 57 metres above Lauriston Place. It is a cluster of five steel-stacks, neatly bracketed together, one stack serving each of the four new boilers and the fifth serving the incinerator. The chimney-cluster thus evolved was acceptable to the Royal Fine Art Commission for Scotland. Its slim, clean-cut lines clearly demonstrate the advantage of basing the design of such a structure on objective, scientific study and the achievement of functional efficiency. In 1980, a *Commendation* of the chimney design was received under the Structural Design Awards Scheme administered, on behalf of British Steel, by the Constructional Steel Research and Development Organisation.

Towards the end of 1973 'severe national economic problems' had again caused the Government of the day to impose delays on hospital building projects, but the Board of Management were relieved to be told, in January 1974, that the Secretary of State for Scotland (Rt. Hon. Gordon Campbell, later Lord Campbell of Croy) did not consider it necessary to defer the start of Phase 1 of the Royal Infirmary scheme, the importance of which he recognised. Even so, a further fifteen months passed before the Lothian Health Board, on 10 April 1975, were able to authorise the placing of the main contract for the building of Phase 1. By that time the approved cost (excluding equipment) had risen to £7,835,000.

Coming almost exactly twenty years after the original proposal for the rebuilding of the Royal Infirmary, the start of building was an auspicious occasion and the Board expressed 'their great satisfaction that authorisation to proceed with this major development had now been received'. Nor were they unmindful of the efforts of their predecessors in office, the fruits of whose labours they were now

K

about to reap and they recorded their 'appreciation of the work of the members of the former Board of Management for the Royal Infirmary of Edinburgh and Associated Hospitals and the former South-Eastern Regional Hospital Board and agreed that this appreciation be conveyed to them'.

In June 1975 Sir Robert Matthew died, having lived only just long enough to see building begin on the project he had nurtured for so long. His firm of Robert Matthew, Johnson-Marshall & Partners continued to be in charge, the project thenceforward being directed by their Associate, Mr. Percy Murray, who had been concerned with the Royal Infirmary re-building scheme since 1960.

Accommodation in the building as completed and handed over to the Health Board in mid-1981 was allocated as follows:

Level 1 (Chalmers Street): Post-mortem suite including special accommodation for 'high-risk' examinations; workshops and boilerhouse.

Level 2 Works Department offices; changing-rooms for non-resident staff.

Level 3 (Lauriston Place): Mainly blood-transfusion premises (the blood-bank remaining in the main Medical building); additional changing-rooms.

Level 4: Three out-patient clinics—for skin diseases, E.N.T. and genito-urinary medicine.

Levels 5, 6 and 7: Residential accommodation for nurses, including those from the nurses' west home, to be demolished to make way for the building of Phase 2.

Phase 2 will be smaller than previously planned and there will probably be a larger number of Phases. Because of changing circumstances and the many advances made in hospital and medical practice the general brief for the complete scheme had to be revised, a process likely to be an on-going one. How the brief for each Phase is eventually adjusted and put into practice will be for a future historian of the Royal Infirmary to tell.

Meanwhile, in addition to the tribute paid by the Lothian Health Board to their predecessors, quoted above, credit is due to the Board of Management, the Regional Board, the Lothian Health Board and the University for the vigour with which, during all the years of planning for the future, they pursued a parallel policy of almost continuous improvement and up-grading of the existing hospital so as to keep pace, as nearly as the limitations of the old building would allow, with changes and modern advances. Their pursuit of that policy is the subject of Chapter 5.

Princess Alexandra Eye Pavilion

So far as plans for replacement of the main building of the Infirmary by a modern hospital were concerned the decade of the 1960s had ended in disappointment; not one brick (or concrete block) even of Phase 1 of the re-building scheme had been laid. But there was a brighter side to the picture. The new Eye Pavilion, work on which had begun in 1965, received its first patients in August 1969 and was formally opened on 1 October 1969 by H.R.H. Princess Alexandra who also graciously consented to her name being given to it.

Progress on the new building had been due only partly to the urgent need (as it seemed at the time) for demolition of the old, 1903, eye pavilion to clear the way for the main re-building scheme. It was due rather more to the fact that the University Department of Ophthalmology required up-to-date facilities for teaching and research and had funds available from which to make a substantial contribution to the cost of a new building. It was due also to the drive and per-severance of Professor George I. Scott, the Infirmary's Senior Ophthalmic Surgeon.

The contribution of the Infirmary to progress in the science and practice of ophthalmology was of long standing. In the late 19th century Dr. Douglas Argyll Robertson, a flamboyant figure, had pioneered the use of physostigmine, an extract of the calabar bean, in the treatment of certain types of glaucoma (having first tested it on his own eyes). Dr. Arthur H. H. Sinclair, Senior Ophthalmic Surgeon from 1920 until 1932, was in 1930 the first in Britain to introduce to the operation for cataract the technique of intracapsular extraction which soon became a standard procedure; and Dr. H. M. Traquair, his successor from 1932 until 1941, devoted a large part of his life to clinical perimetry, the study of patients' visual fields, with valuable results. Doctors E. H. Cameron, C. W. Graham and J. R. Paterson who followed them each made contributions to advancing techniques in their specialty.

Dr. George Scott, a senior ophthalmic surgeon, became the first incumbent of the Forbes Chair of Ophthalmology, to which he was appointed in 1954, and which he occupied until his retiral in 1972 when he was succeeded by Professor C. I. Phillips. Like Dr. Traquair, Professor Scott was interested in perimetry but he was equally concerned with wider medical aspects of ophthalmology. During his years as Professor, his Department's research projects related largely to the eye complications of diseases of the nervous system, hypertension and diabetes or, put more generally, 'disease of the eye in a sick body'.

In the consideration of clinical functions for which provision should be made in the new building, it was noted that 'to-day in Great Britain cataract accounts for over 40 per cent of blindness in those over seventy years of age; glaucoma for about 20 per cent, diabetes for 20 per cent and senile degenerative change at the back of the eye for fifteen per cent'. These were figures which, in an ageing popula-tion, were a cause of considerable concern and they pointed strongly to the advan-tages to be gained by providing the University Ophthalmology Department with modern research equipment in close association with up-to-date patient accom-modation and facilities.

A site was found in garden ground attached to Chalmers Hospital just across Chalmers Street from the site intended for the 'Phase 1' building of the Infirmary reconstruction and plans for the eye pavilion were prepared by the Edinburgh architectural firm of Alison & Hutchison & Partners. Because of the limited size of the site, the building had to be a tall one, six storeys high above the level of Chalmers Street with one floor below that level. The total cost of the building was £700,000. As this was the first (though detached) part of the new hospital the modern accommodation it provides deserves to be briefly described as giving a foretaste of the Infirmary of the future.

The ground floor contains the out-patient department, including an accident and emergency room with an operating theatre. Here also are comfortable waiting accommodation, a cafeteria staffed by Royal Infirmary Volunteers and several staff offices. The University Department of Ophthalmology occupies the whole of the first floor. The second, third and fourth floors each contain a 24-bed ward divided into two six-bed and two four-bed bays and four single rooms, the bays providing a feeling of privacy while still being easily supervised from a nurse's station. One of the wards is adapted for the care of children, with bright decoration and a play-room. There are also day areas and dining-rooms for patients. The fifth floor contains the main operating theatre and also residential accommodation for three doctors. The lower ground floor contains lecture rooms and houses the heating plant and other equipment; a tunnel under the roadway provides a link with the main hospital.

In the brochure produced for the opening of the new pavilion, the following description was given of some of the procedures for which it was equipped:

> Recent advances have brought great changes . . . For some years the light coagulator has been used to produce controlled burns within the eye, in treatment of retinal detachment and other conditions of the retina such as occur in diabetes. New methods of surgery using intense cold, even down to $-70°C$ (i.e. cryo-surgery) are now used in retinal surgery and in cataract extraction. The increasing fineness of stitches and needles, together with the use of operating microscopes, makes possible delicately-controlled work which would not have been contemplated a few years ago . . .

In its first full year of operation (1970-71) the new pavilion dealt with 2,500 in-patients and about 40,000 out-patient attendances compared with 2,100 in-patients and 33,600 out-patient attendances in the last full year of the old eye department (1967-68).

Three years after the opening of the new pavilion an Argon 'laser' (from the words 'light amplification by stimulated emission of radiation') was installed, the initial cost of which (about £14,000) was met by the Scottish Home and Health Department. It was then the only such instrument in any hospital outside London. The white light coagulator had been in use since 1968, enabling certain retinal and other injuries to be treated without subjecting the eye to open operation; some defects not amenable to that treatment could now be dealt with by the 'laser', producing tiny burns at the spot required with pinpoint accuracy. Along with other advanced instruments and aids to surgery it helps to maintain the Eye Pavilion's place as one of the most up-to-date as well as one of the busiest eye departments in the country.

5

1960 and After

Medical Renal Unit and Transplant Surgery

The importance of a multi-disciplinary approach to patient care was demonstrated during the 1960s in many areas of patient management; in none more clearly than in the use of renal dialysis for patients suffering from kidney failure and in the emergence of kidney transplantation.

A healthy kidney regulates the composition of the blood and maintains the right chemical balance in the body's fluids. Acute kidney failure can occur as a result of severe accidents, especially those involving crushing injuries, severe infections and in certain types of poisoning. Chronic kidney failure may be caused by several naturally occurring diseases. Both can be treated by dialysis using an 'artificial kidney'—a machine which does the work of the kidneys outside the patient's body by allowing the blood to pass over a membrane on the other side of which is a specially prepared dialysing fluid, and in doing so to lose waste products and re-adjust the level of some of its constituents. In acute kidney failure the process is a temporary one required only until the natural kidney recovers and resumes its normal function; in chronic failure the patient may have to undergo intermittent dialysis indefinitely, spending several hours attached to the machine twice a week but, for the rest of the week, pursuing a more or less normal life. Success in this field depends upon close and continuing collaboration among physicians, surgeons, bacteriologists checking for infection, clinical chemists analysing blood and other specimens, haematologists reporting on patients' blood groups, pharmacists preparing dialysing fluids, and specially trained nursing teams.

This form of treatment was begun at the Infirmary in medical Ward 23, in the eastmost medical pavilion, within the charge of Professor Derrick Dunlop, Professor of Therapeutics. There, Dr. James S. Robson, then Reader in Therapeutics at the University (who became Professor of Medicine in succession to Professor K. W. Donald in 1977) took a keen interest in the problem of kidney disease and especially in haemodialysis. The first Medical Renal Unit in the Infirmary was set up in a small suite of rooms in Ward 23. It was formally opened on 20 May 1959 by the Earl of Wemyss, then Lord High Commissioner to the General Assembly of the Church of Scotland. The ceremony was a simple one, with minimum publicity, but it marked the beginning of an important phase in the Infirmary's history. The annual report for 1958-59 shows that in the first six weeks of the unit's operation nine patients were dialysed and the report for 1959-60 records: 'The artificial kidney unit, established in July 1959, has carried out 65 dialyses on 50 patients and many lives have been saved'.

Interest in this work was shared by the surgeons in Wards 13 and 14 where Professor Michael Woodruff, Professor of Surgical Science was in charge. His special interest was in transplant immunology and surgery and this had taken him to Boston, USA, to study, at first hand, the early work being undertaken on transplantation of the kidney in man. From this and other studies he had concluded that the procedure was 'indicated in cases of hopeless renal failure when an identical twin is available as donor and in addition is justified under certain defined conditions even when a twin is not available'.

In September 1960 a man aged 49, suffering from severe kidney disease was referred to the Royal Infirmary by Dr. R. F. Robertson, then a physician at Leith Hospital who, having learned that his patient was believed to be an identical twin, was astute enough to recognise the possibility that gave of a successful transplant. When it became clear that there was otherwise no hope of the patient's recovery and that his twin was healthy and was willing to give up one kidney for his brother, it was decided that the transplantation should take place. The operation was the first successful transplantation of the human kidney performed in Britain, and thus was a milestone in transplant surgery as well as in the history of the Royal Infirmary. It took place on 30 October 1960 and was fully reported by Professor Woodruff and his colleagues in *The Lancet* of 10 June 1961.

First, it was essential to confirm that the brothers were truly identical twins. They had frequently been mistaken for each other and their eye colour, and other characteristics were similar. Several tests made in the Infirmary supported the view that the twins were identical but that was not enough. Their blood-grouping having been initially tested by Dr. R. A. Cumming, Regional Director of the South-East Scotland Blood Transfusion Service, it was closely studied by the Lister Institute in London; finger and palm prints were examined at University College, London; and serum-proteins were investigated by an expert at the University of Glasgow. The combined result of all these tests showed that, overall, the possibility of the twins not being truly identical was so remote as to be negligible. Even then, a further test was applied by making skin grafts from each twin to the other. They 'took' perfectly. Finally, the healthy brother signed a statement volunteering to give 'one of my own two healthy kidneys to be used as a graft to my brother' and acknowledging that possible risks had been explained to him. The operation on the donor was performed by Mr. James A. Ross and that on the patient by Professor Woodruff. Both operations were completely successful. The donor was moved to a convalescent hospital after two weeks and resumed work three weeks later. The patient was moved to a convalescent hospital after seven weeks and returned to light work in February 1961—fifteen weeks after the transplantation. The patient survived for six years, his transplanted kidney functioning satisfactorily right up to the time of his death which resulted from an unrelated disease.

For the care of the patient during the critical weeks after the operation, a special room in the former clinical chemistry block had been adapted by the Works Department in order to provide, as nearly as possible, complete protection against infection. Because of the elaborate techniques involved, seven senior nurses were needed to look after one patient in the room. The room was used again in July 1961 when a second kidney transplant was carried out, this time between a brother and sister. They were not twins and, unhappily, the operation was unsuccessful. The annual report for 1961-62 records a third transplant, from a father to his son, after which the son was said to be doing well. In 1983 he is still alive—the longest surviving transplant patient in Britain.

The Human Tissue Act of 1961 regulated the use of donated kidneys from persons who had died and by 1968 more than thirty transplants had been carried out at the Royal Infirmary. In 1968 a purpose-built transplantation surgery unit was completed at the Western General Hospital at a cost of £250,000. The cost was met by the Nuffield Foundation on the understanding that staffing and running costs would be paid by the Scottish Home and Health Department for five years, after which those costs would be the responsibility of the Regional Hospital Board. The unit's special purpose was to provide as nearly as possible a germ-free environment for patients receiving organ grafts or other specially vulnerable treatments. It had been designed by Peter Womersley, a Melrose Architect, to meet the meticulous requirements of Professor Woodruff and his colleagues at the Infirmary, including Dr. John Bowie, Senior Bacteriologist, who had a special knowledge of and interest in scientific means of preventing or controlling infection.

The new unit was opened on 31 January 1968 by Sir Peter Medawar, Director of the National Institute for Medical Research and a Nobel prize-winner for his work on acquired immunity to tissue transplants. 'Edinburgh', he said, 'has been chosen for the unit because that is where Professor Michael Woodruff, one of the grand masters of the theory and art of transplantation is to be found. He is a clinical surgeon who was the first to transplant a kidney in this country. Nowhere in the world will patients get better care.' The Professor then explained that the unit was likely to start by admitting about 30 patients in the first year. So, with the advent of specially built premises at the Western General, the need for transplant operations to be undertaken at the Infirmary came to an end. In future, patients from the Medical Renal Unit who needed, and were able to receive, a kidney transplant would be transferred to the Nuffield Unit.

One more organ transplant, though not of a kidney, was carried out in the Infirmary some three months later, on 15 May 1968. This involved the transplanting of a lung and was said to be the first such operation ever accomplished in Europe. It was undertaken in circumstances of urgent emergency by Mr. Andrew Logan, Thoracic Surgeon. A fifteen-year-old boy who had swallowed a mouthful of the weed-killer, paraquat, in mistake for lemonade had been brought from his home to Edinburgh and the Infirmary. Both lungs were affected and the boy was desperately ill.

As the only hope, and that a slim one, it was decided to transplant a healthy lung from an 18-year-old girl who had died just 2½ hours before the operation took place. It was thought that with one good lung the boy might have a chance of survival. The operation and treatment of the patient, in which Professor Woodruff, Dr. Henry Matthew (Physician in the Poisoning Treatment Centre), and their respective medical, nursing and technical teams participated, appeared at first to have been successful. However, after two anxious weeks of intensive care, the patient died, possibly because the transplanted lung had become affected by the poison. Afterwards it was reported that the boy's father, full of admiration for the team who had done everything possible for his son, still felt that the operation had been worth trying and hoped that the experience gained would lead to success in the future.

Throughout the 1960s the work of the Medical Renal Unit steadily increased. At first it was possible to deal only with persons suffering from acute renal failure who, after dialysis treatment, might be expected to recover the use of their kidneys. Early in 1963, dialysis for patients suffering from chronic failure was begun but its development was limited by lack of space and shortage of kidney machines.

At the end of 1966, the Scottish Home and Health Department stated that there were ten dialysis machines in Scotland, five of which were in Edinburgh Royal Infirmary, three in Glasgow and two in Dundee—still far too few to meet the need. At that time 18 patients were receiving regular intermittent dialysis treatment in the Infirmary, some of them in their fourth year of such treatment; all of them hoping for the availability of a transplant which would free them from the machine's demands.

It was then decided that a new purpose-built unit should be provided, 'thus', in the words of a press report at the time, 'maintaining the Infirmary's position as one of the world's pioneers in the treatment of kidney diseases'. A site for the new unit was found, close to the original unit, by demolishing the Medical Superintendent's house (Meadow House) which had been vacated in 1966, modern means of communication having long made it unnecessary for that officer to live within the hospital.

The new renal dialysis unit was designed by Robert Matthew, Johnson Marshall & Partners, on lines prescribed by Dr. Robson and Dr. John Bowie, to incorporate stringent safeguards against infection. The building was completed in 1969. It provided, on the first floor, wards and facilities for haemodialysis for up to thirty patients, and on the ground floor, offices, laboratories and an academic area for the University Department of Medicine to which Dr. Robson, and the unit, had recently transferred from the Department of Therapeutics. The cost of the building and its equipment was nearly £250,000 shared by the Health Service (70%) and the University (30%) on the basis of the 'Pater formula', a method devised by a civil servant of that name for assessing the proportion of costs attributable, on one hand, to clinical requirements and on the other to teaching needs. The new facilities gave fresh impetus to important research work which was being pursued into renal disease and the physiology of the normal kidney.

Meanwhile a new development had begun which enabled the work of the unit to be extended still further. In 1967, following a suggestion by Dr. Robson, the Scottish Home and Health Department made a grant of £8,500 to the Regional Hospital Board to finance a pilot scheme for the provision of kidney machines of a type suitable for use by patients themselves in their own homes. These machines, smaller than those in hospital, were fitted with special warning and 'fail-safe' devices. Not every patient, it was realised, would be physically or temperamentally fitted to control his or her own treatment, but for those who, after a period of training, were able to do so, the scheme proved to be an admirable one. Provision of such machines, which was a responsibility of the hospital service, necessitated the adaptation of a room in the patient's house, including the installation of special services or, if no suitable room was available, the placing of a transportable hut beside the house. These works were then the responsibility of the Town or County Council as local health authority.

His preliminary training having been satisfactorily completed, the first home dialysis patient had a machine installed in his Edinburgh home in September 1967. Within a few weeks he was quoted as being delighted with the new arrangement which not only released time on a hospital machine for use by other patients, but also enabled him to work a full five-day week, using his machine during off-duty hours instead of having to take days off work to attend at the unit. In any emergency he, or his family, could be in touch with the Infirmary by telephone.

By February 1969, three patients were on maintenance dialysis at home. This, however, was still a trial project and it was accepted that any large extension of it would have to await consideration of plans for permanent supervisory and back-up services. Some eighteen months later, in August 1970, tragic circumstances hastened the extension of the home dialysis service. During a period of unusual prevalence of viral hepatitis in eastern Scotland and despite all the precautions then known having been taken against risks of infection, there had been a serious outbreak of the disease associated with the Medical Renal Unit at the Infirmary and the Nuffield Transplantation Surgery Unit during which 21 patients, 12 members of staff and 2 home contacts of patients were affected. Seven of the patients and four members of staff had died. It was feared that kidney patients who had recovered from hepatitis and returned to the Infirmary unit to continue their dialysis treatment might still be a hazard to other patients and staff. So it was decided, as a matter of urgency, to arrange home dialysis for six such patients, all resident in Edinburgh. A request was sent to the Town Council for the required adaptations to be carried out at the patients' homes. On the day the request was received, the Health Committee of the Council authorised expenditure of £5,000 on the necessary work which was put in hand immediately and speedily completed so that the patients, on completing their training, could transfer to home dialysis without delay.

For a time, new patients were not accepted in the Medical Renal Unit and the Nuffield Unit was closed. The Regional Hospital Board appointed a hepatitis advisory committee, headed by Professor Marmion, Professor of Bacteriology, to investigate the causes of the outbreak and advise on precautionary measures for the future. They made several recommendations upon which the Regional Board and Board of Management quickly acted. Those who worked in the Kidney Unit during the hepatitis outbreak well knew the danger of infection to which they might be exposed but they did not allow that to diminish the care with which they continued to look after their patients. It was fitting, therefore, that in the New Year's Honours List of 1971 there appeared the award of the MBE to Sister Marion Herbertson who had been in charge of nursing in the Unit; whose quiet efficiency during the outbreak had been an example to those who worked with her; and whose comment on the Honour was: 'It is a Unit Award'.

Many patients suffering chronic kidney disease who are on dialysis in the Unit or at home are able to lead nearly normal lives between dialysing sessions, attending to their businesses, playing golf, enjoying social occasions. For five days in August 1971 the Medical Renal Unit was unusually quiet, the reason being that seven of the patients—four men and three women—had been taken for a five-day holiday in London. The excursion, believed to be one of the first group outings of its kind, was made possible by the Edinburgh Round Table and other voluntary organisations and by planning and hard work on the part of members of the Unit's staff. Special diets had been arranged with the willing co-operation of the staff of their London hotel and dialysing procedures were adjusted so that the party could enjoy the usual round of sightseeing and theatre-going on their visit. It was an exercise which demonstrated the value of dialysis not only in saving life but also in enabling patients to maintain the quality of their lives. The patient seen in Plate 27 is one of a small élite group of patients in the world who, for nearly twenty years, have been receiving regular dialysis treatment each week while living nearly normal lives between dialysing sessions.

A measure of the growth of the work of the Medical Renal Unit can be gained by comparing the figures quoted earlier—'1959-60: 65 dialyses carried out on 50 patients'—with figures noted in the year 1981. By that time a total of more than 800 patients had been treated in the Unit for acute renal failure, 90 were then being treated in their own homes for chronic renal failure and more than 100 patients were alive after successful kidney transplantation. In its 22 years existence the Unit had taken part in much research into the nature and prevention of renal disease, the latest exploration being into a method of 'peritoneal dialysis' whereby the long-term dialysing process may be conducted by means of a naturally-occurring membrane within the patient's body instead of through an external machine, thus protecting against a possible danger of slowly-developing aluminium poisoning. Over the years, gifts totalling more than £200,000 had been received to help in the purchase of equipment and the funding of research—a figure which clearly showed the extent of public appreciation of the Unit's work.

Clinical Chemistry Department

Early in the consideration of their re-building plans the Board of Management made a firm decision not to use the prospect of future perfection as an excuse, in the meantime, for doing nothing to remedy inadequacies in the old buildings or to extend their facilities. 'In this era of great advances in medical science and know-ledge', they wrote in their 1959-60 Report, 'many projects and developments must be encouraged and carried out now; they cannot be delayed if patients and students are to obtain the maximum benefit from these advances.'

The fourteen years that remained to the Board of Management were, therefore, years of constant improvement, adaptation and addition, carried on under many difficulties, both financial and practical. Besides seeking to remedy inadequacies and to keep pace with new developments, the Board sought to encourage the growing trend of collaboration and co-operation among a range of different disciplines, medical, surgical and scientific. It was, of course, a process that had been going on for many years; collaboration with the University in medical teaching is as old as the Infirmary itself. In the 1960s, however, the extent to which University and Infirmary departments and different departments within the Infirmary worked closely with one another reached a new level. In the process results were achieved which were undreamed of even ten years earlier.

The process was helped by the completion of two building projects in the Infirmary early in the decade. The first of these was the construction of clinical chemistry laboratories which came into use in July 1960. It was a joint venture of the University and the Health Service, both capital and running costs being shared on the basis of the 'Pater formula'.

The new clinical laboratories, constructed at a cost of £61,000, replaced those in the 'Rockefeller' building at the east end of the medical house which (with some later encroachments into adjoining accommodation) had been in use since 1928. The new laboratories were designed by Arthur A. Dixon, Infirmary Architect in collaboration with Dr. C. P. Stewart, who had been the Infirmary's Biochemist since 1923 and Reader in charge of the University Department of Clinical Chemistry since 1946. When he retired in 1962, 'C.P.' recalled that forty years before, practically all the laboratory work was accounted for by seven different analyses. 'Now', he wrote, 'over 40 estimations are "on tap" and are asked for regularly while some 20 more can be provided on special request.' Referring to new post-operative treatments which had arisen from research by biochemists in co-operation with surgeons and physicians and new means of diagnosis which had emerged from such research, he said, 'Progress, it must be stressed, will be secured only through teamwork by the various specialists'. Such teamwork in the Infirmary in the 1960s contributed notably to successes in many fields.

When the designing of the new laboratories began planning of the new Royal Infirmary to arise on the site of the old was under way and such was the feeling of optimism at the time that the Architect was advised to design the new laboratory building for a life of ten years. Fortunately, he did not take that instruction quite literally and more than twenty years later the laboratories are still serving their purpose and are likely to have to continue to do so for some time to come, despite an ever-increasing work-load.

The new clinical chemistry building was opened on 26 October 1960 by Sir Kenneth Cowan, Chief Medical Officer of the Department of Health for Scotland. It is sited between medical wards 25 and 28 with the windows of the main routine laboratory facing south across the Meadows. At each end the accommodation extends into the semi-basements, or 'duckponds' beneath the ward pavilions; and here it may be helpful to pause and recall the origin of the name 'duckponds'.

As explained by Dr. Logan Turner in his book, the term was first applied, about 1885, by a ward sister with a sense of humour. At that time, before the advent of the Jubilee Pavilion, gynaecology beds were on the third floor of the east-most medical pavilion. Such beds were limited in number and to relieve pressure on them, sleeping accommodation for 20 convalescent patients was provided in the semi-basements of two of the other medical pavilions. During the day, these patients remained in the gynaecology ward. Every evening, wearing dressing-gowns and soft slippers they shuffled, in procession, to their sleeping quarters and a sister through whose ward they regularly passed described them as a line of ducks waddling to their duck pond. The name 'duckpond' stuck and, by simple extension, was applied to the semi-basements of all the medical pavilions; the name still remains although the reason for it is now a mystery to many who use it.

When the clinical laboratories were built, the 'duckpond' under Ward 28 was adapted to house a research laboratory, a workshop and store rooms, and that below Ward 25 provided space for a teaching laboratory. In the new building, besides the routine laboratory, several smaller ones were provided as well as a centrifuge room and rooms for flame-photometry, chromatography and other special processes.

One of these rooms has since been equipped for the making of urgent analyses by medical laboratory scientific officers who are on duty, or on immediate call, day and night. From that laboratory, results today are guaranteed within one hour of a request being received from a clinician and can usually be given to him within thirty minutes, enabling him to decide promptly and confidently on the treatment or change of treatment required to deal with the patient's condition as revealed by the analysis. How many lives have been saved, or recoveries hastened, by such speedy responses to emergency calls can only be conjectured.

After Dr. C. P. Stewart's retiral, Dr. L. G. Whitby was appointed in 1963 to be the University's first Professor of Clinical Chemistry and Biochemist-in-Charge in the Royal Infirmary. At that time the number of specimens dealt with for the Infirmary annually was 85,600, involving 176,000 separate analyses; ten years later, the corresponding figures were 185,000 and 585,000 respectively and by then an additional 62,000 specimens were being dealt with for other hospitals. Already in 1967 the Infirmary's Annual Report recorded that the department 'continues to bear the largest routine diagnostic workload for any clinical chemistry laboratory in Britain'. That workload has continued to grow ever since.

Between 1963 and 1979, the number of staff in the laboratories concerned with teaching and hospital services increased from 28 to 48 including an increase from 20 technicians (the former designation) to 32 medical laboratory scientific officers or MLSO's (their present designation). That increase, however, falls far short of what would have been necessary but for the introduction of automation.

It was in 1958 that the first auto-analyser, a single-channel American model, was installed in the old laboratory. It was one of the first such aids to be used in the United Kingdom and according to Dr. C. P. Stewart it was capable, 'with semi-skilled (but intelligent) supervision by one person, of performing 200 estimations of blood-glucose in one day, a task which by the orthodox manual method, would be a tiring one for two skilled technicians'. The auto-analyser of 1958 is still in the department and can still operate effectively, but it appears a primitive contraption of chains and sprocket wheels when compared with the modern equipment beside it.

The first single-channel auto-analyser could do one selected analysis on each of 60 samples in an hour—i.e. 60 analyses per hour. By 1964 a bank of machines was producing 300 analyses per hour. Then, in 1975 the Scottish Home and Health Department jointly with the Department of Health and Social Security installed a 'sequential multi-channel analyser and computer' (SMAC) in the Clinical Chemistry Laboratory in order to assess its value for use in British laboratories. It was the first of its kind in the United Kingdom. Soon it represented the backbone of the clinical chemistry service performing 20 different analyses on 150 samples every hour—i.e. 3,000 analyses per hour.

The following extract from records maintained in the laboratory shows how the installation of these modern aids has made it possible for fewer technicians to undertake more work and (though this is not shown by the figures) to do it more quickly:

Year	No. of specimens	No. of analyses	No. of technical staff
1970-71	230,800	722,300	44
1974-75	221,000	773,900	39
1978-79	251,300	1,131,000	34

The vastly increased volume of data produced by these methods has to be processed and, in order to keep pace with the flow, a computer has to be used. The first, for processing only, was installed in 1965; it was replaced in 1968 by a model linked to the auto-analysers but this did not prove entirely satisfactory. It was replaced by a larger model, for processing only, linked to the analysers by human and not electronic agency, and it operated effectively.

How does all this highly technical equipment help the patient in the hospital bed? The answer is that, by producing a variety of essential information quickly, it enables the physician to make an accurate diagnosis more rapidly than might otherwise be possible. Far from destroying the human element, as computers are so often accused of doing, it enables human skill and understanding to be applied more speedily and confidently than before.

Medicine and Medical Physics

The second major building project of the 1960s was the construction within the Infirmary of a building to house the University Departments of Medicine and of Medical Physics. The cost was again shared, under the 'Pater formula', by Health Service and University and the project marked the beginning of a new era of integration of the work of the Infirmary and the Medical School.

Hitherto the physical presence of the Department of Medicine within the Infirmary—of long standing and importance though it was—consisted of the two professorial wards 26 and 27 and, after 1947, two consultation rooms and a small laboratory in converted staff accommodation above Ward 27. Professor K. W. Donald who succeeded Sir Stanley Davidson as Professor of Medicine in 1959 carried on his work there, including important researches in the cardio-pulmonary field; and he also developed cardiac catheterisation facilities in accommodation at the east end of the medical corridor 'borrowed' from the Department of Radiology. The offices and main laboratories of the Department of Medicine were in the University Medical School building in Teviot Place, conveniently near the Infirmary yet inconveniently separated from it by the public thoroughfare of Middle Meadow Walk. It had long been realised that a major teaching hospital such as the Infirmary should have within it adequate accommodation for University Departments to which its own interests were closely related.

By the time of Professor Donald's appointment to the Chair, it seems to have been recognised that if candidates of high calibre were to be expected to accept such positions in Edinburgh, facilities of the highest quality must be provided. So it was agreed by all concerned that better provision for the Department of Medicine must be made within the Infirmary quickly, despite the shortage of space and despite the fact that a new hospital, containing every facility, was expected to arise on the site in about ten years time. In view of that expectation it was decided that, as for the Clinical Chemistry Department, any new building should be of semi-permanent construction and should be so sited as to be clear of the early phases of demolition of the old buildings.

The University Department of Medical Physics was an infant compared with that of Medicine. A physicist, Dr. C. A. Murison, had been appointed to the radiology department of the Infirmary in 1936 and had moved to the Western General Hospital in 1955 when the main radio-therapy work was transferred to that hospital. Two years later the University and the Regional Hospital Board agreed that there was a need for a medical physics unit that could serve both the University and the hospitals of the South-eastern Region. Such a unit, with Dr. (since 1966, Professor) J. R. Greening as Director, was established at No. 12 George Square, a former University women students' residence. This provision was no more than a make-shift arrangement and it was soon decided that the building envisaged within the Infirmary for the Department of Medicine could, with advantage, be combined with one for the Department of Medical Physics.

The joint building was designed by John Holt, FRIBA, Architect to the South-Eastern Regional Hospital Board. The first turf was cut on the site by Professor George Romanes, Chairman of the Board of Management, on 6 January 1961 and the completed building was formally opened by the Rt. Hon. Lord Craigton, CBE, Minister of State at the Scottish Office, on 6 April 1962. To have completed such a building within fifteen months on a difficult, constricted site, including the provision of a great variety of technical installations, was a remarkable achievement. For their success in doing so the architects, engineers and contractors, and also the administrators at Board of Management, Regional Board and Central Department levels who had smoothed their way from time to time, all deserved and received much praise. The exercise provided, also, a taste of future problems, with the piecemeal demolition and replacement of the old hospital buildings then expected to begin quite soon. While the joint building grew, there were repeated complaints about noise and disturbance and on one memorable occasion a steel beam being swung into position made an unscheduled entry through a ward window, fortunately without causing injury.

Like the clinical laboratory building, the joint Medicine and Medical Physics building is on one floor with a much smaller flat above. Like the earlier building, it is sited between two medical pavilions, in this case between Wards 22 and 25 but, unlike the other, it extends northward to the main medical corridor, its ground floor filling the whole space between the pavilions but having its own small landscaped courtyard in the centre. It overflows into only one 'duckpond', that beneath Ward 22. The cost, including equipment and furnishing, was almost £200,000.

As described in the brochure prepared for the opening ceremony, the Department of Medicine contained offices and laboratories for staff and for research fellows, a symposium room, a library and reading-room as well as consulting rooms and special clinics. The laboratories were designed for a variety of investigative techniques important to clinical diagnosis and the treatment of many diseases met with in the wards of the Infirmary; and also for dealing with more fundamental research. The principal clinical and research interests at the time were listed as being those related to heart and lung diseases, circulation problems, disturbances of kidney function and intestinal, nutritional and blood diseases. An effort had, however, been made to ensure that the laboratory facilities were flexible enough to be adapted to serve new types of investigation and methods of treatment which would undoubtedly emerge in an age of rapidly changing medicine.

The design of the Medical Physics section of the building took account of recent advances in the use of radio-active isotopes for medical diagnosis and research and in the clinical applications of electronics. Five isotope laboratories were included enabling, on the one hand, supplies of radio-active materials received from the UK Atomic Energy Authority to be manipulated safely and, on the other hand, tiny degrees of radio-activity to be measured precisely in clinical investigations. An electronics laboratory was provided for the construction of new and development of existing electronic equipment. An X-ray laboratory facilitated the giving of advice and scientific support to clinical X-ray departments, not only in the Infirmary but in hospitals throughout the Region; and a mechanical workshop was provided for designing and making many forms of equipment by means of which patients could benefit from the rapid growth of electronic prosthetic techniques. A room with temperature control used initially for making measurements in a controlled environment was later found to be of value for housing a computer and another laboratory, designed to provide scientific support for the diagnostic use of X-rays was in later years, converted to make similar provision for the diagnostic use of ultra-sound. Such a wide range of scientific and technical activity, developing through the succeeding years, led appropriately in 1977 to the Department being re-designated 'Department of Medical Physics and Medical Engineering'.

The introductory brochure already mentioned ended with the words: 'The siting of the Department of Medical Physics in the Royal Infirmary will further improve the close collaboration between people trained in physics and those trained in medicine, a collaboration upon which many future advances in clinical research, diagnosis and treatment will rest.' How true these words were has become more evident with each year that has passed.

Cardiology and Cardiac Surgery

The advances in medical cardiology in the 1950s, and the coming of open-heart surgery to the Royal Infirmary in 1961 were followed in the sixties and seventies by important developments in both fields. They were developments in which the partnership between physician and surgeon played a vital part in a period when, to quote Dr. R. M. Marquis, 'co-ordinated medical and surgical thinking became accepted cardiological practice'. Before pursuing these developments it may be useful to note the sequence of appointments of Infirmary staff to senior clinical and academic posts in both cardiology and cardiac surgery after 1960.

The sequence began in 1964 following the retiral of Dr. A. Rae Gilchrist after his distinguished career of nearly 40 years in the Infirmary devoted almost wholly to treatment of heart disease. In his place, Dr. R. M. Marquis was promoted to be Physician in Administrative Charge of the cardiology unit. Next was Dr. D. G. Julian who, having been a senior registrar in the Infirmary, had spent some years in Australia where he had pioneered methods of cardiac monitoring. On his return he was given charge of the Unit's investigative laboratory. The other consultant physician was Dr. M. F. Oliver.

In 1974 Dr. Julian became Professor of Cardiology at Newcastle-on-Tyne University and was replaced at the Infirmary by Dr. H. C. Miller. At Edinburgh University Dr. Oliver, having become Reader in Cardiology in 1973 was appointed to a personal Chair in 1978. In 1979 he became the first incumbent of the Duke of Edinburgh Chair of Cardiology created with the aid of a grant of £350,000 from the British Heart Foundation. On the retiral of Dr. Marquis a few months later Professor Oliver became also Physician in Administrative Charge of the Infirmary's Cardiology Unit, thus firmly consolidating the long-standing collaboration of Infirmary and University in that field.

In the field of surgery, Mr. Andrew Logan who, as a thoracic surgeon, had contributed much to the progress of cardiac surgery in the Infirmary, retired in 1972 and his colleague, Mr. David Wade was joined by Mr. Philip Caves. Two years later, Caves was appointed to the newly-created Chair of Cardiac Surgery in Glasgow University which he occupied until his sudden death in 1978. Both in Edinburgh in 1975 and in the Glasgow Chair in 1978, he was succeeded by Mr. David Wheatley, whose place in the Royal Infirmary was then filled by Mr. Kenneth G. Reid who had come to the Infirmary from the Brompton Hospital in London. That sequence of events was in line with the general trend whereby surgery of the heart, initially practised largely by thoracic surgeons because of their experience in exploration of the chest cavity, was becoming a distinct branch of surgery.

In May 1966, mainly as a result of the energetic partnership of Dr. Oliver and Dr. Julian, there came into operation the new coronary care unit, the first such unit in Great Britain to have been specially designed and equipped for its purpose which was, primarily, to correct the disturbances of heart rhythm and heart action which commonly occur after a coronary thrombosis. The unit was formed within the area of medical Ward 31, on the ground floor, quickly accessible from the west entrance drive—an important consideration in a unit designed to deal with urgent emergencies. It consisted of six (later eight) single-bed rooms, each

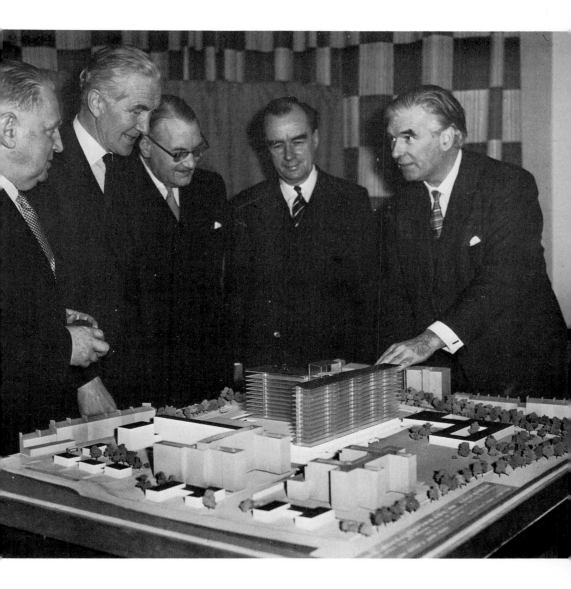

Plate 19   The new Infirmary that might have been — 1961

Professor Robert Matthew, the architect, explains his Scheme 1 to — (left to right) Sir Edward Appleton, Principal of Edinburgh University; Rt. Hon. John S. Maclay, Secretary of State for Scotland; Sir John Dunbar, Lord Provost of Edinburgh and Mr. Charles Gumley, South-Eastern Regional Hospital Board Chairman.

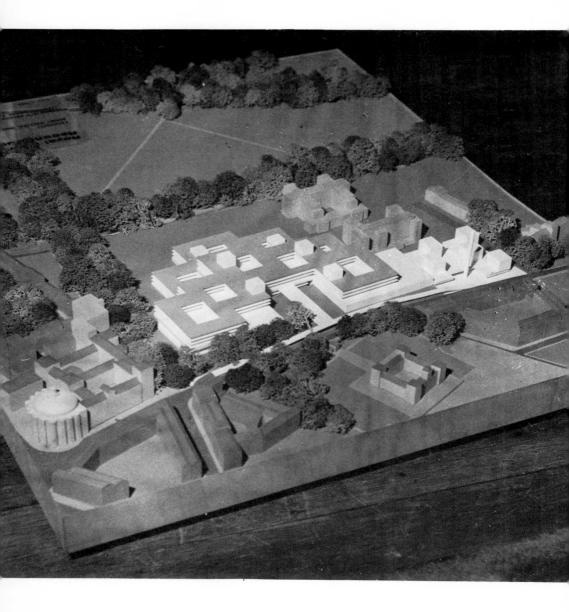

Plate 20   Proposed new Infirmary — Scheme 2, 1965

The model shows a complex of wards and departments grouped round
nine internal open spaces. The Simpson Pavilion and Florence
Nightingale Home remain, on the right. George Heriot's School is in the
foreground and the McEwan Hall to the extreme left of the Infirmary.

acoustically insulated from its neighbours to ensure privacy and quiet and to protect the patients from the sounds of crises in adjoining rooms. Double-glazed windows enabled the patients to be seen from a central monitoring station. Monitors were installed to register various aspects of each patient's condition with display screens at the central station and to give visual and audible alarm signals whenever dangerous symptoms appeared. Electro-cardiograms could be automatically recorded at pre-arranged intervals and also when certain critical conditions occurred. Each room was provided with oxygen and suction points and with a variety of other items of equipment ready for immediate use. Medical staffing was arranged on a rota basis. Other arrangements ensured that experienced nurses would be in constant attendance. Technical and other ancillary staff received special training to meet the needs of the Unit and their interest and support made an important contribution to its success.

At the end of the first year's operation of the Unit it was reported that '23 patients who would otherwise have died from cardiac arrest were successfully resuscitated and discharged from hospital. In addition many other patients have probably had their lives saved by the prompt treatment of disturbances of heart rhythm.' Seventeen years and many hundreds of emergencies later, there must be countless former patients enjoying life among their families who previously would not have survived.

The unique standing of the coronary care unit resulted in its prompt recognition by the World Health Organisation which selected it for the first and second international training courses (in 1967 and 1970) in acute coronary care. Each year the Unit is visited by doctors and nurses from many parts of the world and throughout its existence it has continued to act as a base for research into many aspects of heart diseases and their treatment.

In parallel and in close association with the physician's treatment of heart disorders, cardiac surgery was being developed in surgical wards 17 and 18 and the operating theatre attached to them, near the western end of the surgical house. By 1969 the facilities there had been much improved by the conversion of Ward 17 to form an intensive care area for patients recovering from operations, especially those who had undergone open-heart surgery involving temporary mechanical replacement of the functions of heart and lung by cardiac bypass and assisted ventilation procedures. These facilities included monitoring equipment and the bedside provision of oxygen. They were facilities which greatly helped the recovery of patients though the adaptations had, of necessity, reduced the number of beds available in the two wards.

During 1972 the Regional Hospital Board reviewed the provision in the South-East Region for cardio-thoracic surgery and proposed that, pending the re-building of the Infirmary, such provision should be made as follows:

(a) most cardiac surgery, including provision for infants and children, to be undertaken at the Royal Infirmary;

(b) most general thoracic surgery and perhaps some non-bypass cardiac surgery to be undertaken at the City Hospital; and

(c) some cardiac surgery not requiring bypass facilities, for infants and children, to be undertaken at the Royal Hospital for Sick Children.

To these arrangements the Infirmary Board of Management agreed, but on the understanding that thoracic surgery would continue to be done at the Royal Infirmary in respect of the hospital's own patients.

An important Report on the subject of Cardiac Surgery in Scotland appeared in 1977. This, the 'Kay Report' had been prepared by a Programme Planning Group appointed by the Scottish Health Services Planning Council 'to recommend the extent and location of provision required in Scotland for cardiac surgery, including paediatric cardiac surgery'. The Group's Chairman was Sir Andrew Kay, Regius Professor of Surgery at Glasgow University. The fourteen other members were experienced physicians, surgeons, nurses and administrators, several of whom had first-hand knowledge of the hospitals in the East of Scotland generally and the Royal Infirmary in particular.

In their Report the Group stressed the importance of cardiology being regarded 'as a partnership of disciplines, professional and technical, medical and surgical, in which patients with heart disease have access to the full range of services while their conditions are investigated and treated'. To ensure the availability of these services they recommended the establishment of cardiac centres which would 'afford the opportunity to rationalise the professional, scientific and technical skills required by cardiology and cardiac surgery'.

Among the statistics gathered by the Group they found that, in Edinburgh, the number of cardiac operations on adults had increased from 267 in 1972 to 378 in 1975 and that, within these figures, the proportion involving by-pass procedures had increased from 65% to 87%. On the basis of these and other statistics (including a combined waiting-list estimate for Edinburgh and Glasgow of 300) they considered that the annual demand for cardiac operations on adults in Scotland might be expected to rise to between 1,600 and 2,000. They then recommended that this demand should be met by three cardiac centres (two in Glasgow and one in Edinburgh) each with twin operating theatres and full supporting services. For operations on children they estimated an annual demand for 400 operations which, they suggested, should be met by surgical teams from the adult centres operating within the 'paediatric environment' of the existing Sick Children's Hospitals in both cities.

For the Lothian Health Board these recommendations posed a complex problem because of the basic demand to provide, in the proposed cardiac centre, twin operating theatres if the estimated requirements were to be met. The root of the problem in Edinburgh was that only a single theatre was available to the cardiac surgery unit in the Royal Infirmary and that if a second theatre was to be provided it must be close at hand. For that, no space was available within the existing building and no space remained on the Infirmary site on which a new twin-theatre unit could be built. Seven different suggested solutions were thoroughly explored. Five of them had to be discarded for a variety of reasons and then a sixth was given prolonged consideration. It was that a new twin unit should be built at the Western General Hospital—a proposal which had both strong advocates and strong opponents. At the Western General Hospital though space might have been available for twin theatres, several essential back-up facilities already available at the Infirmary would have to be provided and that would have led to both building and staffing difficulties. So, after much discussion and hard thinking, a consensus decision was at last reached and was approved by the Scottish Home and Health Department.

The decision was that a second cardiac surgery theatre should, after all, be built at the Royal Infirmary as a 'twin' of the existing theatre by the device of constructing it in the form of a bridge, suspended at third-floor level between Ward 17 and the nearest projecting area to the east of it, close to the theatre of Wards 9/10. This was a complicated and difficult solution, requiring ingenious planning and skilful building as well as the provision of efficient protective shields against disturbance so as to enable the existing cardiac theatre to continue in use to its utmost capacity during the building period. Detailed planning of such a project was inevitably a time-consuming process; but in October 1982 work began on the site, with mid-1984 as the intended date for completion.

How, it may have been asked, did that solution fit in with the long-standing plans for complete replacement of the hospital? Given the economic realities of the times, the answer to that question could only be that, whatever re-phasing programme might finally be adopted for the main re-building project, the new theatre would be safe from encroachment for a good many years—fully long enough, in fact, to make its construction worth-while in terms of the work it would do and the lives it would prolong.

Therapeutics

In 1962, Professor Sir Derrick Dunlop retired from the Chair of Therapeutics which he had occupied since 1936. He was succeeded in the Chair by Professor Ronald H. Girdwood, who had been a Consultant Physician in the Infirmary since 1951. He was a member of the Government Committee on the Safety of Medicines and also Chairman of the Executive Committee of the Scottish National Blood Transfusion Association. He retired from his University and Infirmary appointments in 1982.

During the year 1962-63, besides conducting much important research, his Department looked after about 980 patients in Wards 23 and 24 in the Medical House. They also dealt with more than 10,000 out-patient attendances. The work had then been helped by the fact that Wards 23 and 24 had just been modernised. The opening of the new clinical chemistry department in 1960 had released space at the east end of the Medical House but much of that space was occupied by the hospital department of cardiology; while the development of the renal dialysis unit and the introduction into the Therapeutics Department of special accommodation for kidney transplant patients had made large inroads into the space available to the Department.

These problems were eased, but not solved, by some minor adjustments. Then in 1963 two things happened, by coincidence on the same day. It was announced that the Distillers Company were to give a grant of £40,000 to provide facilities for research into congenital abnormalities; and the Professor's attention was drawn to a type of prefabricated construction suitable for building on top of a flat roof. Beside Ward 24 there was a large area of flat roof above the Physiotherapy

Department on the upper floor of the Radiological Department. When that building was erected in 1926 it had been designed, thanks to the foresight of the Infirmary Managers, in such a way as to allow for an additional storey to be added if necessary. So, after 37 years, their foresight, the generosity of the Distillers Company and the recognition of a possible use for a method of prefabricated building all came together to produce at least a partial solution to the Department's difficulties. Within a year there had arisen above the Physiotherapy Department a building of light construction forming a well-equipped Congenital Abnormalities Unit, the provision of benches and other equipment having been funded by the University Grants Committee. The Unit came to be used jointly by the Departments of Therapeutics, Bacteriology, Pharmacology and Surgery. The Department of Therapeutics' share of the accommodation consisted of six laboratories (bringing their total to fourteen), two doctors' rooms and a secretary's room.

Thus the laboratory problems of the Department had been largely overcome, thanks to the co-operation of all concerned. But limitations on space remained and were not more fully eased until, in 1968, the Nuffield Transplantation Unit was opened at the Western General Hospital and, in 1969, the new Renal Dialysis Unit was built on the site of the Medical Superintendent's former house in the Infirmary. Meanwhile the number of patients cared for continued to grow and the Department's programme of research became steadily longer, more complex and more closely associated with research in the Blood Transfusion Service and the Department of Haematology. The wide-ranging nature of the Department's work was finally recognised when, in 1978, their title was expanded to 'Department of Therapeutics and Clinical Pharmacology'.

Geriatric Medicine

An important innovation in the work of the Royal Infirmary was made in 1963 when, for the first time in its history, beds were allocated specifically for elderly patients. Hitherto, provision made by the Infirmary had been for the acutely ill, irrespective of age. Old people, admitted to acute wards because of disease or injury, received the full care and attention required by their acute condition and such extra care on account of their age as could be managed in busy general wards. Many remained in such wards for longer than their medical condition required because of their inability to look after themselves, or to be looked after, at home and because of a continuing shortage of other suitable hospital or residential home accommodation. It was a situation which was neither good for the elderly patients for whom an acute ward was far from being the right environment, nor good for the hospital as, increasingly, beds remained blocked which should have been available for new admissions.

As the proportion of elderly and aged in the general population steadily increased, the hospital problem also grew despite some progress in the 1950s and 1960s by the Regional Hospital Board in providing more long-stay beds in other hospitals and by local authorities in providing new residential homes. Extension of the home help and 'meals on wheels' services also helped by enabling many elderly patients to return home who could not otherwise have done so. These extra facilities, however, were not keeping pace with the growing needs. Meanwhile, the study of problems of the elderly and of the process of ageing was gradually emerging, to become a new specialist branch of medicine.

As a first step towards dealing with the problem as affecting the Infirmary, twelve beds in Wards 45 and 46 in the dermatology pavilion were made available as an assessment unit in which the condition and the needs of elderly patients could be studied while arrangements were being made at their homes which might enable them to return there or while admission to other accommodation was being sought. In July, 1963, the first twelve patients (six men and six women) were admitted. Doctors, nurses and physiotherapists, helped also by voluntary workers, all collaborated to provide rehabilitation measures aimed at developing each patient's capabilities so far as possible. During the Unit's first year, 97 patients were admitted, some from general wards but most direct from their homes. At first sight, from the hospital's point of view, this was disappointing, as greater relief of pressure on the general wards had been hoped for, but it was pointed out that several of those admitted direct to the Unit would otherwise have had to come into hospital anyway. So the relief gained was greater than the figures alone might suggest.

Small though the Unit was, it soon became a valuable part of the Regional Hospital Board's comprehensive geriatric service which was gradually being built up and which included beds at Longmore and Liberton Hospitals, then part of the Edinburgh Southern Hospitals Group.

The small number of beds in the Infirmary Unit limited its benefits, especially as several of its patients had to remain there for two years or even longer before other suitable provision could be made for them. Then, in 1966, a new opportunity occurred, through circumstances quite unconnected with the Unit. In December, 1965, as an early move in the 'decanting' process which had been planned to permit of demolition work in preparation for the phased re-building of the Infirmary, the in-patients of the Ear, Nose and Throat Department had been transferred to the City Hospital where new, up-to-date accommodation had been provided for them. But already, it had become clear that the re-building programme was going to be considerably delayed and that several years were likely to elapse before it would become necessary to demolish the buildings which stood in the path of its second and later phases. So it was agreed that, in the meantime, the vacated accommodation in the ENT Pavilion should be used for several purposes including the extension of provision for the elderly.

In that pavilion Wards 37, 38, 39 and 40 were allocated for the purpose and it was decided that the 42 beds there should be reserved for elderly women patients transferred from acute medical wards. These greatly eased the pressure on those wards. Most of the patients moved, however, required a prolonged period of care and so the four wards, instead of continuing simply as temporary relief accommodation, soon became an active geriatric unit. There everything possible was done to maintain the comfort and interest of the patients and to help them to become as active and self-sufficient as their age and physical condition would allow. From the outset physiotherapists played an important part in the work of the Unit. Then, in 1970, an occupational therapist was appointed. The appointment of others followed later. A comfortable day-room was provided and members of the Royal Infirmary Volunteers helped in several ways to make the patients' stay in hospital as pleasant as possible.

About this time increasing importance was being placed on the teaching of geriatric medicine to students in view of the certainty that, in later years, they could expect to find a growing proportion of older people among their patients. One outcome of this was that, in 1970, the unit was designated as a sub-department of the Department of Medicine for the purpose of undergraduate teaching and Dr. Neil Macmichael, who had been in clinical charge of the unit since its inception, received a University appointment as Honorary Lecturer. These were developments which generated new interest and enthusiasm among the staff of the unit at all levels and, it was reported, proved 'not only acceptable to the students but they ask for more'.

After Dr. Macmichael's retiral in 1973 the assessment beds, along with beds at Longmore Hospital, came under the charge of his colleague, Dr. Hugh MacLeod. Responsibility for the longer-stay beds (later, in association with a similar unit at the City Hospital) was undertaken by Dr. James Williamson who, in 1976, was appointed by the University as their first Professor of Geriatric Medicine. Once again the Royal Infirmary was playing its part, as a great teaching hospital, in an advancing branch of medical knowledge.

Ear, Nose and Throat Department

The year 1965 was a year of change for the Department of Otorhinolaryngology or, more familiarly, the Ear, Nose and Throat Department. It was the year in which their provision for in-patient treatment was transferred to the City Hospital, only out-patient facilities remaining at the Infirmary. Special provision for out-patient treatment of 'ENT' patients had existed in the Infirmary for 82 years and beds had been allocated to the specialty for 74 years—i.e. since 1883 and 1891 respectively. The separate 'ENT' pavilion had been in use for 62 years, since it was built in 1903.

In 1929 the two surgeons in charge of the wards in the pavilion were Dr. J. S. Fraser and Dr. J. D. Lithgow. Both were distinguished practitioners in their special field. Their most famous precursor in that field in the Infirmary had been Dr. A. Logan Turner. Having served as Surgeon-in-charge for the normal period of 15 years (1906 to 1921) he had been persuaded, exceptionally, to continue as 'surgeon-consultant' for a further three years, before retiring in 1924 to become a consulting surgeon. For ten years after 1924 he was a member of the Board of Managers. He died in 1939 and is remembered widely for his professional skills and even more widely as the author of a standard text-book of his specialty, a 'Life' of his father, Sir William Turner who was Principal of Edinburgh University from 1903 until 1916 and the *Story of a Great Hospital—the Royal Infirmary of Edinburgh, 1729 to 1929*.

J. S. Fraser died in 1936 and J. D. Lithgow retired in that year. They were followed by George Ewart Martin who continued as surgeon-in-charge until 1950. Logan Turner's main interest had been in the nose and throat and he was said to have been the first in Britain to practise bronchoscopy—the use of instruments to obtain internal views of the windpipe. Ewart Martin carried that work much further and became a leading exponent in Europe of broncho-oesophagoscopy.

Three who followed him as surgeons in charge of wards until they retired were Dr. Ion Simson Hall (1946-1961), Dr. J. P. Stewart (1950-1965) and Dr. A. Brownlie Smith (1961-1970). As assistant surgeons in the 1930s Simson Hall and Brownlie Smith were associated with the development in Edinburgh of the operation of fenestration—the opening of a tiny 'window' in a bone of the inner ear to overcome deafness due to otosclerosis. The operation had first been undertaken in Stockholm by a Swedish surgeon, Gunnar Holmgren, in 1917. Thereafter it had been done in this country only a few times, the last being in 1923, before Dr. Brownlie Smith performed it on a patient in Edinburgh in 1937. In the following years a special technique for the operation was perfected by Dr. Simson Hall; and, later, Dr. Brownlie Smith evolved an improved 'slim-line' microscope for use in such operations which had the obvious advantage that it could be used during the operation and not just to facilitate examination beforehand. The fenestration operation was widely practised until it began to be replaced, about 1953, by the procedure known as 'mobilisation of the stapes' (i.e. a bone of the middle ear). By 1958 it was almost entirely superseded by stapedectomy, or removal and replacement of the bone. Disappearance of the fenestration procedure was also in part due to improved standards of asepsis and advances in chemotherapy and the use of antibiotics.

The Board's annual reports for the early 1960s record that much time was being spent on the other two operations mentioned and on reconstructive surgery of the middle ear 'although not to the detriment of interest in rhinology and neck surgery'. While these surgical procedures were continuing, Dr. R. B. Lumsden (Assistant Surgeon, 1950; Surgeon 1965 to 1967) was patiently investigating the use of ultra-sound in the treatment of Meniere's disease of the ear, a cause of fluctuating deafness and distressing attacks of vertigo; a study which was continued after his retiral by Dr. G. D. McDowall.

The change that took place in 1965 was made in December. Quietly and without fuss, the whole in-patient section of the ENT Department moved out of the Pavilion to accommodation which had been prepared for them at the City Hospital. There, they found facilities more in keeping with modern requirements than could be provided in the old pavilion. The reason for the move, however, was not to obtain better facilities (though these were much appreciated) but, as noted in an earlier chapter, to prepare for demolition of the old pavilion which stood in the path of phase two of the Infirmary re-building scheme as then envisaged. There the pavilion still stands, used now for a variety of purposes, its fate postponed to an indefinite date. The out-patients section of the department remained in its old quarters for a few more years. In 1969 the Eye Department moved westward from the adjoining Moray Pavilion into their fine new Princess Alexandra Pavilion. That gave the opportunity for the Moray Pavilion to be upgraded and converted to meet the needs of ENT out-patients. In 1971 the out-patient department moved in and found many improvements, including three sound-proof rooms for the better testing of patients' hearing. Facilities for research into voice disorders had been provided and on the top floor there were a seminar room and clinical-teaching rooms. With the additional space provided it was possible to transfer the hearing-aid centre from Cambridge Street and thus to develop a fully-integrated service for that branch of the work. This was of special importance as new types of hearing-aid were becoming available, which could be selected and adjusted by expert audiometricians to meet individual needs. In May 1983 the out-patient department moved from the Moray Pavilion to the 'phase 1' building of the projected new Infirmary where even more up-to-date accommodation had been prepared for it.

For some years treatment and research in the field of laryngeal disfunction had been undertaken. Research into the causes of speech defects and means of correcting them was developed, notably by Dr. Malcolm Farquharson (Assistant Surgeon 1945; Surgeon 1973-1976) in fruitful co-operation with the University Department of Phonetics. In line with trends elsewhere the work of the ear, nose and throat practitioner was becoming progressively sectionalised, each expert concentrating on his own highly-specialised branch of work but all co-operating whenever these overlapped or merged.

Urology Department

In the Surgical House an important development occurred in 1967 though it had been foreshadowed forty years before. This was the establishment, officially, of a Department of Urology. Mr. Henry Wade who, in the twenties and thirties, was in charge of Wards 15 and 16, had already become specially interested in that subject and had then and afterwards increasingly been regarded as an expert in the field. He had obtained from the Managers authority to establish, in association with the two early radiologists, Dr. Hope Fowler and Dr. Woodburn Morison, a small theatre in which patients suffering from urological complaints could have their condition investigated. The theatre was provided with special apparatus including X-ray equipment and was then known as the 'electric diagnostic theatre'—'electric', however, was later dropped from its name.

As time went on the diagnostic theatre underwent much development and change and arrangements were made for it to be used on certain days by other surgeons for investigative purposes. After Sir Henry Wade's retiral it came under the charges, successively, of Mr. R. L. Stewart and Mr. J. R. Cameron, both general surgeons who were also interested in urology, and they, with the support of other members of the surgical staff, worked gradually towards the establishment of a separate department. After the retiral of Mr. Cameron, their work finally bore fruit when, in 1967, Mr. Thomas I. Wilson (who had been one of Henry Wade's clinical tutors in the 1930s) was appointed Surgeon in Administrative Charge in Wards 15 and 16. The two wards and their main operating theatre were upgraded. The diagnostic theatre had been redesigned in 1964 and re-equipped with sophisticated apparatus and instruments for investigation and clinical research. Soon afterwards, seven 'day beds' were provided in a small ward converted from office accommodation. There, patients under investigation or receiving minor surgery for urological complaints could be comfortably accommodated for a brief recovery period. In the main wards, in 1970, thirty beds were allocated for the new department's in-patients, the remaining ten being made available for general surgery, an arrangement which encouraged useful collaboration among the surgeons concerned. A second urological surgeon, Mr. Peter Edmund, had been appointed in 1968 and on Mr. Wilson's retiral in 1973, he succeeded him.

Meanwhile, in 1971, the unit had been officially accredited as a centre for the training of urological surgeons. Thus the special branch of surgery, pioneered in the Infirmary by Sir Henry Wade so many years before, received full recognition with a clinical and teaching department wholly devoted to it.

Accident and Emergency Department

For generations, the part of the Royal Infirmary best known to the general public was, almost certainly, the Surgical Out-patient Department—the 'SOPD'—at the east end of the surgical house, close to the east gate. To it came daily a stream of patients on foot, in cars, taxis and ambulances; and to its present-day successors, the Accident and Emergency and the Surgical Consultation Departments, they still come, but now in separate streams. The old SOPD dealt with two groups of patients intermingling with one another to the disadvantage of both.

The first group were those referred by general practitioners and some coming of their own accord, for surgical consultation or to receive minor surgical treatment in the department's operating theatre which had been built in 1904 in the space between the first and second surgical pavilions. The second group were those urgently in need of attention as the result of accident or sudden illness, some of whom might also require minor surgery in the department.

There was no appointments system (for those in the second group there could not be) and patients in the first group tended to arrive in large numbers between nine and ten o'clock each morning in the hope of being early in the queue for attention. They often had to wait for up to two hours, and sometimes longer, until a doctor was able to see them, the length of their wait depending to a large extent on the number of accident or emergency cases arriving in the meantime, who obviously had to be given priority. The Royal Infirmary Summary Report for the years 1948 to 1958 contains an interesting comparison between the volume of work in the SOPD in the 1930s and that in the 1950s (the 1940s having been omitted as untypical). It shows that the numbers of patients dealt with were as follows:

	New Patients	Return Visits	Total
Annual average 1933-37	30,466	76,894	107,360
Annual average 1953-57	34,383	43,917	78,300

The drop in the number of return visits seems surprising until one reads the explanation that the decrease is 'owing to the less frequent dressings required in the antibiotic era'. After 1957 the number of new patients continued to rise annually until in 1963-64 (the last full year of the SOPD in its old form) the numbers were:

New patients 41,324; Return visits 37,584; Total 78,908.

One of three post-war projects which had been decided upon by the former Managers in 1946 was the improvement of the SOPD at a cost of £12,450. But post-war times were difficult times and, eighteen years later, the conditions in which the patients and their relatives or friends were received and had to wait still differed little from those in the old charitable institution days, with wooden benches to sit on and dreary tiled walls to look at. A report on a survey of twelve out-patient departments in the Infirmary undertaken in 1954 had commented under the heading 'Reception arrangements'—'these range from the frankly squalid in the SOPD—a department which is fifty years old—through varying stages up to the excellent facilities in the orthopaedic out-patient department and the newer departments'. The word 'squalid' in that context must be read in the knowledge of pre-National Health Service and especially pre-war circumstances when the use of hard wooden benches was regarded as necessary to facilitate frequent vigorous scrubbings in the interests of hygiene and for the avoidance of infection. By 1954, however, improvement in the waiting conditions was long overdue. As for congestion in the Department—that, as one of the consultants in the SOPD pointed out, was partly due to the fact that the number of senior surgical staff there was still the same as it had been in pre-National Health Service days and it was only after repeated pressure from the Board of Management that the Regional Board agreed to increase the number of Registrars from two to three. Probably because of that increase a second survey, carried out in September, 1956, showed that the percentage of patients having to wait for 'one hour or more' had dropped from 13.6% to 5.3%.

In 1960, about 40% of first visits to the Department were of patients referred by general practitioners for consultation and treatment, without appointment. That, combined with the unpredictable arrivals of accident cases, must have made any orderly arrangement of the work of the Department extremely difficult. It was then that plans began to be made to split the Department into two, separating the consultation and minor surgery patients from the accident and emergency patients. Planning for the complete re-building of the Infirmary having already begun, it was decided that plans for division of the SOPD must be on a fairly modest scale, as the life of the building in which it was situated was then thought likely to be short, perhaps fifteen years at the most. The first step was to separate the two groups of patients. By 1963, a surgical consultation suite was completed by the conversion of Ward 2 nearby which had been vacated by oral surgery. To that new suite patients referred for consultation or pre-arranged surgery were directed and an appointments system was introduced for such patients who would be seen there by the staff from the ward unit concerned with their type of complaint.

In 1964, conversion of the old SOPD accommodation, including the theatre, into an up-to-date Accident and Emergency Department was begun. The Architects for the conversion were Messrs. Robert Matthew, Johnson-Marshall and Partners, advised by two surgeons with much experience of casualty work, Mr. T. J. McNair and Mr. W. McQuillan. In the same year, Mr. McNair became Surgeon in Administrative Charge of the Department and remained in that position until 1967, developing the unit until it became a highly efficient accident and

emergency centre. Despite the urgent need for the new facilities and their importance in improving efficiency and also in improving the public image of the
hospital service, the Board of Management had still been unsuccessful in their
efforts to persuade the Regional Board to give the project a sufficiently high
priority in the building programme for the Region. So the cost of the work,
amounting to £47,000, had after all to be met from the Royal Infirmary's
endowment fund.

So as to enable the work of the Department to continue without interruption
(though not without inconvenience), the conversion work was done in four
phases. The first phase, including long overdue improvements to the reception
and waiting areas, was completed and brought into use early in 1965. Among
the new arrangements, the separation of 'walking cases' from 'trolley cases'
speeded up the progress of patients through the Department and helped to reduce
waiting-time while an appointments system for return visits enabled such visits
to be spread more evenly throughout each day. In view of the rising toll of road
accidents, bringing ever more pressure on the Department, these improvements
came none too soon as is evident from the following figures comparing the
volume of work in its first full year as a separate unit with the volume seven years
later (the figures rounded in each case to the nearest 100):

Year	New Patients	Return Visits	Total
1965-66	40,000	24,200	64,200
1972-73	56,700	20,500	77,200

The reduction in the number of return visits shown by these figures was due not
only to the benefit of antibiotics but also to the introduction of a more stringent
policy of referring patients to their general practitioners for follow-up attention,
whenever practicable.

The whole scheme was completed in 1967 and the re-organised Department
with its more comfortable rooms and modern decor was officially opened in
June of that year by Professor George J. Romanes, Chairman of the Board of
Management. An important advance was the inclusion of a well-equipped resuscitation room and two X-ray installations, one in the resuscitation area for examination of skull, spine, chest and abdominal injuries and a separate one for simpler
and more routine examinations. Facilities were provided for rapid communication
with the surgical neurology, orthopaedic, coronary care and other units, thus
enhancing the collaboration which already existed with these units. The improved
link meant that, in addition to the general skills within the Department, highly
specialised attention in many branches of medicine and surgery would be more
readily available to every patient requiring it.

This close association with other departments was of special importance in the
fields of surgical neurology and orthopaedics as the increasing volume and speed
of road traffic led to increases in the number and severity of accidents involving
serious head injuries and fractures. As Professor John Gillingham who, after 1962,
succeeded Professor Dott in the University and as Surgical Neurologist in charge

of Ward 20, frequently pointed out, it was a trend tragically made worse by the failure of so many road users to take the simple precaution of fastening their car seat-belts. It was, indeed, fortunate that elective neurosurgery (from 1962 also directed by Professor Gillingham) had been transferred in 1960 to the Western General Hospital, because otherwise it is difficult to see how Ward 20 could have covered the growing volume of emergency work. As it was, that ward became an essential feature of the Royal Infirmary's position as a Central Accident Hospital.

Similarly, the Orthopaedic Department became a vital part of the Accident Service. During 1958, the year in which Professor James succeeded Professor Mercer as head of the Infirmary's orthopaedic service, the number of operations carried out in the orthopaedic theatre had been 800. Thereafter, as the number of accident cases brought to the Infirmary steadily increased, it became necessary to limit the orthopaedic work there to a trauma service only, all non-traumatic and reconstructive orthopaedic surgery being concentrated completely at the Princess Margaret Rose Orthopaedic Hospital. How essential that division of work was is demonstrated by the continuing growth in the volume of orthopaedic accident work at the Infirmary in later years. In 1965, 2,500 operations were carried out there; by 1978 that number had increased to 3,200 and the service treated 2,600 in-patients and 4,000 out-patients.

Meanwhile, to return to the main Accident and Emergency Department, an important aid to its efficiency had been installed in 1968, the year after its opening. This was a direct radio link between the Department and ambulances of the Scottish Ambulance Service, enabling reports on a patient's condition to be made by the attendant and first-aid advice to be given to him while the ambulance was speeding towards the hospital. In the following year a closed-circuit television link with the Surgical Neurology Department at the Western General Hospital was provided. Other improvements and innovations included the organisation of a round-the-clock secretarial service, enabling patients' records to be rapidly completed and letters reporting on their conditions to be sent to the patients' general practitioners within 24 hours.

For major accidents involving several badly injured people, some of whom might be trapped in wreckage, the new lay-out of the Department incorporated space near the entrance for the storage of hampers containing 'crash equipment' ready to be loaded, at a moment's notice, into ambulances or police cars. In 1980, these 'major accident' arrangements were brought to a further stage of efficiency by Dr. Keith Little who in 1978 had been appointed the first consultant in accident and emergency medicine. He and his colleagues devised a flying-squad van, containing anaesthetic apparatus, sterile surgical packs and other special equipment, so that emergency surgery and other urgent treatment could, if necessary, be carried out at the scene of an accident. The van, manned by an ambulance service driver and carrying a medical and nursing team of three or more, is linked by radio with the Department and with ambulances and carries personal radios for use by the team at the accident scene. This flying-squad van cost £15,000. It was paid for by members of the public who had responded generously to an appeal launched by the *Edinburgh Evening News* to mark the 250th anniversary of the

Royal Infirmary in 1979; an appeal that was an echo of the 'Evening News Shilling Fund' appeal made by that paper on behalf of the new Simpson Memorial Maternity Pavilion, more than forty years before.

Medical Out-patient Department

The transformation, in 1967, of the old surgical out-patient department into an up-to-date accident and emergency unit had an immediate beneficial effect on the medical out-patient department which was situated further down the east entrance drive and extended into part of the ground floor of the old, 1738, George Watson's Hospital building. The MOPD had long suffered from a complaint similar to that of the SOPD—the mingling of emergency and non-emergency cases, though the problem was less severe because people injured in accidents did not usually figure among those arriving at the medical department. Even so, the average number of emergency arrivals was about 2,000 annually.

Until 1956 there had been no appointments system in the MOPD. Those attending for non-emergency consultation had to share a drab and crowded waiting-room with others suffering from acute conditions requiring urgent attention. That had been partly remedied in 1956 when the appointments system was introduced; and at the same time a programme of renovation began to improve waiting conditions. Real improvement started in 1968 when the transformed accident and emergency department was able to relieve the MOPD of emergency medical cases by day, the SOPD having previously accepted such cases only during the night.

For many years referrals to general medical clinics had been diminishing, their place being taken increasingly by referrals to specialist clinics. During the 1930s specialist clinics had been established in neurology, chest diseases and psychiatry. By the 1970s there were also specialist out-patient services in asthma and bronchitis endocrinology, gastro-enterology, haematology, hypertension, renal medicine and rheumatology. To meet these and other needs better accommodation was necessary and between 1974 and 1976 the department was reconstructed and extended by the provision of an upper floor and the conversion of a former lecture theatre. By these means modern consulting suites were provided, as well as a bright and comfortably furnished reception and waiting area for patients, described as being equal to that of a good-class hotel.

Poisoning Treatment Centre

Close to the East entrance gate on the ground floor of the Surgical House, was Ward 3 which, in 1962, became the Infirmary's Poisoning Treatment Centre under the administrative charge of Dr. Henry Matthew. Since the opening of the new Infirmary in 1879 there had been a secure ward, known as the 'incidental delirium ward', so named because it was the ward to which were transferred patients who were so delirious or fractious as to cause serious disturbance to their fellow patients. For more than fifty years Ward 3 had filled that role and the staff there were trained and experienced in the care of such patients. From time to time they also looked after prisoners and others brought in by the police. Security was provided by doors which, from inside, could be opened only by using a key.

As the use of sedatives, tranquillising drugs and antibiotics developed, the need for segregation of delirious patients almost disappeared; but, ironically, the growing availability of barbiturates and other drugs brought with it a new problem. In the early years, a secondary function of Ward 3 had been to care for patients suffering from poisoning, accidental or self-inflicted, and as the number of such cases resulting from the use and misuse of drugs increased, the ward gradually became a poisoning treatment unit in fact, if not in name. 'Ward 3' continued in its old accommodation close to the Accident and Emergency Department until 1970 when, because of the need to expand that Department, it was moved to an upper floor of the old eye pavilion which had then recently been vacated.

The changing function of the ward had begun to come about long before the Ministry of Health and the Scottish Home and Health Department, in 1962, advocated the setting-up of district and regional centres where, for poisoning cases, special facilities for medical treatment, laboratory investigation and psychiatric assessment of patients could be undertaken. Ward 3 then became, officially, the Infirmary's Poisoning Treatment Centre, continuing under the administrative charge of Dr. Henry Matthew, until his retiral in 1974, and thereafter of Dr. A. T. Proudfoot, as Consultant Physicians.

The Scottish Home and Health Department's concern for the setting-up of such centres arose from the remarkable upward trend in the post-war years in the number of poisoning cases throughout the country. So far as affecting the Royal Infirmary the trend was dramatically illustrated by a graph prepared by Dr. Matthew and published in the Scottish Medical Journal in January, 1966. It showed that the number of patients suffering from poisoning admitted annually had increased from 80 in 1945 to 730 in 1964. In 1967 the centre was recognised as the Regional Poisoning Treatment Centre for South-east Scotland. By 1970, the annual number of admissions was approaching 1,200. In 1980 there were nearly 2,000.

Although such treatment centres could not have been expected to halt that trend, they could—and did—greatly diminish its effects by making efficient treatment promptly available, thereby easing much distress and, in serious cases, saving lives. It was estimated by Dr. Matthew that some 80% of those admitted to the Centre would be suffering from 'self-poisoning', a term he preferred to 'attempted suicide' since in many cases the intention of such patients (consciously or subconsciously) is not self destruction but to utter 'a cry for help' at a time of emotional crisis. Some would purposely take less than a lethal dose or so arrange things that they would be found in time. Some were even known to have telephoned for an ambulance before becoming unconscious. A much more recent estimate puts the proportion of self-poisoning cases at nearer 95% of the total. But during the 1970s the experience of the Treatment Centre had been that the pattern of drug-taking in such cases had changed. Barbiturates featured less and the use of minor tranquillisers such as valium, librium and related drugs had become more frequent. In consequence, people were less likely to be unconscious and seriously ill after over-dosage, whether intentional or accidental. On the other hand, the number of patients admitted after taking drugs 'for kicks', including those taking cannabis and LSD and injecting narcotics and barbiturates, had increased.

There are doubtless many reasons for these trends in modern times and sociological assessments of them have been the subject of several studies. For the purpose of this history it is sufficient to note the readiness of the Infirmary Board of Management to cope with the problem as soon as the serious nature of the trend was recognised and at the same time to note the success with which the work of their Poisoning Treatment Centre has been pursued ever since.

When the Centre was officially set up, there was already close co-operation with bio-chemists in the Department of Clinical Chemistry, where a section specialises in problems of clinical toxicology, and with the Department of Anaesthetics in dealing with patients suffering from respiratory failure. Once the condition brought about by poison has been cured or alleviated, it is equally important to discover and, if possible, help to remove the cause of its being taken in the first place. There has therefore always been fruitful collaboration with psychiatrists in the University Department of Psychiatry ('Department of Psychological Medicine' until 1964) under the leadership, successively, of Dr. W. I. N. Kessel, Professor G. M. Carstairs and Dr. (later Professor) Ian Oswald. Social workers, too, play an important role and may find it necessary to keep in touch with patients of the Centre and their families for long periods. The team approach to the Centre's work has always extended, also, to all members of its staff and not least to the ward porters who provide a stabilising influence by helping to calm those patients who, under the influence of alcohol and drugs, are less restrained in their behaviour than they might be.

The staff of the Centre have always been willing to share their knowledge with others. For example, statistics gathered in the Centre were used extensively by the Medical Research Council in the study of the epidemiology of psychiatric illness. Collaboration has sometimes extended to work with other teaching hospitals, a notable example being the research undertaken jointly with staff at Guy's Hospital, London, which led to the publication of a pioneer paper on the rational assessment of the severity of paraquat poisoning from consideration of the concentration of the poison in the patient's blood. Though not significantly advancing treatment, the study was effective in putting assessment on a scientific basis.

Scottish Poisons Information Bureau

The reputation for expertise in their special field gained by Dr. Henry Matthew and the staff of Ward 3 was such that, in 1963, a Poisons Information Bureau, which had been operated for a short time by the Edinburgh University Department of Forensic Medicine, was transferred to the Poisoning Treatment Centre which was then given the additional designation of Scottish Poisons Information Bureau, with Dr. Matthew (later, Dr. Proudfoot) as Director. It was—and still is—one of four such centres in the United Kingdom, the others being in London, Cardiff and Belfast. At each an index is maintained of several thousand substances used in agriculture, industry and medicine and in the home, along with information about their composition and their poisonous effects. Any hospital or doctor confronted with a case of poisoning or suspected poisoning may telephone the Bureau and receive information about the substance taken and advice about specialised treatment. In practice, about two-thirds of all calls received by the Bureau are from hospitals and, although its area is officially Scotland, about one-tenth of the enquiries are from England. Some come from further afield, even so far away as Hong Kong.

In the first full year of its operation, the Bureau received 315 enquiries. Four years later there were more than a thousand calls and in 1970 almost two thousand. The number received in 1982 was 5,480. These increases are no doubt partly related to the growth in the number of poisoning incidents; they also reflect growing confidence in the advice given. Early in the life of the Bureau, it was reported that a large proportion of the enquiries related to instances of possible poisoning in children. 'A vast variety of substances were incriminated', the report continued, 'ranging from common salicylates, laburnum seeds and household bleach to the inside of a golf ball.' Though there is always satisfaction in being able to give a helpful answer to a worried enquirer, perhaps the most satisfying occasions of all to the staff of the Bureau have been those on which they have been able to reply that the substance swallowed was not poisonous after all.

The Scottish Bureau has only one full-time member of staff. Otherwise it is operated by the medical and nursing staff of the Centre. By 1981, the Bureau's poisons index filled sixteen large unwieldy volumes. The information contained in them included the names of products, their ingredients, their toxicity, any special features and methods of treatment of anyone poisoned by them—all meticulously and laboriously cross-referenced. The mass of information presented an obvious case for transfer to computer storage and so the Bureau, in conjunction with the Lothian Health Board's Computer Services Unit, embarked upon an exercise to find the computer system most likely to satisfy its needs. The aim was to provide a process whereby all products containing the same toxin, or causing similar effects, could be instantly cross-related to entries for clinical features and treatment. After exhaustive trials a suitable system was devised and it was formally inaugurated in April 1983 by Mr. John Mackay, Scottish Office Minister for Health and Social Work. The first computerised poisons information service in Britain, it had cost £80,000 to instal, financed largely by the Scottish Home and Health Department as being a new health care development and partly by the Lothian Health Board. The installation enables hospital casualty units, and general practitioners registered as authorised users, to obtain instant access to the computer by telephone at any time of day or night and to have the information they require displayed on a television screen. Once again a computer is playing its electronic part in providing a sure and rapid service; a service which may often be a life-saving one.

Radiology

An account was given in earlier chapters of the origin of the Royal Infirmary's X-ray Department, its development during the 1930s as a combined centre for both diagnosis and therapy and its division, in October 1946, into separate

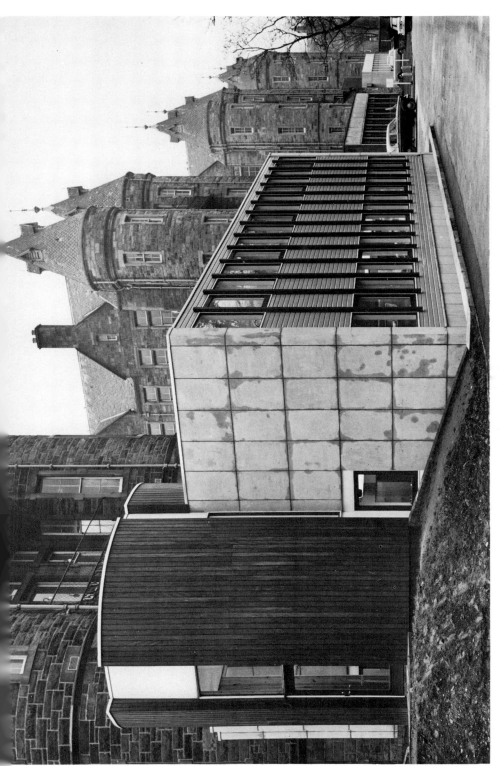

Plate 21   New buildings of the 1960s

Haematology Department, 1967, beside ward 31; beyond are — Clinical Chemistry Department, 1960, between wards 25 and 28; Medicine and Medical Physics Departments, 1962, between wards 22 and 25.

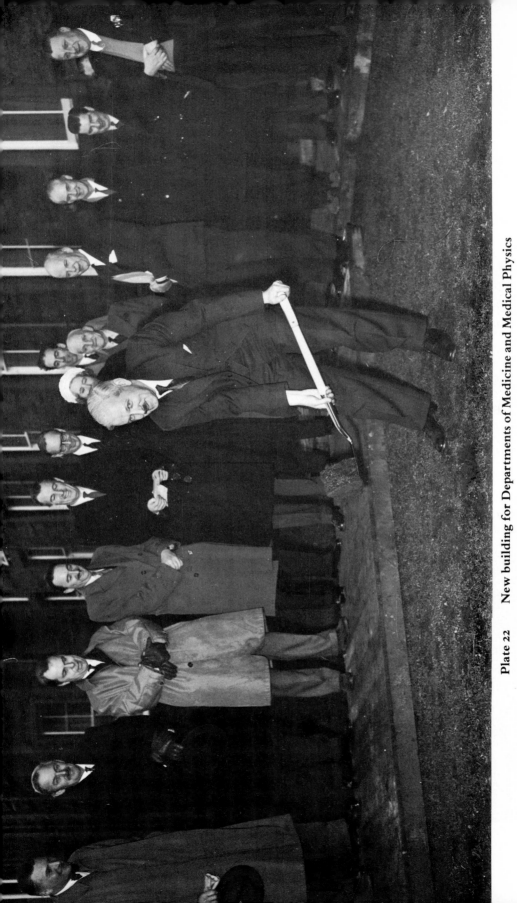

Plate 22   New building for Departments of Medicine and Medical Physics

Professor George J. Romanes, Chairman of the Board of Management cuts the first turf—January 1961, watched by (left to right): 1: T. A. Jeffryes, Dept. of Health. 2: A. A. Hughes, Dept. of Health. 3: Professor Iohn Brotherston. 4: Dr. I. R. Greening. 5: Professor K. W. Donald. 6: Dr. S. G. M. Francis, Med. Supt. 7: Miss Hunter, Asst. Lady Supt. of Nurses. 8: Dr. D. C. Simpson. 9: Dr. E. C. Fahmy. 10: Tom Hurst, Secy. and Treas. 11: William Russell, Regional Engineer. 12: G. D. Robb, Dep. Secy. and Treas. 13: G. Scott, Clerk of Works.

departments with Professor McWhirter continuing as Director of the radio-therapy service. Before taking up the story of the present Infirmary Department of Radiology as it developed from 1960 onwards, it will be desirable to give some account of the ten difficult years during which the two separated departments each sought to develop their work within the same area as had previously been used by the combined department. That two departments need more space than one is usually true, even if the total volume of work remains the same. In this case the need was even greater because the volume of work was steadily increasing. The number of radio-diagnostic examinations grew from 42,000 in 1947 to 76,000 in 1957 and the complexity of many of the examinations also increased. In a comprehensive report to the Board of Management in 1954 it had been pointed out that about 20,000 of the examinations annually were being done by the Department's staff in outlying units, including the Simpson Pavilion, and some 50,000 within the Radio-diagnostic Department. The work done centrally represented (on the basis of a six-day week) the use of about 500 films daily, probably one film every twenty seconds at peak periods. That was at a time when the processing of each film took about half an hour, for it was before the intro-duction of automatic processors. The problem of containing all that work within the available space grew from year to year.

In the former combined Department Dr. John P. McGibbon had been Senior Assistant Radiologist since 1942 and had gained a wide reputation as both prac-titioner and teacher. Since childhood he had suffered from effects of poliomyelitis and this, combined with the effects of other illnesses, prevented him from accepting appointment as Director of the new Radio-diagnostic Department. He remained in that Department, however, and continued to make an outstanding contribution to its work. The esteem in which he was held was such that after his death as the result of an accident in 1952, a Memorial Lecture was founded in his honour by the Scottish Radiological Society and is still delivered annually.

In 1945, Dr. W. S. Shearer had joined the combined Department as an assistant radiologist. An Edinburgh graduate, afterwards qualifying in Radiology, he had practised his specialty in Manchester for eight years and during his war-time service had been a specialist radiologist, mainly in the Middle East. He was appointed Director of the new Radio-diagnostic Department and continued in that post during its first ten difficult years.

It is fair to say that, in deciding to divide the old department into two, the Board of Managers had not intended both to occupy the old accommodation indefinitely. Their intention had been to house the Radiotherapy Service in a new building within the grounds of the Infirmary and to allocate the whole of the existing X-ray accommodation to radio-diagnosis. However, there was a problem. Space might possibly have been found in the grounds for a new building to accom-modate the type of 250,000-volt machines and other equipment then in use for radiotherapy; but, during and immediately after the war—partly as a by-product of radar research—great advances had been made in the production of more powerful X-ray equipment. These advances had culminated in the successful production of a type of linear accelerator capable of developing 4-million volts and producing X-rays with a more deeply penetrating effect than ever before.

M

The Treasury, giving way to the urgent demands of the Ministry of Health and the Department of Health for Scotland agreed that, to serve the needs of the whole country, five such linear accelerators would be provided; and on the advice of the Medical Research Council it was decided that they should be allocated to London, Liverpool, Manchester, Newcastle and Edinburgh on condition that suitable buildings would be available in good time to receive them. For Edinburgh, the Secretary of State promptly accepted that condition.

Clearly there was no space at the Infirmary on which to erect a building large enough to accommodate the linear accelerator with its necessary protection, its ancillary equipment and associated beds. Beside the Western General Hospital ample space was available and there, it was agreed, a Radiotherapy Institute would be built to accommodate one 4-million volt linear accelerator, one (later, two) 2-million volt machines and several less powerful pieces of equipment, some transferred from the Infirmary. Initially, the Institute treated patients from all over Scotland, but later only those from the South-Eastern and Northern Hospital Regions, the needs of the others being met in Glasgow.

By 1957, radiotherapy in-patient treatment had been transferred, only one machine being retained at the Infirmary to be available for certain emergency treatments. (By the time it reached the end of its serviceable life, occasions for its use had become so infrequent that the machine was not replaced.) The new Institute was opened on 5th July 1957 by Sir Ernest Rock Carling, Chairman of the International Commission on Radiological Protection. The Royal Infirmary Summary Report for the years 1948-1958 contains the following description: '[At the Western General Hospital] two units in the supervoltage range have been provided and the apparatus of conventional voltage is of the latest type. There are 110 beds in the Department and an operating theatre for the insertion of radium. Patients—of whom there are over 2,000 new ones every year—can now be offered all the most modern forms of treatment, including treatment by radio-active isotopes.' Some misgivings had been expressed by members of the medical staff of the Infirmary when the removal of radiotherapy from their hospital was proposed. Perhaps partly because of their concern, but also for the convenience of patients, it was agreed that although all treatments would be carried out in the new Institute, the clinical examination of new patients and of patients reporting back after treatment would continue to be undertaken in the X-ray department of the Infirmary. This meant that not all the space formerly used for radiotherapy would be available for radio-diagnosis, though there would be some welcome relief of congestion.

Sadly, before there had been time for him to experience fully the advantages of the new arrangements, Dr. Shearer died suddenly in August 1957. After a year during which Dr. D. W. Lindsay, Senior Radiologist, was Acting Director Dr. Eric Samuel, who had been an Associate Professor in the University of Pretoria became Director of the Radio-diagnostic Department of the Royal Infirmary in September 1958.

Soon after Dr. Samuel's appointment some reduction in the number of out-patient attendances for diagnosis resulted from the opening of investigative centres in other parts of the Region but any reduction in the volume of work this might have caused was much more than offset by the growing number of examinations per patient being asked for by clinical staffs or being undertaken because of new trends in the development of radiography. This was a point vividly demonstrated by a graph prepared by Dr. Samuel for the period from 1930 to 1963. It showed, among other facts, that during those thirty-three years, while the total numbers of patients admitted annually to the Infirmary had risen by 35% (from about 20,000 to 27,000) the number of radiological examinations had increased by 566% (from 15,000 to 100,000). The increase had been steep from 1940 onwards, showing only two brief periods of reduction, one in the early 1950s when there had been a shortage of X-ray film and one in the later 1950s when a wave of concern about radiation hazards had occurred.

Along with the growing volume of work in the Department there came a growth in its complexity. The annual report for 1959-60 records that, during the year, tomography (focussing on selected layers of the body), selective angiography (involving injection of an opaque medium into arteries or veins to show them more clearly on the X-ray film) and other techniques soon to become almost commonplace had been practised for the first time.

In the following year two new technical developments began. Closed circuit television enabling X-ray films to be viewed at a distance and thus of particular value for teaching was successfully introduced and an experimental machine for the automatic processing of X-ray films was tried. It had been supplied as a prototype by the Department of Health for Scotland and, after some modification by the makers, two such machines were installed in July 1961. They were said to be the first used in Scotland and they enabled X-ray films to be ready for inspection 6½ minutes after exposure, instead of 30 minutes as required by the former manual process, a reduction welcomed by the staff but even more by patients awaiting the results. In later years the processing time was reduced to 90 seconds and other improvements eliminated the need for a dark-room. Eventually twelve automatic processing machines were installed in the Department and its outlying units.

Removal of the Department of Medicine to their new building in 1962 enabled the Department of Radio-diagnosis to extend into part of the vacated accommodation, giving some much-needed relief from the congestion which still hampered their work.

By the very purpose and nature of the work, the practice of radio-diagnosis involves collaboration with almost every other medical and surgical department for, with few exceptions, whatever injury or ailment is being dealt with, the clinician will need, at some stage, to see what damage has been done to bone or tissue or how a patient's organs are functioning. Special equipment is, therefore, used by radiologists in 'offshoots' from the main Department who bring their specialised skills to the service of surgical neurologists, orthopaedic surgeons, obstetricians and other medical colleagues throughout the hospital. Such collaboration had been growing and extending to new fields ever since radiology began but in no period did it develop more rapidly than that from 1960 onwards.

Nowhere was this collaboration closer or more valuable than in the field of cardiology. In the planning by the Department of Cardiology of their pioneering coronary care unit, radiologists pooled ideas and advice with cardiologists and other specialists in a joint operation. There, in 1966-67, the most up-to-date equipment for cardio-vascular investigations was installed, including provision for high-speed X-ray cinematography in two planes simultaneously. At about the same time a mobile image-intensifier and television unit was developed in the Infirmary, primarily for use in connection with the insertion and monitoring of cardiac pacemakers. The unit proved so successful that it was made commercially available and came to be widely used.

Mammography, for the detection of breast cancer, was pioneered by Dr. Samuel in the 1960s, Edinburgh becoming one of the main centres for that work, later carried on in collaboration with Professor Forrest of the Department of Clinical Surgery. A different research project undertaken in 1965 and 1966 produced interesting results but was found to achieve little that could not be more accurately done by other means. This was a trial of thermography, using 'thermo-vision', a means of investigation by studying radiated heat generated by the body. Because its results were not entirely satisfactory its use was phased out. It might, however, have provided a means of investigation which could be used in circumstances where it was desirable to avoid even the slightest risk of harm from the use of X-rays. That was soon afterwards achieved in another way by the use of 'ultra-sound', a technique involving the beaming towards selected organs or areas of the body of vibrations with a frequency far above the range of human hearing and studying the resulting echoes as these are displayed on the screen of a highly sensitive receiver.

Professor McWhirter retired in 1970 after 35 years connection with the Infirmary during which he had gained world-wide recognition of his work. There followed a period of changing function and varying nomenclature. Dr. Eric Samuel was appointed to the Forbes Chair of Medical Radiology and continued as Director of the Infirmary Department of Radio-diagnosis. At the same time, a new Chair of Radiotherapy was created by the University. (The clinical field it dealt with, but not the Chair, was re-named 'Radiation Oncology' in 1981 when a separate Chair of Medical Oncology was instituted, concentrating on the use of chemo-therapy in cancer treatment.) The first incumbent of the Chair of Radiotherapy was Professor William Duncan whose clinical work, though centred mainly on the Western General Hospital, includes continuation of the consultation clinics at the Infirmary which had always been, and still are, an important focal point in the radiotherapy service.

After Professor Samuel retired in 1978 Dr. Thomas Philp, who had been a member of the radiological staff of the Infirmary since 1949, became Consultant with administrative responsibility for the Infirmary Radio-diagnostic Department which later came to be called the Department of Radiology. In 1979, Dr. J. J. K. Best, an Edinburgh graduate who had specialised in radiology in Manchester became Professor of Medical Radiology at Edinburgh and Honorary Consultant in the Infirmary, with a special interest in medical imaging.

The term 'medical imaging' had arisen in recognition of the fact that methods of visualising the condition and performance of organs of the body had moved beyond the use of conventional X-ray photography to include also the technique of ultra-sound, already mentioned, and increasingly sophisticated methods of isotope scanning. Under these methods radio-active isotopes are introduced into systems of the body and their movements and concentrations are detected by scanning parts of the body with a scintillation counter or a gamma camera, the results from which, recorded either as marks on paper or as a photographic image, convey invaluable information to the clinician. Such methods developed rapidly during the 1970s when scanners of different types, including a head scanner for use in locating and identifying brain damage, were introduced to the Department. Then came the introduction of computer methods of recording, analysing and instantly displaying the results of such scanning. By 1979, the techniques had advanced to the point of producing whole-body scanners whereby, with the patient reclining inside a large cylinder, the scanner can be made to rotate around him, taking a rapid sequence of pictures which show many cross-sections from a variety of angles from which the computer produces three-dimensional details of great precision. This was an immense technical advance, the full value of which has no doubt yet to be assessed. Such a non-invasive examination may well tell the clinician necessary facts which could previously have been learned only by surgical operation.

When the Lothian Health Board in 1979 authorised the installation of a whole body scanner in the Radiology Department at a cost of £500,000, the problem of its accommodation might have been a serious one, for the scanner with its ancillary equipment, viewing rooms and other facilities takes up a lot of space. A solution, however, was at hand close to the Department in the century-old shape of the East Medical Lecture Theatre with its high ceiling and steeply-tiered rows of wooden benches from which generations of medical students had looked down on to their lecturers standing below. To divide the space into two storeys by inserting a new floor midway between old floor and old ceiling was the obvious answer. The upper space was then used to form a lecture room designed and equipped to meet modern requirements while the lower half of the old lecture theatre became the 'computerised axial tomography' section of the Department. There a diagnostic service came into being, to provide for the needs of the Fife, Lothian and Border Regions, bringing the Infirmary into the forefront of yet another branch of scientific medical practice.

Meanwhile, with the expansion of angiography and nuclear medicine, the Radiology Department had begun to move beyond the realm of exploration and examination into the field of interventional techniques, in a sense blurring the sharp division between diagnosis and therapy. As a by-product of the practice of angiography it had been found possible, for example, to use the technique in such a way as to halt points of bleeding as a pre-operative procedure, thus easing the surgeon's task or, in certain circumstances, superseding open surgery entirely. Conversely, vascular continuity could sometimes be restored where a blockage had occurred. With the introduction of these techniques the Royal Infirmary became a leading centre of interventional radiography.

This account of progress in the field of radiology has concentrated on the work of a succession of radiologists. Another dedicated group of experts also played their part. They were—and are—the radiographers, skilled in controlling the increasingly sophisticated equipment used in the Department. Their contribution is part of the story of the para-medical professions which is told in Chapter 7.

Operating Theatres and the Theatre Service Centre

Early in the 1960s a programme was begun for improvement of the main operating theatres in the Infirmary most of which, despite modification from time to time, did not match up to the rising standards of that time. In pre-war years the theatre attached to Wards 7 and 8, used by Sir John Fraser and that for Wards 15 and 16 used by Sir Henry Wade, had been modernised in accordance with the ideas of their day and during the first decade of the National Health Service some upgrading of the wards 9/10 theatre had been undertaken; but otherwise little had been done.

The first theatres to be dealt with in the new programme were the one attached to Wards 11/12 near the west end of the surgical house and the theatre of Wards 17/18 immediately above it. In 1960 a scheme was adopted under which, in each of these, the former students' large open gallery was removed, providing valuable additional space, the lower part of which was used for the construction of anaesthetic and recovery rooms and of preparation annexes while the upper part accommodated nurses' changing-rooms and an air-conditioning plant. That plant was a significant part of this and other reconstruction schemes. In the not-so-distant past, theatres had had windows which could be opened or closed and during the war proposals to brick up some of them as a protection against blast had been opposed because of the ventilation problem that would have caused. By now, window-less walls and air-conditioning to protect against infection, were an indispensable part of theatre design.

In the 11/12 theatre a small gallery, seating up to ten students, was provided. Unlike the former large gallery which had been open-fronted in the traditional form, the new one was glass-fronted thus protecting the operating area but still giving a clear view of the proceedings.

The work of alteration made it necessary for each theatre to be closed for several months during which time operations were conducted in other theatres. Although this was inconvenient, the temporary change caused surprisingly little reduction in the volume of work undertaken, thanks to the willing co-operation of the normal theatre users.

The Wards 13/14 theatre was also reconstructed in the early 1960s. It, too, had its student gallery removed. The theatre was completely cleared and re-built to provide a larger operating space and an anaesthetic and recovery room as well as segregated 'sterile' and 'dirty' supply and return areas and automatic entrance doors with an airlock system. The air-conditioning equipment for these and other theatres had been carefully designed and adjusted in consultation with bacteriologists to ensure as far as humanly possible that only clean air would be directed towards the operating area and contaminated air always carried away from it.

Among other theatres rehabilitated in greater or lesser degree during this period and in the early seventies were the diagnostic theatre (as described earlier)

colleagues could have complete confidence in the sterile condition of the instruments and other articles they used.

Accommodation for the service centre had been found in the main part of Ward 4 in the surgical house. Ward 4 had served many purposes in past years. For long it was the 'spare ward' to which patients could be moved when another ward was being overhauled; it had sometimes been the 'disaster ward' to which injured miners were admitted and, in two wars, it was named 'the soldiers' ward'. In pre-National Health Service days it often accommodated sales of work on behalf of Infirmary funds. Now its main ward area was converted and equipped for the theatre-service experiment and there, as well as in extensions added later, the service centre remains. The southern end of the ward which had contained its side-rooms and other ancillary accommodation was converted, in 1967, to house the Department of Anaesthetics, a welcome move for that Department from the three small attic rooms which they had previously occupied.

When the theatre service centre began to function experimentally in August 1964 it served three general theatres—those for Wards 7/8, 11/12 and 17/18. The experiment drew much praise and little criticism; in fact, the chief fear expressed by those who benefited from it was that after the experiment ended they might have to revert to the old arrangements. Instead, in the years that followed, the service provided by the centre spread rapidly. By 1967 it was serving all the general surgery theatres and the thoracic surgery theatre, supplying the requirements of nearly 700 operations every month. In 1968 it began to supply the three gynaecology theatres and the Simpson Memorial Maternity Pavilion.

It was soon found that distance alone is no bar to the benefit that may be derived from such a system. That was clearly demonstrated in 1969 when the service was extended to the newly-opened Princess Alexandra Eye Pavilion and when by the early 1970s the centre was serving also operating theatres at Chalmers Hospital and as far away as the Western General Hospital, including the Nuffield Transplantation Surgery Unit.

Through all this time the theatre-service centre frequently received visitors from other parts of the country—nearly 250 of them in 1967—many of whom returned to their own areas to set up similar systems. That many succeeded in doing so is evident from the Infirmary Report of 1969-70 which records that 'Visitors continue to come from overseas to see the Theatre Service Centre, e.g. from the United States, Australia, Lebanon, Greece, Israel, Switzerland and Sweden. Visitors from England are now few because many Theatre Service Centres have already developed there.'

Blood Transfusion

The story of the development of blood transfusion in Edinburgh and South-East Scotland up to the point of its re-organisation in 1940 to meet the anticipated needs of wartime has already been told. In the post-war years, instead of diminishing as many had expected, the demand for blood rapidly increased. Even by 1953 Dr. R. A. Cumming, who had been appointed Regional Director of the Service in 1947, had reported that the annual supply of blood to the Royal Infirmary had risen within a few years from 8,000 pints to 20,000 pints and that between 500 and 600 patients each month were receiving transfusions. (In 1946 the monthly average had been 200.) He ascribed the increase to four main causes:

(1) the growing demand for blood in the treatment of road accident cases;
(2) improved methods of blood preservation and storage;
(3) the fact that research had largely eliminated the danger of incompatible transfusions; and
(4) the growing use of blood derivatives and plasma fractions as distinct from whole blood.

The transfusion of rhesus-negative blood to save severely affected 'rhesus babies' in the Simpson Pavilion—a procedure introduced in the 1940s—was just one of several new needs which had to be met.

The increasing demand led to the organisation in 1955 of a round-the-clock service for the supply of blood. It led also to an urgent need for enlargement of the blood transfusion centre near the west end of the medical house. In 1961 the enlarged centre was completed and it was then described as 'one of the finest and most progressive centres in the country'. It had three main sections: the regional blood bank from which the Royal Infirmary and other hospitals in south-east Scotland were supplied; laboratories for blood-testing and for research; and a national blood products unit supplying blood fractions for clinical use not just in the region but throughout Scotland. The donor centre was in the same area of the Infirmary.

The report of the Royal Infirmary Board for 1960-61 explained that although the Blood Transfusion Service supplied the whole region, a large proportion of the blood was used in the Royal Infirmary for whose patients almost 10,000 compatibility tests were being carried out annually, more than half of them as emergencies. The introduction of renal dialysis in 1959 and of open-heart surgery in 1961 with its requirement for extra-corporeal circulation through the heart-lung machine, brought still larger demands for specially-prepared blood. To meet these demands, with their need for fresh blood, it was necessary to have the co-operation of selected donors who often had to attend at short notice, sometimes during the night, a requirement reminiscent of the early years of transfusion practice when individual donors were called for patients as and when required.

During the 1960s the work of the Service became more complex year by year and the range of research undertaken in its laboratories increased greatly. The growing use of separate blood-components to meet particular needs made the provision of more space for the blood products section essential. For a time that was achieved by a re-arrangement of laboratories within the existing area. Further relief was not obtained until 1973 when the donor organisation and blood withdrawal sections moved out of the Infirmary into converted shop and house premises nearby, at the corner of Lauriston Place and Archibald Place. That had the added advantage of providing more space and greater comfort for those on whom the whole system depended—the voluntary donors.

For the blood products unit, however, the space vacated was still not enough. The unit was becoming an increasingly important part of the organisation of the Scottish National Blood Transfusion Association and before long it became clear that larger, purpose-built accommodation must be provided if there was to be room for the extensive laboratories and equipment necessary to meet all the demands upon it. A site was found at Liberton on the south side of the city beside Liberton Hospital (then within the Edinburgh Royal Victoria Group of Hospitals). In the planning of the new building and its equipment Mr. J. G. Watt, Scientific Director of the existing unit and his colleagues played an important part and, in 1974, the work was transferred to the new Centre, Mr. Watt continuing as Scientific Director there. In that new fractionation centre plasma from all over Scotland is converted into a variety of products required for patients throughout Scotland. Besides increasing the clinical safety of transfusion the process enables each patient to receive only the blood constituent he or she requires, leaving others available to benefit other patients. One donation, therefore, may be used for several patients.

Transfer of the Scottish Fractionation Unit to Liberton released more space at the Infirmary for use by the South East Scotland Blood Transfusion Association as laboratories and blood bank. In the year in which the Unit moved out, three other important events in the life of that Association took place. Dr. Robert Cumming, OBE retired after 27 years service as Regional Director, during which he had guided the Association as it grew from the fairly primitive organisation of the 1940s into a highly scientific organisation renowned for its contributions to research as well as for its primary service to patients. He was succeeded by Dr. John D. Cash who had been his Deputy Director. When Dr. Cash left to take up another appointment in 1979 his place was taken by Dr. Brian McLellan.

The year 1974 was also that in which Miss Helen M. White, MBE retired from the post of Regional Organising Secretary after 38 years service to the cause of blood transfusion in south-east Scotland. During that time she and her helpers, travelling tirelessly about the region, exhorting, recruiting and organising, built up the panel of donors from a few hundred to more than 70,000 names and saw the annual number of donations of blood increase from 560 to more than 60,000.

The third event of 1974 was that, as part of the National Health Service re-organisation, the blood transfusion service came under the wing of the newly-formed Common Services Agency which became responsible for its administration and funding. Day-to-day running, however, remained with the Association—and prime responsibility for its success continued to be, as always, in the hands of the great band of voluntary blood donors in Edinburgh, in Fife and in the Lothian and Border Regions; more than 80,000 of them by 1979.

In August 1982, the blood withdrawal laboratories and donor organisation moved into accommodation planned for the purpose in the new 'Phase 1' building. There the laboratory staff found improved working conditions and the donors find themselves in spacious, comfortable surroundings which help to make each session a pleasant, sociable occasion.

Medical Records

Not all the advances made in the Infirmary during the 1960s were in the realms of medical, surgical or scientific techniques and not all required extensive new building works to be undertaken. Some called mainly for persistence and sustained effort to bring them about. One such advance, made slowly and painfully, eventually brought many advantages. This was the introduction and development of a central system of medical record keeping and, allied with that, the centralisation of admission arrangements. It may well be said that nothing now contributes more to the smooth running of the clinical work of the Infirmary than do these systems. They did not come easily and in order to understand the difficulties that were surmounted in bringing them about, it is necessary to turn back, briefly, to the time before the advent of the National Health Service.

Traditionally, as in many hospitals, the records of a patient's treatment and progress were kept separately by each medical or surgical charge or department. At one time, each patient in a ward was allotted a page in a large register in which his or her history and details of treatment were entered by the ward staff. When, inevitably, this became too cumbersome, a system of patients' case-sheets was adopted. This was an improvement, but as different wards favoured different styles of case-sheet, recorded the information in their own distinctive ways and retained the case-sheets in their own hands, the difficulty of tracing the medical history of a patient who had been treated at varying intervals in several wards or departments was considerable; yet such knowledge may be of great importance in diagnosing a condition and prescribing for it.

The need for an improved system of records had been recognised by the former Board of Managers shortly before their term of office expired. In November 1947, following a medical records conference in Oxford which had been attended and reported upon by a member of the surgical staff, the Managers appointed a special committee to examine the arrangements in the Infirmary and suggest improvements. Six months later the committee reported; but by then the date for the transfer of the hospital was only a few weeks away. So all that the Managers were able to do was to send copies of the report to the Regional Hospital Board and the Department of Health for Scotland, both of whom were then too busy with other aspects of re-organisation to take any immediate action on it.

Rather more than a year later the Regional Board commissioned a report from the Nuffield Bureau of Health and Sickness Records. Their expert, having visited the Infirmary, strongly recommended the introduction of a 'unit' system whereby, for each patient, records of all admissions to and contacts with the hospital would be brought together and be available to any clinician when required. As by-products of the system, he pointed out, such central records would be of value in clinical and epidemiological research, in planning future provision and sometimes for legal purposes. He also advised the appointment of medical records officers at hospital level (in large hospitals), at group level and at regional level.

The Board of Management's reaction to the report was sceptical. 'The whole structure and organisation of the Royal Infirmary for the past fifty years', they said, 'has been based on a policy of de-centralisation.' That was clearly a policy many of them had no wish to change; but officially they based their objection mainly on their view that space was not available within the hospital for a central records department. In 1950, however, urged on by the Regional Board, and by a visit from the Secretary of State for Scotland and the Chief Medical Officer of the Department of Health, they agreed to the appointment of a medical records officer whose duties would include taking steps to introduce some measure of centralisation.

A records and appointments office was opened in 1951 but it dealt with only a few departments and when the Medical Records Officer submitted her first report recommending a fully centralised system, she was told only that 'there is a lot to be said for each charge retaining its own records for a period of two or three years . . . '. During the following year she must have been successfully converted by the advocates of 'no change' because in her final report before resigning in 1952, she wrote that 'for geographical and other reasons a complete appointments and medical records system such as has been contemplated is not practicable in the Royal Infirmary'. There, for the time being, the matter seems to have been left.

In 1955 it was conceded that the current records system was 'somewhat haphazard'. Gradually, however, appointments systems were introduced. By 1959 such arrangements were operating for the medical, cardiology and orthopaedics departments and in the following year, the ophthalmic and skin out-patient departments were said to be 'almost ready to launch themselves into this project'. In that year, 1960, it appeared that real progress was at last beginning to be made. Two things occurred—a Group Medical Records Officer, Mr. J. C. Pepper, was appointed and a medical records committee was established. The committee was chaired by Dr. J. C. H. Dunlop who, as Associate Obstetrician and Registrar of Records in the Simpson Pavilion was, for 20 years, responsible for the production of comprehensive and highly praised clinical and statistical reports on its work. The other members of the committee included senior consultants in medicine, surgery and radiology.

Even such a prestigious committee was nearly defeated. In November 1962 its members bitterly complained that their efforts and those of the Medical Records Officer were being brought to nothing by lack of financial support. 'For many years' they wrote, 'it has been recognised that the records system in the Royal Infirmary is antediluvian.' They and the Records Officer, they continued, had been appointed expressly to remedy this and yet almost every attempt to improve matters was thwarted by a failure to make the necessary funds available. The committee chairman even threatened to resign if the position did not improve.

Although the immediate response to this protest was a negative one, on the all-too-familiar ground that, financially, times were difficult, the protest seems to have had some effect. In the following year the Regional Hospital Board engaged a firm of management consultants 'to assist in introducing a comprehensive medical records service with a balanced staffing structure' and, acting on the firm's advice, they authorised the appointment of a Deputy to relieve the Records Officer of routine work and enable him to concentrate on planning and organisation.

At about the same time Mr. Pepper left to take up another appointment and it fell to his successor, Mr. N. Pedelty, to undertake the planning and development of the system. The new officer was a prominent member of his profession, becoming in 1964, National Chairman of the Association of Medical Records

Officers, then still quite a young organisation, having been founded in 1948, but an active and enterprising one. He was appointed also to the Sub-Committee on 'Development and Standardisation of Hospital Medical Records in Scotland' set up by the Secretary of State's Standing Medical Advisory Committee. That Sub-Committee, chaired by Professor J. Walker, Professor of Obstetrics and Gynae-cology at St. Andrews University, were required 'to consider medical records systems in Scottish hospitals, their present and potential functions and the possibility of standardisation . . .'

While the Walker Sub-Committee were gathering and considering informa-tion, progress began to be made in the Infirmary in the evolution of an improved records organisation. This included the introduction of a mechanical 'Addresso-graph' method of printing essential registration details on each patient's documents and on labels which could be used on other forms for the same patient and on containers for medicines prescribed for him. At the same time a mechanical master-index of patient admissions was introduced. These arrangements relieved medical, nursing and other staff members of much of the clerical work they previously had to do.

Any sound medical records system must include a readily understood means of providing a unique identification number to be used on all the records relating to any one patient. While ways of achieving this were being explored, it was learned that an effective system was in use in Denmark and Mr. Pedelty was authorised to visit the County Hospital in Copenhagen to see it in operation. There he found that each patient's date of birth was incorporated into his or her record code; and he was assured that the system had worked well for six years. On his recommendation, supported by the Medical Superintendent, Dr. Francis, the system was adopted in the Infirmary. This was the first use of the method in Scotland though it was later found to have been used earlier in an English hospital. With some modification it is still in use for the Infirmary records of the 1980s.

The Report of the Walker Sub-Committee was published in 1967. Its 24 main recommendations covered almost every aspect of medical record-keeping, from the all-important maintenance of confidentiality to methods of management, from the design of case-note folders to the sizes and qualities of paper suitable for different kinds of records. By 1971 the Board of Management were able to report that the recommendations had been accepted and that substantial progress had been made in putting them into effect.

Mr. Pedelty had left for an appointment elsewhere in 1969, so it fell to his successors to superintend much of the modernisation of the records service. Most of all, however, the transformation of the system was due to the work of an active advisory committee set up by the Board of Management in December 1967. As an earnest of their commitment to the project, the Board appointed the Convener of their Medical Committee, Mr. Donald McIntosh (Surgeon) to be Chairman of the Advisory Committee, the other members of which were Dr. Andrew Doig (Physician) and Dr. M. G. Pearson (Obstetrician), who were appointed on the recommendations respectively of the Physicians and the Gynae-cologists in the Infirmary. Under that Committee's guidance the centralisation and modernisation of the admission and records arrangements began to produce valuable results. It was clear to them that a necessary accompaniment, if not pre-requisite, of any new system must be a central admission point to which patients would go to register their arrival at the hospital. At that place their appointment notices could be presented, their numbers allocated and their records start their progress through the system while the patients were being directed to the appro-priate ward. At the same time any questions by the receptionist to clarify entries in the admission form or by a patient or patient's relatives on matters of hospital procedure (but not on clinical matters) could be asked and answered.

It was obviously desirable to have the admission point in or close to the records department. The Advisory Committee were insistent, also, that it should have a re-assuring atmosphere and, as Mr. McIntosh put it, should be at least as welcoming as the reception area of a good hotel. With difficulty, arrangements were made to occupy accommodation beside the existing records department, entering from the lower surgical corridor, near the east entrance drive. The whole department was redesigned and extended to provide additional filing space on the floor below and to incorporate a library in which medical staff undertaking survey and research work could consult records without removing them from the department. At one end, separated from the main area by receptionists' desks, there was room for a small but comfortably furnished waiting area for patients. This was a foretaste of what might be expected on a more spacious scale in the new Infirmary. Its immediate effect was to soften the worry and reduce the bewilderment felt by those arriving in hospital, especially those doing so for the first time.

The improved and extended department came into operation in 1971. In the meantime, the phased centralisation of the patients' records holders continued. Although, by 1979, a few departments had still not come fully into the centralised system, all their records were accessible through the central master-index. Other improvements continued to be made. Among the most important was the 24-hour service introduced in 1969 whereby, in an emergency, a patient's records of previous admissions and attendances can be produced at any time of day or night. Another was the introduction, for statistical and research purposes, of a disease index based on a recognised international coding system, through which a researcher can be assisted in tracing records relating to the treatment of whatever disease he may be studying.

Since 1948, Scottish hospital records have been legally the property of the Secretary of State for Scotland and periods for which they must be preserved are regulated by statute. The basic rule, under the Public Records Act of 1937, requires retention for six years after a patient's discharge from hospital but later legislation specifies much longer periods for some special groups of records. Thus the Limitations Act of 1975 requires extended periods of retention for records of patients in certain types of employment—e.g. miners—so that they may be available in the event of late development of an industrial disease; and the Con-genital Liabilities Act, 1976 requires obstetrics records to be preserved for thirty years.

The storage of such records obviously presents a massive problem. In 1970 it was found possible for a large basement area under the Florence Nightingale

Nurses Home to be made available for the storage of older records, only those in current use or of recent date being retained in the records library.

By that time, every proposal for improvement of the records service was being looked at in the light of the possible application to it of computer methods. A computer organisation—the Edinburgh Medical Computer Unit—was established jointly by the Scottish Home and Health Department, the Regional Hospital Board and the Royal Infirmary Board of Management and housed in part of the former Simpson Memorial Hospital building in Lauriston Place. It, however, was used almost exclusively for laboratory and scientific purposes. The application of that computer to in-patient records began in 1973 but only for the preparation of statistical information required by the Scottish Home and Health Department. More comprehensive use of a computer by the medical records department, to provide information which would assist the day-to-day running of the hospital did not become possible until after the Health Service re-organisation of 1974. The newly-established Lothian Health Board then became partner in a Scottish Health Service consortium whose more up-to-date computing unit was accommodated in former Executive Council premises in Drumsheugh Gardens, Edinburgh. There, in November 1975, a Computer Assisted Records System began to operate, initially for the Royal Infirmary, but later to serve other hospitals. In accepted computer fashion, the name of the system was abbreviated to CARES an acronym which aptly emphasises its purpose of aiding patient care by helping to maintain and improve the quality of the hospital's services. This it does, not only by producing statistics of value in long-term planning but also by issuing, every morning, up-to-date information about bed-occupancy in each ward, and on other matters, which is immediately available to departments needing it as a basis on which to organise their work for the day.

Later, a start was made with the lengthy task of transferring to computer storage the information contained on the master-index cards of which, by 1979, there were nearly 600,000. Not only does computer storage save space, it saves time and effort in maintaining and consulting the index. It also eliminates the dangers of wrong filing of cards and the confusion of one card with another which could have serious results if the record is wanted in connection with the treatment of a patient. Having once been given the correct information the computer, when asked to display it, can produce that information and no other.

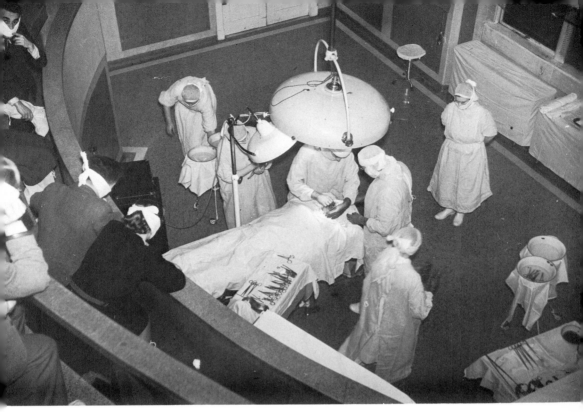

Plate 23   Wards 15/16 operating theatre in 1943
The view from students' open gallery

Plate 24   Wards 11/12 operating theatre in 1983
Viewed from students' glass-fronted gallery. Pre-set trolley-top
tray on right; modern anaesthetic equipment on left

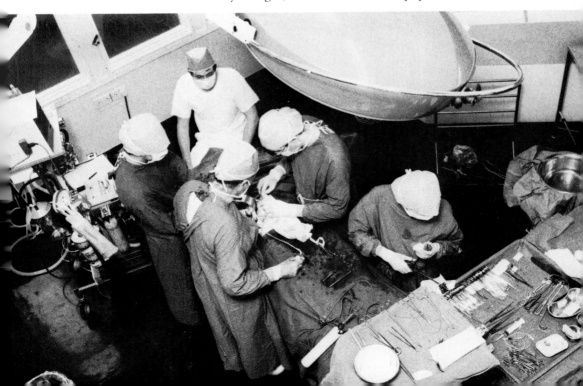

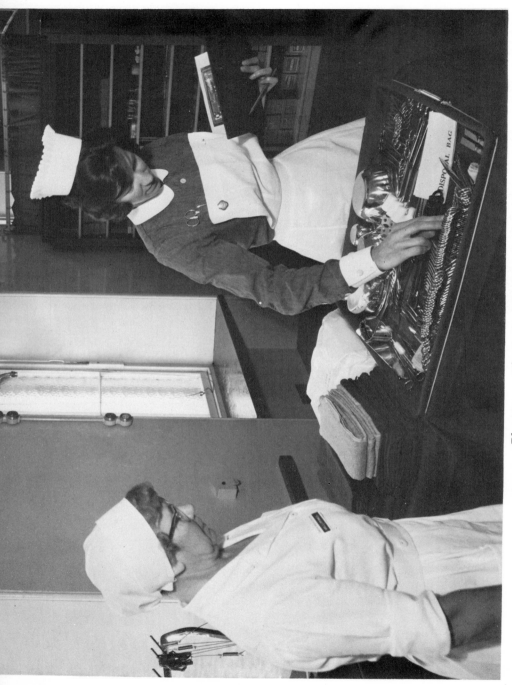

Plate 25   Theatre Service Centre

The Edinburgh pre-set trolley-top tray system in operation soon after installation in 1964. Sister S. D. A. Scott, first Supervisor, who was closely involved in the initiation of the system, is checking a tray, watched by a Tray Assembler.

6

Re-organisation

Chalmers Hospital—and an innovation

For a quarter of a century—from 1948 until 1974—the administrative grouping of hospitals in south-east Scotland remained almost unchanged. In the late 1950s one small Board of Management had been discontinued and its two hospitals added to other Groups and in 1969 a second Board was discontinued and its single hospital similarly transferred but these changes did not affect the Infirmary. Meanwhile, in 1968, the Regional Board had begun a general examination of the need for re-grouping to take account of changes in the uses of some hospitals and the advisability of eliminating very small Groups which did not easily fit into modern administrative arrangements and accounting systems. After much discussion and consultation they decided that, among other adjustments, the Edinburgh Central Hospitals Board of Management should be disbanded and that their three hospitals (Royal Edinburgh Hospital for Sick Children, Princess Margaret Rose Hospital, and Chalmers Hospital) and Clinics should be allocated among other Boards. On 1 April 1970, under that arrangement, Chalmers Hospital in Lauriston Place became part of the Royal Infirmary Group. That also was no more than a local adjustment of the original health service pattern of administration. The formation of a radically different overall pattern was not far off; but before describing its introduction it will be well to look briefly at Chalmers Hospital and at an important innovation which was in preparation there at the time of its transfer to the Infirmary Board.

The origin and history of Chalmers Hospital were briefly described in an earlier chapter. In 1953 there had been added to it as an annexe the Hospital for Diseases of Women in Archibald Place immediately west of the Infirmary but that small out-dated hospital was demolished in 1968 to make way for Phase 1 of the Infirmary re-building scheme. In 1970 Chalmers Hospital had 64 beds (34 surgical and 30 medical) in four wards and was described as a 'general non-teaching hospital which does not cover the full range of work within the main specialties'. It had an operating theatre in a wing at the rear, static and mobile X-ray equipment and a well-equipped physiotherapy department; and its out-patient clinics dealt with more than 20,000 attendances annually. It was a comfortable, homely hospital offering its patients a quieter, more restful environment than can be provided in a large hospital such as its new 'parent'.

Chalmers Hospital had always been able to call on the Infirmary in cases of urgent need. From 1970 it was brought fully within the ambit of the Infirmary and quickly found its place and proved its worth there while still retaining the Chalmers 'atmosphere'. To cement the merger its telephones were now linked to the Infirmary switchboard which had just been modernised and transferred to new premises in the former garden behind the Queen Mary Maternity Home. The multitone call system was also extended to include staff at the newly adopted hospital.

At the time of transfer a new storey was being built above the operating-theatre block at Chalmers Hospital to form a general practitioner unit of 18 beds bringing the total to 82. The new unit was being provided in pursuance of a policy, then being widely advocated, of bringing general practitioners more fully into partnership with the hospital service. This would be the first such unit in Edinburgh to offer them general hospital facilities as distinct from the obstetrical facilities which had been available to general practitioners in the Queen Mary Home since 1958.

After some delays in building, the new GP unit was opened on 5 June 1974, having cost £54,500 of which £30,000 was met from former Chalmers Hospital endowment funds. Having been begun on the initiative of one Board of Management and completed by another, it was brought into use by the Lothian Health Board which had superseded both. Contracts regulating the terms and conditions of use of the new accommodation had been entered into with some fifty doctors practising in the Edinburgh area. These family doctors were then able to arrange for their own patients to be admitted for investigation and treatment by them in the knowledge that the diagnostic facilities of the hospital, the skill of the nursing staff and specialist advice when required would all be available to them. The unit included a treatment room to which patients could be admitted on a day basis. A Committee composed of representatives of the participating doctors and a con-sultant was formed to assist in the administration of the new unit.

The New Pattern—1974 and After

From this history, so far, it will not have escaped notice that, during the first 26 years of the National Health Service much time was spent by the Infirmary Board of Management and their officers in discussing, and often arguing, with the Regional Board and then in awaiting that Board's decision as to whether projects might or might not be allowed to proceed. Several important projects, in fact, were eventually allowed to go ahead only because the Board of Management agreed to meet the whole cost, or a substantial part of it, from their endowment funds. That system of dual control, perhaps justifiable when the Health Service was new, had also become the cause of difficulty elsewhere in Scotland where there were few hospitals with enough endowment funds to enable their local Boards to adopt the Infirmary Board's solution quite so readily. The difficulty caused by the two-tier system of control was one reason why reform was necessary.

There was also another reason. While the hospital service had two tiers, the National Health Service as a whole had three branches. There was the hospital service provided by Regional Boards through the Boards of Management (initially 16 and latterly 13 in the South-Eastern Region). Primary medical care, provided by general medical practitioners, and general dental, pharmaceutical and ophthalmic services were administered by Executive Councils of which there were four serving the Region; and community health care, including protection from infectious diseases, was provided by eleven local health authorities in the Region. That made a total of 32 (latterly 29) authorities in three separate groups. The needs to be met by the three branches of the health service were closely inter-linked but, despite much effort and goodwill at many levels, co-ordination and co-operation among the authorities providing them were too often inadequate.

After much consultation and debate, the National Health Service (Scotland) Act 1972 was passed with the object of bringing the three branches of the Service under one controlling authority. With effect from 1 April 1974, regional hospital boards, boards of management and executive councils were disbanded and responsibility for community health services was removed from local authorities. Henceforth, all National Health Service functions in Scotland were to be exercised by 15 new all-purpose Health Boards, acting on behalf of the Secretary of State for Scotland. This greatly simplified the structure, achieving at one stroke a more than tenfold reduction in the number of statutory bodies and of board and committee members. Some activities of the Health Boards were to be carried out on their behalf by a new organisation, the Common Services Agency, in the management of which the Health Boards would be represented; and provision was also made for the establishment in each Board's area of Local Health Councils to provide liaison between the Boards and those receiving their services and with the general public.

To offset the greater range of responsibilities placed upon the new Boards, the geographical areas to be served by them were smaller than those of the former Regional Hospital Boards. Thus the south-eastern region, stretching from Fife to the English Border, would in future be divided among three Health Boards whose areas and names would be the same as those of the three Local Government Regional Councils of Fife, Lothian and Borders which under the Local Government (Scotland) Act of 1973, were to become operative on 16 May 1975.

The Royal Infirmary of Edinburgh, under this new arrangement, was the largest of nearly forty hospitals within the ambit of the Lothian Health Board, whose area embraces the four local authority Districts of the City of Edinburgh, Midlothian, East Lothian and West Lothian. It is important to remember, however, that this new administrative pattern did not diminish the 'catchment' area of the Infirmary to whose wards, departments and clinics patients would continue to come from all over south-east Scotland and further afield if it was the hospital most able to treat their ailment or most convenient to them. National Health Service boundaries continued to be administrative limits, not barriers to patients.

So, in 1974, the Royal Infirmary came under the management of one statutory Board only, instead of two placed one above the other; but whereas the members and officers of the former Board of Management had been able to concentrate their interest and their loyalty on the Infirmary (with its few associated hospitals), devoting their energies to seeking to maintain its position in the forefront of the hospital service, the new Board had not only to direct the affairs of some forty hospitals and many clinics, but also to control the other branches of the Health Service throughout their area. The change, removing the body directly interested

in the Infirmary and with long accumulated corporate knowledge of its organisation and its special needs, was seen by many as sadly diminishing the status of the
Infirmary, leading to a lowering of morale at many levels. This seemed all the
more regrettable in view of the Infirmary's standing as a famous teaching hospital.
These were natural reactions. Whatever doubts existed, however, there was
general agreement that, within the new pattern of administration, the work of the
hospital must proceed as vigorously as ever in the best interests of its patients.
The hope was that, in time, the change, perhaps with modifications, would be
seen as having been a necessary step in the evolution of a fully integrated hospital
and health service in which the Royal Infirmary, through its variety of skills,
would continue to play a leading part.

While the statement that, after 1974, one statutory Board instead of two
controlled the affairs of the Infirmary is true, it is an over-simplification. The
Lothian Health Board Area is the second largest in Scotland in terms of both
population (about 750,000) and health resources and it was one of ten large
Scottish Areas which it was deemed advisable to divide, for administration purposes, into Health Districts. At first sight division into four Health Districts
coinciding with the four local government Districts in the Lothian Region might
have seemed logical, making for easy communication between health service and
local government on matters of common interest. But neither Midlothian nor
East Lothian had a major hospital in their area, and over many years, the people of
Midlothian had depended on the Royal Infirmary as their main hospital while
those in East Lothian were increasingly dependent on the Eastern and Western
General Hospitals on the north side of the city. So a division of the Lothian Area
into three Health Districts was decided upon, ensuring that each had a major
hospital within its ambit.

With the approval of the Secretary of State, the City of Edinburgh, for
health service administration only, was split in two by an imaginary line drawn
along Princes Street and extended, with some undulations, to east and west. The
part of the City south of that line was joined to Midlothian to form the South
Lothian District with the Royal Infirmary as its principal hospital, while the part
to the north of the line was joined to East Lothian to form the North Lothian
District, its main hospital being the Western General. The area of the local
government District of West Lothian, with Bangour Hospital almost at its centre,
was able to stand by itself as the West Lothian Health District.

While the new structure of Health Board and Health Districts was coming
into being, new concepts of consensus management and of consultation procedures
in Health Service administration (and also in local government) were being
evolved. Stated as simply as possible, these procedures were based on the principle
that the Health Board should make decisions on major policies and planning and
on the broad allocation of resources, leaving the carrying out of such policies, and
their application to day-to-day management, to senior officers meeting in
Executive Groups in which their separate fields of knowledge and experience
could be jointly applied. Directives on the application of the Board's decisions
would henceforth be given by the Lothian Area Executive Group (Secretary,
Chief Administrative Medical Officer, Treasurer and Chief Area Nursing Officer),

Meanwhile the Infirmary's maintenance costs had soared from just under £1 million in 1951 to more than £7 million in 1974. In short, the whole pattern of hospital activity had altered, outgrowing the capabilities of an administrative system designed to meet simpler needs. To cope with the new circumstances a new kind of administrative machine was needed, its methods based on up-to-date concepts and techniques of large-scale management. That, in the main, was the reason for the adoption of the new management system. Critics of the new system as it began to operate should, perhaps, have reflected that the former system had had over two centuries in which to evolve, the last thirty years of which had seen unprecedented developments. It would have been strange if the old pattern had been able to deal effectively with so many new circumstances and equally strange if the new system had emerged perfect overnight.

In accordance with the Act of 1972, the Lothian Health Board took over responsibility for the three branches of the National Health Service within the Lothian Area on 1 April 1974. The South-Eastern Regional Hospital Board and the Royal Infirmary of Edinburgh and Associated Hospitals Board of Management had each held their last meeting on 29 March; the Edinburgh and the Lothians and Peebles Executive Councils had also held their final meetings during that month.

The new Lothian Health Board consisted of a Chairman and 22 other members all appointed by the Secretary of State for Scotland after consultation (as required by the Act) with the outgoing authorities, with the four local authorities in the Area whose Health Service functions were transferred to the new Board (Edinburgh Town Council and the County Councils of Midlothian, East Lothian and West Lothian), with the University of Edinburgh and with numerous organisations representing medical and allied professions or otherwise concerned with the health of the community. Among the members of the new Board then appointed three, immediately before the change-over, had been members of the Regional Board, one had been a member of the Royal Infirmary Board of Management, seven had been members of other Boards of Management and seven had served on one or other of the two Executive Councils within the Lothian area. At least five had formerly been or still were local authority members. The new Board, therefore, inherited a wide range of National Health Service knowledge and experience.

To ensure continuity, appointments to the Board had been made several months in advance. A nucleus of members had met on several occasions from June 1973 and the full Board had held three meetings in February and March 1974. These meetings dealt with preliminary planning of the new arrangements and the making of appointments to key posts in the Board's administration.

For a Board faced with such a major re-organisation, involving the welding together of several functions previously separately administered, the choice of first Chairman is important. The holder of such a position should, if possible, have some experience of the administration of each of the services to be taken over. As it happened, the Chairman of the out-going South-Eastern Regional Hospital Board, Mrs. (later, Dr.) Catherina T. Nealon, had had just such experience and she was appointed Chairman of the Lothian Health Board with effect in 1973.

Mrs. Nealon's public service in Edinburgh began in May 1949 when she was elected as a Town Councillor for Pilton Ward whose residents she represented for

25 years. Her main concern during the whole of that time was for the promotion of welfare and public health. She was a member of the Council's Health Committee for 21 years, the last two of them as Chairman. For 22 years she served on the Edinburgh Executive Council of which she was Vice-Chairman for nine years. She had been a member of the Royal Infirmary Board of Management for four years (1952 to 1956) and of the South-Eastern Regional Hospital Board for nine years, five of them (1969 to 1974) as Chairman. Thus, for a total of twelve years she had served simultaneously on bodies concerned with the three branches of the Health Service—local health, primary medical care and hospitals—which were to be combined.

In 1977 Mrs. Nealon received from the University of Edinburgh the Degree of Doctor *honoris causa*. At the medical graduation ceremony held on 29 June of that year her laureation address was given by the Vice-Principal, Professor S. B. Saul, who described the award of the Degree as one of the highest honours the University could bestow. It was being conferred, he said, as a tribute to one 'who had devoted herself unstintingly to the public good through public work'.

Two years later, in 1979, Dr. Nealon's record of public service was further recognised when she was awarded the Honour of CBE. That was the year of the 250th Anniversary of the Founding of the Royal Infirmary, in the celebration of which she took a keen interest. Dr. Nealon continued as Chairman of the Lothian Health Board until the completion of her second term of office in March 1981.

7

Fifty Years of Change

Teaching of Medicine

Since its foundation, the Royal Infirmary has had two complementary purposes—the treatment of patients and the training of doctors. In the past, both in the old Infirmary and in the Lauriston Place building, much teaching of medicine was done by lectures to serried ranks of students in large lecture theatres. That is a method now less favoured but still with a part to play, for, to quote the late Sir Derrick Dunlop, 'there are many principles that can be taught as well to 100 people in a lecture theatre, and with a great saving of teaching time, as to five in a tutorial'. The teaching of smaller groups in wards and clinics also existed from the start but many such 'smaller' groups were, by modern standards, much too large. Accounts have been given of students in the 1930s crowding and jostling to secure admission to some of the more popular clinics and bedside teaching sessions; popular because of the brilliance or sometimes just the style of the physician or surgeon concerned. There were times, it is said, when some of those in the rear ranks had to stand on beds in order to see what was being demonstrated, or else just remain in the background picking up what scraps of information they could manage to hear.

Arrangements for the teaching of students in the Infirmary were formalised in an agreement between the Infirmary Managers and the University in 1913 and a supplementary agreement of 1917. The former provided, among other things, for all members of the honorary staff to participate in medical teaching. The latter sought mainly to regulate arrangements for the instruction of women medical students whose numbers had increased markedly during the war. Hitherto, women students had been taught by two members of staff and in two wards only. Thenceforward, in terms of the 1917 Agreement, the teaching of women students was to be shared by all, but they were still not taught quite on equal terms with men. Lectures on general medicine and some specialties were given to mixed classes but lectures on surgery and bedside clinics, held in the surgical wards continued to be organised separately for men and women; clinics in the surgical out-patient department were not open to women students at all. Why this was so, when nurses were there as a matter of course, defies logical explanation, but it was not until 1936, following demands by the Students' Representative Council's Medical Faculty Committee that the Managers agreed to allow women students to attend clinical surgery classes on equal terms with men, 'this to come into effect as soon as possible'.

By 1927 it had been accepted that the old agreements were out of date and a special committee was appointed by the Managers to negotiate two new agree-ments—one with the University and one with the Governing Board of the joint School of Medicine of the Royal Colleges of Physicians, and of Surgeons, of Edinburgh.

An important clause in each Agreement was the following:

All students attending the Infirmary for clinical teaching, whether students of the University, students of the School of Medicine or unattached students, shall, so far as possible, have free choice of the particular clinic which they desire to attend. Such choice shall be subject to the maximum as to number attending any clinic which may be prescribed . . . and to any other arrangements as to allocation which may be made . . .

The Agreements were concerned with procedures for appointment and working conditions of members of the University academic staff and the Infirmary's honorary staff participating in the teaching of students in the Infirmary. They also provided, in some detail, for the setting up within the Infirmary of Clinical Boards for Medicine, Surgery, Gynaecology, Ophthalmology, Ear, Nose and Throat and Diseases of the Skin. These Boards were to arrange, among other things, for:

(a) the division of clinics into Senior and Junior Sections;
(b) the joint or separate teaching of male and female students in the clinics; and
(c) the allocation of the students among the several clinics.

In doing so, they were to give effect, so far as reasonably possible, to each student's choice of clinic, 'provided always that the number of students attached to a clinic at any one time shall not exceed forty, unless with the special consent of the [Infirmary] Board'.

By present-day standards the limit of forty students at any clinic seems much too high. It has to be remembered, however, that the number of medical students admitted by the University in the early 1930s was about 250 annually. Theo-retically, therefore, there could then have been up to 750 University students seeking ward experience during the last three years of their medical course, though in practice that number was unlikely ever to have been reached. This was because, the Medical Faculty's entrance requirements being less demanding then than they have since become, a significant proportion of those admitted would not succeed in reaching the later years of the course. There were also students from the Royal Colleges' School of Medicine (discontinued in 1948) to be accommodated. For all those students, only the Royal Infirmary and the Royal Hospital for Sick Children were available for clinical instruction in the main branches of medicine and surgery although there were other hospitals providing instruction in infectious diseases, tuberculosis, obstetrics and mental disorders. From the University Session 1933-34, however, beds were also available for general clinical teaching at the municipal general hospitals and they provided some relief to the Infirmary.

In later years the admission requirements of the Medical Faculty became more stringent. The number of those embarking annually on the medical course became smaller, but because of the higher entrance standards almost every applicant admitted was likely to be able to pursue the course to a successful conclusion. In the 1960s and 1970s, while the annual number of applicants varied between 1,800 and 2,400, only those showing the highest ability were admitted, between 125 and 165 annually. In 1979, the number was 150. While student numbers were falling, the number of possible opportunities for general clinical experience increased, until there were at least eight hospitals in and around Edinburgh, besides the Infirmary, in which such experience could be obtained. Students, therefore, could be spread more thinly among the available wards and clinics.

In comparing conditions in later years with those of the past it should also be remembered that in the 1930s less regard was given to the wishes or feelings of those patients whose ailments and forms of treatment were the subject of bedside or out-patient clinical instruction. Having accepted the charity of the hospital, they were then expected (unless severely distressed by the thought of it) to accept as normal the intrusion into their privacy of large groups of medical students. Today, bedside teaching is given to very small groups only, and only if the patient has no objection.

Before 1946 each student, having intimated his choice of clinic for instruction had to pay for a 'hospital ticket'. This could be a 'perpetual ticket' for which the charge was £12, covering the 'clinical years' of the course. Alternatively, the student could obtain a ticket for one year (£6 : 6s.— £6.30); six months (£4 : 4s.— £4.20); three months (£2 : 2s.— £2.10); or one month (£1 : 1s.— £1.05); in which cases, as soon as the sum of the separate payments reached £12 : 12s. (£12.60), the student would receive a perpetual ticket. These fees were paid to the Infirmary and between 1930 and 1945 the average annual income from that source was about £4,400. In 1946 that system was replaced by a payment from the University Grants Committee, distributed by the University to appropriate hospitals in proportion to the contributions they had made to medical teaching. After 1948 no such financial arrangement was necessary because, since then, in terms of the National Health Service (Scotland) Act 1947 it has been one of the duties of the Secretary of State 'in providing hospital and specialist services, to make available such facilities for undergraduate and post-graduate clinical teaching and research as he considers necessary to meet all reasonable requirements'.

To enact that such facilities are to be provided is easy. To provide them effectively and keep them up-to-date is more difficult. Ten years later, in 1957, the Royal College of Physicians of Edinburgh prepared a Report on Teaching Facilities in Scottish Hospitals in which, in a section on Edinburgh they wrote:

> When the Edinburgh Royal Infirmary was built 80 years ago . . . it incorporated many features for clinical teaching that have proved of continuing benefit to the Medical School. It has three large and several smaller lecture theatres and a room for tutorials and side-room work is attached to each medical ward . . . With the passage of time and the great increase in scope of undergraduate and especially postgraduate teaching, many aspects of these teaching facilities have become out-dated so that they are now unworthy of a great medical institution. Thus there is no modern lecture-theatre . . . and there is no reading-room in the hospital either for students or teachers.

Some, if not all, of the defects to which that report referred were remedied when the new premises for the Department of Medicine came into use in 1962.

In July 1964 Sir John Bruce (Professor of Clinical Surgery, 1956-70) who was then Surgeon in Administrative Charge of Wards 7/8, wrote to the Board of Management reminding them that 'virtually nothing has been done to assist either teaching or research since I was a student over forty years ago'. Either as a rapid result of that reminder or, more probably, because plans were already well advanced, the Board were able to include the following statement in their Report for the year 1964-65:

> The interior of the old surgical lecture theatre, with its steeply sloping horse-shoe gallery and uncomfortable seating was completely stripped out during the Summer vacation of 1964 and the theatre re-modelled to present-day requirements.

The provision of a lecture-room equipped with comfortable seating and modern visual aids was of undoubted value in undergraduate teaching. Its position near the hospital's central entrance made it useful, also, for the holding of occasional conferences and for post-graduate teaching in which the Infirmary had also co-operated for many years.

In the twenty years between 1959 and 1979, the Medical Faculty of the University twice made important changes in the curriculum for the MB, ChB Degree which affected arrangements for clinical teaching in the Infirmary and other hospitals. The main effect of the changes, from the hospital point of view, was the wholly desirable one of reducing the number of students in wards and clinics while, at the same time, giving the senior students a more positive role to play as members of ward or unit teams. The first change, introduced in the early 1960s and fully operative by 1966 extended the length of the Degree course from five years to six, of which the last three were the 'clinical years' in which students received clinical instruction and worked in wards and clinics during all except their final 'revision term'. On completion of the first six year course the medical and surgical departments in the Infirmary reported favourably on it.

The second change became fully operative in the year 1978-79. It restored the length of the course to five years. The new pattern pursued further the idea of providing practical experience in wards and clinics by enabling senior students to participate in small numbers, as members of clinical teams, in medical and surgical wards and in a wide variety of special departments, different hospitals and other spheres of work, thus enlarging their insight into such problems as those associated with care of the elderly, general practice and community health, as well as the more traditional hospital-based disciplines. Under this system as few as two students may be attached to a ward functioning almost as junior house officers, spending the whole of each day in the ward and, on emergency receiving days, remaining on duty till midnight. They also play a clinical role under supervision during the absence of house officers on leave. Thus the senior students learn individually, under guidance, by taking an active part in the work of the ward rather than by listening and watching, in groups, to formal explanations and demonstrations, though these have not disappeared. This was, in a sense, a return to the old idea of medical 'apprenticeship' but in a more fully developed form, enabling students to progress through a sequence of short attachments to a variety of departments in several hospitals working, in each case, as members of the ward or unit team.

House Officers and the Residency

Having successfully graduated, the erstwhile medical students must obtain approved appointments as House Officers. Until the Medical Act of 1950 came into operation in 1953 the normal period of such service (not then a statutory requirement) was six months. Since then they have had to serve for at least twelve months, six in medical and six in surgical wards (with the more recently permitted alternative, in some cases, of spending part of the time in a health centre). During their time 'on the wards' the residents bring their acquired knowledge to the service of the hospital and in return gain valuable professional experience; to have had such experience in a great hospital like the Royal Infirmary brings an added accolade.

For all the generations of house officers before 1948 their service was unpaid. One who remembered those days explained the position thus: 'Though he got his keep, the houseman worked without pay for 24 hours a day for seven days a week, with a few interrupted hours for sleep. It was an eagerly sought appointment!' They do not now have to give their service free and their hours on duty and on call are organised to allow off-duty periods and weekend and holiday leave on a rota basis. Their numbers were nearly doubled when the Medical Act came into force in 1953. For a while that lessened the work each had to do, but not for long. As the number of patients has increased and many new tests and treatments have come into use, the House Officers' work has become even more intensive and taxing than before.

The Residency, which is the House Officers' home, is at the heart of the Infirmary. In a sense it *is* the Infirmary's heart for from it House Officers circulate daily and nightly through the arteries (or corridors) of the hospital, to the wards to which they are attached. The building in which the Residency is situated is much older than the rest of the Infirmary, being part of the old George Watson's Hospital of 1738. As a place of residence it is thus far from modern in design and until the 1950s its accommodation was austere; but it has been well maintained and improved since then and it undoubtedly has 'character'. It contains dining-room, sitting-rooms and 26 bedrooms on three floors, residents beyond that number being accommodated elsewhere in the hospital and in nearby houses. The Residents' Mess is supplied with food from the main hospital kitchens immediately below. It was long presided over by a succession of Residency butlers. One who served in that capacity for several years, until his retiral in 1967 after 41 years service in the Infirmary, was Mr. Bob Morris, a popular figure, whose farewell oration at the end of each group's period of residence was always enjoyed. Plate 31 shows him with some of the silver acquired by the Mess over many years. The silver, which makes its appearance on special occasions, includes cups given by outgoing groups of residents, and other items presented by residents to popular Chiefs on their retiral and later returned to the Mess. There is also a handsome bowl given to the residency by Professor Harvey Cushing, American pioneer of brain surgery, when he visited the Infirmary in 1925. Among other treasured possessions are many dining-room table-top leaves on which the signatures of hundreds of residents have been inscribed—a practice begun in the old Infirmary and continued ever since.

In the memories of medical men, especially those who were House Officers in pre-National Health Service days, the Residents' Mess holds a very special place. Much more than today, it then had the character of a club and the friendships and camaraderie engendered within its walls were long-lasting and deeply cherished— so much so that in 1895 an Edinburgh Royal Infirmary Residents' Club was formed to 'promote good fellowship, interchange of confidence and unity of aims between past and present Residents and, so far as possible, to further the interests of the Royal Infirmary and of medical education in Edinburgh'. In 1898 Lord Lister attended the Residents' Club Dinner the menu for which, signed by him, is still displayed in the dining-room. The Club flourished for half a century but barely survived the second world war.

For the conduct of residents two sets of rules (additional to those regulating their professional duties) were long ago drawn up. There were, first, official rules prescribed by the Board of Managers last century and revised from time to time. They included regulations for the appointment on a rota basis of Mess President, Vice-President and Secretary. There were also other, lengthier rules drawn up by the Residents themselves to control almost every aspect of their social behaviour. As they stood in 1944 these Mess Rules ran to many pages and can only be touched on. They provided for elections to numerous honorary offices of the Mess— enough to ensure an appointment for everyone. These included 'Faither' of the Mess (the oldest member), The Babe (the youngest), Mess Bard, Mess Lawyer, Mess Orator and some with titles of a distinctly medical, surgical or mildly improper flavour but with few functions, or none, attached to them. Today the only surviving appointments are Mess President, Mess Secretary and Mess Treasurer.

Legends abound of the exuberant behaviour of residents, usually at the end of their term of service when, not unnaturally, a sudden surge of high spirits signalled release from unrelieved toil. On such occasions the singing at a late hour of loud, sometimes bawdy, choruses within earshot of wards and the running of trolley races along corridors are among the excesses that are recalled as earning a rebuke from the Superintendent next day, followed by payment, usually willingly made, for any damage caused. In more recent years such boisterous frolics are less frequent, partly because the granting of holidays and off-duty periods has reduced the strain of each tour of duty and partly because more house officers are married and live outside the hospital, occupying their Residency rooms only when on call; and, not least perhaps, because the presence among them of women residents provides a restraining influence.

The first woman resident doctor was appointed in 1920. However, she and her early successors, though accommodated in the Infirmary, did not live in the Residency. By 1945 a few women doctors had been allowed to live within it but, even as late as that, the President of the Mess wrote to the Managers expressing strong disapproval of women being permitted to infiltrate the Residency which, he insisted, 'is traditionally and constitutionally a male one'. The Managers wisely remained unmoved by his protest.

Until the early 1960s the household care of the Residency was the responsibility of a succession of housekeepers, some of whom are remembered for their 'mothering' of the residents—even darning socks and sewing on buttons. Since then such minor tasks have been left to the residents to manage for themselves while cleaning and 'hotel services' generally have become routine functions of the hospital's domestic department.

Many special occasions have been enjoyed within the Residency. Some were Royal visits and a table-top is still displayed which was signed, in July 1920, by Their Majesties King George V and Queen Mary and by HRH Princess Mary, The Princess Royal; and another, signed by HRH The Prince of Wales (later King Edward VIII). An occasion specially remembered by medical men and women who were residents in 1961 is that on which HRH Prince Philip, Duke of Edinburgh in course of a private, informal visit to the Infirmary dined with the residents as their Guest of Honour. At the centre of one of the table-tops preserved in the Residency his signature remains as a permanent record of that visit.

Nurses and Nursing Education

In the fifty years covered by this history no group of Hospital Staff experienced greater changes than the nurses. After many almost static years during which their system of training, duties and conditions of service scarcely altered there came a series of changes affecting the lives of them all, from the youngest recruit to the most senior nursing administrator. These changes eventually brought about the full recognition of nursing as a profession but without diminution of its long-held status as a vocation; and they led also to its recognition as a branch of academic study with its own Professorial Chair of Nursing Studies in the University of Edinburgh—the first such Chair in Great Britain, established in 1972.

In the Royal Infirmary, as in hospitals everywhere, the leading figure in matters concerning the nursing staff was the Matron, known in the Infirmary from 1872 as Lady Superintendent of Nurses, a title which continued for exactly 100 years, until the re-structuring of the system of nursing administration took place in 1972. The Lady Superintendent's position was one which called not only for all-round knowledge of both the practice and the teaching of nursing, but also for a high degree of tact, understanding and firmness. She was responsible for the recruitment, training, deployment and direction of the nurses and, in the days when all nurses in training were resident in the hospital or its attached Homes, this included a large measure of responsibility for their behaviour and their general welfare even when off-duty. To each new 'intake' of probationers (i.e. student nurses) she acted *in loco parentis*, a role which many of their parents welcomed in the 1930s when the idea of young single women living away from the parental roof was less easily accepted than it is now. In addition, until 1960, the Lady Superintendent had direct responsibility for the domestic staff of the hospital;

thereafter she exercised that function through a Domestic Superintendent until, in 1968, the Domestic Superintendent became head of a separate department under the general administrative control of the Secretary and Treasurer, thus finally relieving the Lady Superintendent of responsibility for domestic services.

The Lady Superintendent was head of the Royal Infirmary School of Nursing which had been founded in 1872 with advice from Florence Nightingale and the help of a group of nurses from her School of Nursing at St. Thomas's Hospital, London. Since then, the fame of the Royal Infirmary School had steadily increased. By the 1930s a preliminary training school had been started and the School itself provided all the teaching required to satisfy the General Nursing Council's three-year syllabus—both practical training in the wards under guidance of the ward sisters and tutors and attendance at lectures on subjects prescribed by the Council. The three-year course led to recognition as a Registered General Nurse; at the Infirmary nurses were expected to complete a fourth year, entitling the successful candidate to receive the Royal Infirmary School's own badge, introduced in 1917. It depicted a pelican feeding her young with her own blood, symbolising the nurse's dedication to the service of others. So holders of the badge had come to be known, world-wide, as 'Pelicans'.

The nurses' prize-giving ceremonies, held annually in May, were by long tradition attended by the Lord High Commissioner (the Sovereign's representative at the General Assembly of the Church of Scotland), always a distinguished public figure, who addressed the nurses and who (or whose wife) presented the prizes. On 20 May 1969 that tradition was outshone when The Queen attended the General Assembly in person and later in the day Prince Philip, Duke of Edinburgh came to the Infirmary and presented the prizes to the nurses. It was a happy occasion. Even the Board's annual report threw off its mundane manner to record that Prince Philip's speech to the nurses 'delighted and inspired his audience and the effect of his visit caused a glow within the whole hospital'. The Prince also visited the nurses' classrooms and talked with nurses and tutors about their work, making it a day long to be remembered by them.

From 1929 onwards there were six Lady Superintendents of Nurses in the Infirmary. Miss E. F. Bladon who was appointed in 1925 had received her early training in the Infirmary and had been Deputy Lady Superintendent for several years. She retired in 1931. During her years in office she played a part in improving facilities for the teaching of nurses, including the conversion of the red-brick former laboratory block in the west roadway (now the cafeteria) into lecture-rooms which continued in use till 1956. She was a supporter of anything tending to foster a sense of fellowship among the nurses and in 1927-28 the Infirmary Nurses' magazine *The Pelican* began publication; in 1936 it became the organ of the Royal Infirmary of Edinburgh Nurses League, linking ex-trainees of the Infirmary all over the world.

Miss E. D. Smaill followed. She also had been a Royal Infirmary trainee. She had had wide nursing experience, first in Bulgaria during the Balkan wars of 1912/13 and then in France during the first world war. Afterwards she was one of the pioneer local authority Health Visitors in Edinburgh and she had been Assistant Lady Superintendent in the Infirmary since 1922. Taking charge at a

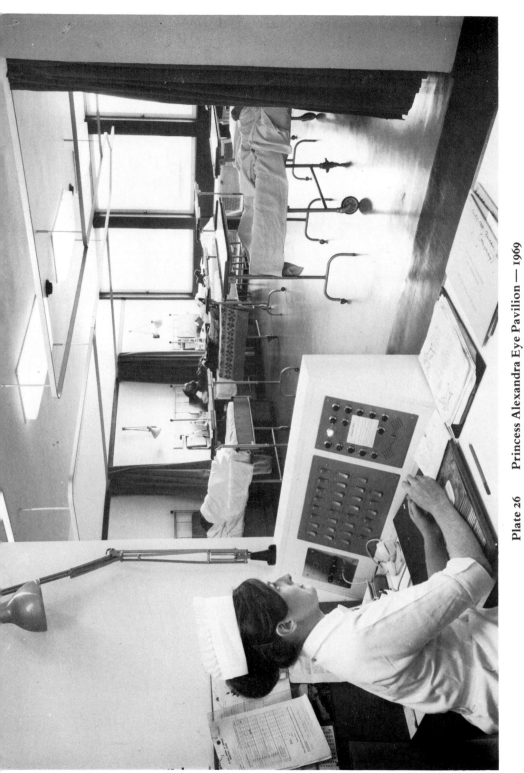

Plate 26   Princess Alexandra Eye Pavilion — 1969

A ward seen from the nurses' station

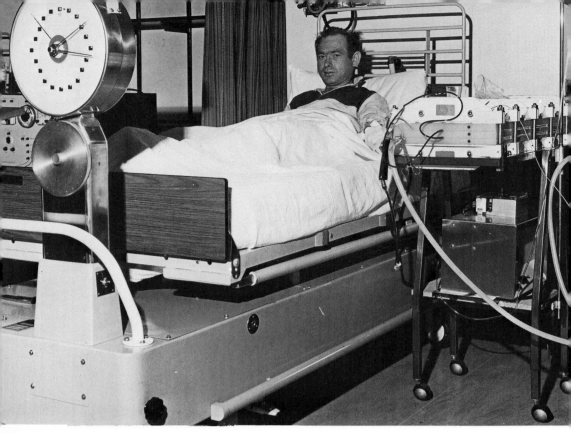

Plate 27   Renal Unit

A dialysis machine in use in 1969

Plate 28   Medical Records Department

Patients' reception area, opened in 1971

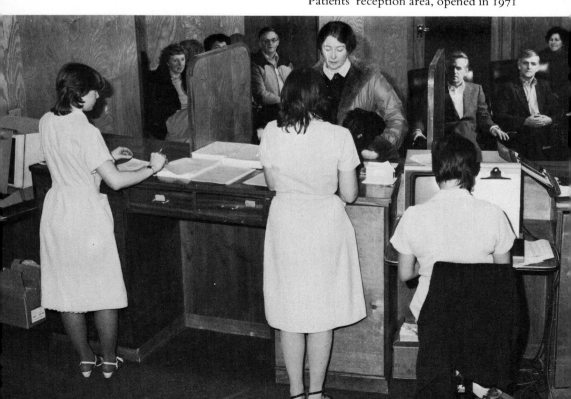

time of important developments in the treatment of patients she was much in-volved in the nursing aspects of the use of radium and radiotherapy and the growth of the dietetic department and school. Early in 1939 it fell to her to organise the first occupation of the new Florence Nightingale Nurses' Home and to co-operate with the Matron of the new Simpson Memorial Maternity Pavilion, Miss J. P. Ferlie, OBE, in bringing the Pavilion into use. No sooner were these matters dealt with than Miss Smaill was plunged into the problems of organising the nursing services of the Infirmary on a wartime basis. She retired in 1944. In 1938 she had been awarded the OBE for her services to nursing; and in 1947 she was made an Honorary Doctor of Laws by the University of Edinburgh 'in virtue of her outstanding merit'.

Miss Smaill was a member of several Government committees, including the important Committee on Nursing appointed by the Department of Health for Scotland under the chairmanship of Lord Alness which reported in 1938. Although there had been earlier reports on aspects of nursing, this seems to have been the one which set in motion the trend towards improving the conditions of service of nurses and especially nurses in training, in Scotland. Evidence was given to the Committee on behalf of the Infirmary by Professor-Emeritus Lovell Gulland (Board Member), Lt-Col A. D. Stewart (Superintendent) and Miss M. C. Marshall (then Assistant Lady Superintendent of Nurses). A Sub-Committee also heard the views of probationers from seven hospitals, including the Infirmary, on the condi-tions under which they worked. The Committee's report does not refer specifically to the Infirmary but it gives some insight into the life of a student nurse at that time; for example:

Hours of duty were said to be between 52 and 60 weekly and up to 70 when on night-duty. (In the Infirmary, since 1921, the norm for day-duty had been a 56-hour week.) The Committee urged hospitals to work towards a 48-hour week, an aim which was achieved in the Infirmary in 1948.

Probationers, who all 'lived in' and had meals provided, received starting salaries of £18, £20 or £22 yearly. In what now seems to be a remarkable under-statement, the Committee said 'These sums leave very little margin' for expenditure on such things as fares home for holidays, out-door clothes and amusements. The starting salary, they recommended, should be 'in the region of £30'. (Staff nurses should have £75 to £90 yearly and Sisters £100 to £130, with more for long service.)

Nurses still had to do a lot of domestic work—the Committee had been told of some who, in their third and fourth years, were required to scrub out lockers and polish brasses—and they recommended that nurses should be called on to do only such domestic work as could properly be entrusted only to nurses. How the dividing line was to be drawn was not explained.

Off-duty times should be notified to nurses well in advance and not at the last minute as frequently happened; 'off-duty conditions in nurses homes should be more homely' and 'the policy of locked doors at 10 p.m. or 10.30 p.m. should be abandoned'.

o

Assuming that Miss Smaill concurred with her colleagues in making these recommendations (and no dissents are recorded) nurses in the Royal Infirmary clearly had the benefit of working under a Lady Superintendent of enlightened views for that time.

In 1944 Miss Margaret C. Marshall returned to the Infirmary to succeed Miss Smaill whose senior assistant she had formerly been. Her first experience of nursing had been as a VAD during the first world war. Then, after an interval, she had trained at the Royal Infirmary, gaining the Affleck Medal for distinction. Her later progress, as Matron of Beechmount Hospital in the 1930s and from 1939 as Principal Matron of the Emergency Hospital Service in Scotland and first Chief Nursing Officer of the Department of Health have already been described. In 1947 she was awarded the OBE. She retired in 1955. Twenty years later the honorary degree of Doctor of Laws was conferred on her by the University of St. Andrews in recognition of her distinguished career and her continuing activity in voluntary work, especially on behalf of the blind and the elderly.

In the years immediately following Miss Marshall's appointment as Lady Superintendent, war-time restrictions and post-war controls still posed many problems. Shortage of trained nurses continued until the Services were able to release a number of Sisters who returned to the Infirmary wards. Determined efforts were being made to reduce the hours worked by nurses. In 1944, although the 56-hour week which had operated since 1921 continued, it was found possible to allow one day off each fortnight instead of one and a half days each month—a small concession but none the less welcome. By 1948 Miss Marshall was at last enabled to organise nurses' duties on the basis of a 48-hour week, as had been recommended ten years before. Even then, the change was made in the face of many difficulties, not least being the provision of residential accommodation for the extra nurses required in order to reduce the hours worked. The problem was not satisfactorily solved until the introduction in the mid-1950s of the practice of allowing probationer nurses who wished to do so (and whose parents approved) to live outside the hospital—a privilege at first granted to those who had completed their first year's training and later permitted after six months.

Both Miss Smaill and Miss Marshall were firm believers in keeping every branch of work for which they were ultimately responsible under close observation and both made a practice of visiting every ward and every department, including kitchens and laundry, regularly every week. It was a time-and-energy consuming operation and on one occasion Miss Smaill calculated, with the help of a pedometer, that her tour of the hospital had involved a walk of five miles. Like her predecessor, Miss Marshall also served on several nursing committees and advisory bodies and on the introduction of the National Health Service she was appointed a member of the South-Eastern Regional Hospital Board, Scotland on which she served for three years.

On Miss Marshall's retiral in 1955 she was succeeded by Miss Barbara H. Renton, also a Royal Infirmary trainee and Affleck medallist. After varied experience in England Miss Renton had been, briefly, Assistant Matron in the Simpson Pavilion. During the war she was Matron of Bangour Emergency Hospital and then, for ten years, Matron of the Victoria Infirmary, Glasgow. Her time in the Royal Infirmary, however, was short as she resigned after $3\frac{1}{2}$ years, on her marriage.

Miss Renton's short tenure of the Infirmary post coincided with the beginning of important developments in the training of nurses. Just before the opening of their new teaching unit in 1956, the 'block system' had been introduced, releasing groups of nurses in turn from their ward work to undertake uninterrupted periods of study—a change of great benefit to the nurses but calling for skilful organisation of their duty and study schedules. This was further complicated by General Nursing Council amendments to training requirements leading to a series of changes in the times allotted to different branches of nursing. As these changes were being made, it came to be realised that the time allowed for nurses to gain ex- perience in operating-theatre work was insufficient. To remedy this it was decided to introduce a theatre course which would enable those with a special interest in that work to obtain an extra qualification. The first theatre management course of nine months was accordingly instituted in October 1957. A post of Theatre Superintendent had been created, the duties of which included the planning of the course in consultation with surgeons and bacteriologists, and its organisation and supervision. Appropriately, the first Theatre Superintendent was Miss Anna Gordon who had had long experience as Theatre Sister in the Wards 7/8 Theatre and who as already described acted as Theatre Sister at Buckingham Palace when Professor Learmonth operated on King George VI in 1949.

Miss M. H. Cordiner became Lady Superintendent in 1959. In one respect her appointment broke with tradition—her early training had not been in Edinburgh, but in Aberdeen and Glasgow. She came to the Infirmary from Bristol where she had been Matron of the Royal Hospital and Principal of Nurse Training for the United Bristol Hospitals. Miss Cordiner held a qualification in nursing administra- tion which must have been of value as the pace of adjustment and change quickened during her eight years at the Infirmary.

In 1959 a 44-hour week for nurses was adopted experimentally in two medical wards and led to the predictable conclusion that its general adoption throughout the hospital would be impossible unless preceded by a sufficient increase in staff. The trial, however, was valuable in that it seems to have convinced the Regional Hospital Board that the Board of Management's demands for authority to engage more nurses were justified. The annual report for 1961-62 showed a total nursing staff of 923, compared with 770 in 1959-60. The higher figure was made up as follows:

Trained nurses (full-time 272; part-time 46)	318
Nursing auxiliaries (full-time 63; part-time 106)	169
Student nurses	436
	923

As a result of the increase in numbers, the 44-hour week (or, more correctly, an 88-hour fortnight) was introduced throughout the hospital, but it was not the growing numbers alone that had made the change possible. Three other factors contributed. First was the increasing tendency for both qualified and student nurses to live outside the hospital; the second factor was the new practice of employing part-time nurses, many of whom had previously had valuable nursing experience and brought welcome skilled help to the wards; and, thirdly, the employment, from 1960, for the first time in the Infirmary, of assistant nurses or nursing auxiliaries who, after a brief period of introductory training helped in the wards. These were women who, while wishing to work in caring for the sick (and many having great aptitude for doing so) either did not want to embark on a full training course or did not have the necessary basic qualifications to enable them to do so.

The Royal Infirmary had been slow to accept the employment of such assistants, for there were still those among the Board members and staff who feared that to do so might dilute the high standards of nursing for which the Infirmary had long been renowned. It could equally have been (and doubtless was) argued that by providing basic care and relieving the student nurse of some of her simpler but time-consuming routines, the help given by assistants in the wards would enable her to become more quickly skilled in the more technical aspects of nursing, thereby helping to *raise* standards. A report to the Board of Management in 1966 by a nurse education advisory committee headed by Sir Derrick Dunlop noted that ward assistants when first employed had not been well received, but added: 'However, they have now become an indispensable part of the ward team and are likely to become increasingly necessary'.

Some years earlier, the General Nursing Council, recognising the need for a modified form of training had prescribed a teaching programme leading to enrolment as 'State Enrolled Nurse'. It was a two-year course with less emphasis on theoretical study than the course for State registration. The first such course was begun in the Infirmary in January 1963 and the first six pupils successfully completed that course in 1965, receiving the hospital certificate and a specially adapted 'Pelican' badge.

In spite of what had seemed to be an easing of tension resulting from the employment of some additional staff, a crisis occurred early in 1963 demonstrating dramatically that the increase was still insufficient. Suddenly, after consultation by the Medical Superintendent and the Lady Superintendent of Nurses with members of the clinical staff, and committee approval having been obtained, 106 beds in the gynaecology, ophthalmology, ear, nose and throat and dermatology wards were taken out of use, releasing some thirty nurses for transfer to ease the strains elsewhere in the hospital. The beds were 'closed' on 26 February and remained so for five weeks.

Not surprisingly, such an unusual and drastic step caused an outcry from several quarters and the Regional Hospital Board appointed a Committee of Inquiry (the majority of whose members were from other authorities) to investigate all the circumstances. Many reports, minutes and statistical records were studied and more than thirty 'witnesses' were interviewed. It was explained to the Inquiry that the nursing staff had been under severe strain for a long time and only their loyalty and devotion to duty had prevented a more serious breakdown. There had been many reasons for this, including the increasing volume and complexity of work, developments in nurse-training requirements and the introduction of the 88-hour fortnight. The volume of work had grown largely because of the 'quickening turn-over of patients'. Its complexity had increased markedly through the introduction of special units—for renal dialysis, respiratory resuscitation, thoracic surgery and others. These, involving intensive care of patients, required highly-skilled nursing and a high nurse-to-patient ratio. The situation had been worsened by the winter influx to the medical wards of elderly patients with respiratory troubles. For all these reasons, repeated requests for increases in the establishment for nurses had been made but they had failed to persuade those in higher authority to make the necessary resources available or to take effective steps to have patients diverted to other hospitals. This, it was said, had caused a feeling of frustration at many levels.

From the outset it had been planned to re-open the beds on 1 April 1963 because it was expected that the general improvement of weather would by then have reduced both the demand for medical admissions and the incidence of fractures due to falls on ice or snow. (According to press reports it had been the coldest winter in Edinburgh for 48 years.) The five weeks' relief of pressure, it was believed, would enable the nursing staff to 'recover their equilibrium'. And so it came about; the 106 beds were brought back into use on the expected date.

Towards the end of 1963 a Regional Hospital Board work-study team, with the help of a senior member of the Infirmary nursing staff seconded to work with them, began a detailed examination of the nursing organisation in the hospital. As their study progressed, experimental duty rotas were introduced in several wards and departments. At the same time, other studies were being pursued into such matters as the supply of linen to wards, secretarial services and the duties of domestic staff, all of which had a bearing on the work of nurses. Little more than a year later it was reported that 'the recommendations of the work study team have been studied and generally accepted. Implementation is in progress, the 42-hour working week for nursing staff has been introduced, fewer 'split' duties are worked and the long period of night duty for junior nurses has been eliminated'. Although the full number of nurses recommended by the work-study team was more than could be authorised, some increase was possible. That increase along with measures of rationalisation and reorganisation had not only removed the likelihood of a repetition of the circumstances which caused so much concern in February 1963; they had also made it possible for the nurses' standard weekly hours of work to be reduced from 44 to 42.

As it happened, these internal adjustments easing pressures in the Infirmary coincided with the beginning of a series of events which led to far reaching changes in the pattern of nursing organisation in hospitals throughout the country. First, in 1963, the General Nursing Council for Scotland issued a new syllabus calling for 'wider basic training' for student nurses working for their general nursing certificate. The new syllabus was approved by the Secretary of State for Scotland and its adoption became obligatory on 1 January 1964. It increased the number of weeks student nurses would have to spend in their study blocks. There would also have to be an end to the practice of allowing nurses, during study-block periods, to work in wards for short morning and evening shifts and on Sundays. Periods of secondment to other hospitals for experience in special branches of nursing were increased. Such secondment, instead of being confined to infectious disease hospitals and children's hospitals as before must, in future, include periods of psychiatric nursing and obstetrics and also attachment to a public health department. Explaining these and other changes to the Board of Management, Miss Cordiner said that they would increase from 49 weeks to 61 weeks the period for which each student nurse would be away from the Infirmary wards during her three year training. This would make the student nurse a 'less stable element in the ward team'. Stability would therefore have to depend on the employment of a higher proportion of qualified staff, both registered general and state-enrolled nurses, and on the 'wiser use of auxiliary personnel'. To make all this possible, she estimated that it would be necessary to increase the total staff to 1,066 nurses made up as follows:

Trained nurses	386
Nursing auxiliaries	150
Student nurses and pupil enrolled nurses	530
	1066

The next event was the publication in April 1964 of the Report of the Committee, chaired by Sir Harry Platt, Bt, FRCS, which had been set up by the Royal College of Nursing in one of several attempts to reconcile the needs of ward nursing with those of nursing education. Among the Platt Committee's forty members, distinguished in many medical, nursing and educational fields were two Honorary Consultants with long experience in the Royal Infirmary and a wide knowledge of its nursing organisation and problems. They were Professors Emeriti Sir Derrick Dunlop and Sir Walter Mercer.

As part of the Platt Committee's plan to disentangle the education requirements of student nurses from their services in hospital, while recognising the educational value of these services, recommendations were made about the establishment of schools of nursing which would be independent from individual hospitals. From the seeds sown by these recommendations, modified by those of the Committee on Nursing under the chairmanship of Professor (later Lord) Briggs in 1972, there eventually emerged in 1976 the new South Lothian College of Nursing and Midwifery to take the place of the Infirmary's own school. Other recommendations provided support for ideas on the composition of ward nursing teams and on the allocation of their duties, towards the adoption of which the Infirmary and other hospitals were already moving.

In December 1965, while Miss Cordiner, her Deputy and her Assistant Lady Superintendents were still engaged in adapting the nursing organisation in the Infirmary to meet the requirements of wider basic training and other recent recommendations, yet another weighty volume was thrust upon them; this time, one that has had a profound effect on the whole pattern of nursing administration. This was the Salmon Report prepared by a Committee appointed jointly by the Ministry of Health and the Scottish Home and Health Department with a remit to advise on senior nursing staff structure (ward sister and above) of which the Chairman was Mr. Brian Salmon, CBE, then Vice-Chairman of the Board of Governors of the Westminster Hospitals Group. They had been a small Committee of only ten members, a more manageable size than Platt's forty, but their recommendations were more revolutionary.

Because of the complexity and far-reaching nature of the Salmon recommendations, their application required a long preliminary period of study, discussion and trial. As a result, they were not put into effect nationally until July 1972. Their purpose was well described in the Royal Infirmary's Annual Report for that year as being: 'to provide the best possible patient care through effective management of the skills and resources available to nursing. The method of achieving this will include the provision of further supportive services to those who work close to the patient, the establishment of clear and speedy lines of communication and the clarifying of the levels at which decisions are taken and responsibility rests.'

Miss Cordiner resigned as Lady Superintendent in January 1967 and so had only been able to take part in the first year's discussions on the Report. She had, however, been responsible for or participated in many other advances during her eight years in office, including the development of the theatre service centre and the introduction of post-registration courses in the theory and practice of nursing in thoracic, renal, respiratory-resuscitation and coronary care special units. On her resignation the Board of Management acknowledged that it was 'largely due to her wide foresight that the progressive schemes now in hand have come into being'. In 1967 she received the Honour of OBE.

During Miss Cordiner's time there had been a break with tradition by the transfer of the Lady Superintendent's house from the heart of the hospital to its periphery. The house adjoined the Chapel and had direct access to it—a reminder that both had once been part of the old George Watson's Hospital School when the house had been occupied by the Headmaster. Despite the stout walls of the house its successive occupants could never fully escape from the atmosphere and bustle of hospital activity. In the past this had doubtless been taken for granted but it did not conform to the ideas of the 1960s; and, besides, office accommodation for the nursing department was in urgent need of expansion. So, in 1965, a house (since demolished) was made available for the Lady Superintendent at the south end of Chalmers Street, to the west of the Simpson Pavilion, and the former house became the administrative headquarters of the Infirmary's nursing service.

A milestone was reached in 1968 when the first male student nurses under a combined mental nurse/general nurse scheme began working in the wards of the Infirmary. Three years later the first male nurse entered on the full three year general nursing course. He qualified in 1974. By 1979, among 616 student nurses taking that course 31 were men.

The Lady Superintendent of Nurses appointed in 1968—the last to occupy that position and to hold that title—was Miss M. F. Cullen who had been Deputy Lady Superintendent since 1962. Like Miss Barclay, the first Lady Superintendent a century earlier she was a 'Nightingale', having received her training in St. Thomas's Hospital, London.

The Salmon Committee had recognised that, with the increasing pace and complexity of hospital work and the extension of nursing skills from simple (yet still all important) patient care to embrace complicated scientific techniques, it was essential in large hospitals to define and maintain clear lines of authority and communication. Their recommended system, therefore, provided a chain of authority leading upwards from Ward Sisters, each responsible for a Ward, to Nursing Officers, each supervising a Unit (group of wards) each of whom would be responsible to a Senior Nursing Officer supervising an Area (group of units). Above that level there were to be Principal Nursing Officers, each in charge of a Division (e.g. general nursing; maternity nursing; nurse-teaching). The whole organisation was to be controlled by a Chief Nursing Officer, corresponding nearly (not exactly) to the former Lady Superintendent. She would be the spokesman on nursing and related matters in policy discussions among other chief officers and at Board meetings.

After acceptance of the recommendations by the Minister of Health and the Secretary of State for Scotland it was decided, in 1967, that time should be allowed for a series of pilot schemes to be undertaken before the new organisation was put into general operation. The South-Eastern Regional Hospital Board organised such schemes in four hospital groups, but the Royal Infirmary Group was not one of them. The Infirmary Board of Management nevertheless embarked on their own 'mini-scheme' by adopting, for a trial period, a variant of the Salmon structure in the surgical house.

Meanwhile the work of the wards continued under the familiar pressures of seeking to provide an efficient service within the limits imposed by permitted 'ceilings' of expenditure which seemed never to be quite high enough. Yet despite these difficulties, it was possible on 1 January 1972, to comply with the requirement of the Nurses and Midwives Whitley Council that the working week for nurses should be reduced to forty hours. Six months later, on 1 July 1972, the 'Salmon' organisation was adopted in hospitals throughout the country and, for the Royal Infirmary of Edinburgh and Associated Hospitals Group, Miss M. F. Cullen became Chief Nursing Officer.

The re-organisation covered not only nursing services but also nurse-teaching. It was a fitting coincidence, therefore, that the centenary of the founding of the Royal Infirmary of Edinburgh School of Nursing occurred also in 1972. It was on 7 October 1872 that Miss E. A. Barclay had established the School; and on 7 October 1972, the Board of Management gave a formal lunch and an evening reception to celebrate its centenary. On the following day a service of thanksgiving was held in the Kirk of the Greyfriars; and for three weeks an exhibition depicted the history of the School and of nursing generally, with displays of documents, photographs and equipment, including examples ranging from early types of poultices to modern intensive-care monitoring machines. Nor were the interests of younger nurses forgotten, for the Board's report records that 'a Centenary Discotheque, to which all student and pupil nurses were invited was a great success, the patients being cared for by the trained nursing staff working at unusual hours in the absence of students'.

A booklet—*The Story of the Royal Infirmary of Edinburgh Nurse Training School, 1872-1972* was published, written by two former Lady Superintendents, Miss M. C. Marshall and Mrs. B. H. Quaile (formerly Miss Renton) and a former

Nurse-Tutor Miss A. I. Peterkin. It gave a comprehensive illustrated account of the School's development, enlivened by reminiscences gleaned from former students and teachers. As a permanent record it became of greater value than its authors had anticipated when, four years after its publication, the Royal Infirmary School was superseded by the South Lothian College of Nursing and Midwifery, with headquarters in Chalmers Street where the School had latterly been based. The Royal Infirmary continued to be the principal hospital in which students of the College would obtain their practical experience but, in future, other hospitals in South Lothian District (previously attached to other hospital-based schools) would also participate.

From the viewpoint of the Infirmary, the transition from hospital school to district college marked the end of an era, although the fact that the College Director of Nurse Education, Miss Muriel Shinie, and other first occupants of posts in the College had been members of the former School of Nursing staff provided a re-assuring measure of continuity. One clear sign of the change was the discontinuance of the issue of the much-prized Royal Infirmary 'Pelican' badge. In its place new badges were designed to be awarded to nurses qualifying from the College. These retain the motif of a pelican with her young, above the words 'South Lothian' and doubtless, with the passage of time, they will acquire for their wearers a prestige comparable with that conveyed by the former badge. Similar badges, inscribed 'North Lothian' and 'West Lothian' were designed for the new Colleges of Nursing and Midwifery based, respectively, on the Western General Hospital and Bangour Hospital.

One group of nurses and former nurses deeply regretted the disappearance of the old 'Pelican' badge. They were the members of the Royal Infirmary of Edinburgh Nurses League. The League had always been open to nurses from the Infirmary School who, after registration, worked for at least one more year in the Infirmary and membership continued to be open to those who did so after completing the college course. Soon after the former badge had been discontinued, members of the League responded enthusiastically to a suggestion that they should issue a badge of their own to new members and this was done. Their badge again incorporated a pelican motif and also carried the name of the League, thereby making clear the wearer's link with the Royal Infirmary of Edinburgh.

The year 1972, besides marking the centenary of the Royal Infirmary School of Nursing saw another milestone in the study of nursing—the establishment in Edinburgh of the first University Chair of Nursing Studies in Britain. Since 1962 the University had provided courses leading to the Degree of MA with Nursing Studies (later discontinued) and the Degree of BSc (Social Science—Nursing) as well as diploma and certificate courses in nursing studies. Now, the Director of the Department of Nursing Studies, Miss Margaret Scott Wright, MA, PhD, SRN, became the first Professor. As a Boots Research Fellow in Nursing, between 1957 and 1961, she was not unknown in the Infirmary, having conducted surveys of nursing methods there during that time.

Students taking nursing courses in the University are required to undertake periods of practical hospital nursing. Many do so in the Royal Infirmary and some graduates later return to its wards as staff nurses and ward sisters. They have provided another link between Infirmary and University to add to those long existing through the Faculty of Medicine.

To return, now, from the academic to the organisational aspect of nursing: by an inconvenient piece of legislative timing, just when the new Salmon pattern was settling into shape, the re-organisation of the National Health Service came into operation on 1 April 1974. This meant that the Royal Infirmary, instead of continuing as the principal hospital in its Group, became one (though still the largest) among some twenty hospitals in the South Lothian District of the Lothian Health Board. To ensure effective co-ordination of all nursing and nurse-teaching in the new Board's area, another new senior nursing structure had to be devised. In that structure, the post (only two years old) of Chief Nursing Officer at the Royal Infirmary, responsible to the Board of Management, was superseded by that of Divisional Nursing Officer (General Nursing) for the Royal Infirmary Sector of the South Lothian District, the Sector incorporating the Eye Pavilion and Chalmers Hospital. That officer was now responsible, through a District Nursing Officer and the (Lothian) Area Chief Nursing Officer, to the Lothian Health Board.

At about the same time as the new organisation began Miss Cullen resigned, and on leaving, she received from the Consultants an unprecedented compliment, the gift of a sterling silver rose-bowl in appreciation of her services to the Royal Infirmary. Her Principal Nursing Officer for general nursing, Miss M. S. Laing, was promoted to be South Lothian District Nursing Officer and in 1976, Miss J. L. P. Robertson from the Eastern General Hospital became Divisional Nursing Officer for the Royal Infirmary Sector, the post she continues to hold.

The advantages to be brought about by these organisational changes were intended to be two-fold. First, they were to relieve those closest to the patient from extraneous duties, leaving more time for bedside nursing and for attention to an increasing range of equipment and scientific appliances provided for the patients' benefit. Secondly, by relieving those in the most senior positions from time-consuming attention to detail, they would free them to consider broad policy and to apply up-to-date management methods. One example of the use of such methods may serve. In 1977 a 'patient dependency survey' was carried out by nursing staff in collaboration with the Lothian Health Board's work study department. By applying currently accepted criteria as to the extent to which different types of patients depend on nursing services, it was possible to work out on a statistically sound basis the optimum number of nurses for each department and for each hospital.

From the results it was found in 1978 that, for a 40-hour week, the Royal Infirmary Sector should have such number of full-time and part-time nurses as would be equivalent to 1,268 full-time nurses, including student nurses. The Health Board, because of cost limitations, were able to finance only 85% of that requirement. Nevertheless the system had provided an objective guide, instead of the earlier subjective estimates, on which to allocate available provision among wards and departments. In 1981 the nurses' standard working week was reduced to $37\frac{1}{2}$ hours, bringing them at last into line, in that respect, with most other professional people. The required number of nurses on the 'full-time equivalent' basis, then rose to 1,344, to which it was still necessary for the 85% rule to apply.

This account has, of necessity, been much concerned with changing organisational and administrative matters. Yet despite all the changes that have been described, a nurse's fundamental concern continues to be for the care and cure of each individual patient. Often such caring is carried well beyond the demands of duty and many examples of that could be given. To conclude this account, however, one outstanding incident must suffice. It took place on 12 January 1971, not long after Ward 3—the Poisoning Treatment Centre—had been transferred from the Surgical House to an upper floor in the old Eye Pavilion which had been vacated after the opening of the Princess Alexandra Pavilion. The minutes of the meeting of the Board of Management on the day of the occurrence tell the story. They record that the Lady Superintendent of Nurses reported to the Board:

> that, earlier in the day, a mentally disturbed woman patient had climbed out of a high window in the bathroom attached to Ward 3 and on to the glass roof of the balcony and had been in danger of falling forty feet to the ground. A staff nurse in the Ward had seen the patient's foot break through the glass roof and had immediately run to the other turret of the Ward and had climbed through the window on to the roof of the balcony. She had spoken to and calmed the patient while gradually working her way over the glass roof to the patient whom she had held until the Fire Brigade was able to take them off the roof with the aid of a turntable ladder.

The minute continues:

> The Board noted the outstanding courage displayed by the Staff Nurse, who wished to remain anonymous, and unanimously agreed to record in the minutes its deep appreciation of her brave action.

It was later reported that the staff nurse concerned, Mrs. L. A. Robertson, had been awarded the Queen's Commendation for Brave Conduct. The Commendation was formally presented to her by the Lord Provost, the Rt. Hon. Sir James McKay, at a ceremony in the City Chambers which was attended by her family, by representatives of the Board of Management and of the South-Eastern Regional Hospital Board and by Dame Muriel Powell, Chief Nursing Officer of the Scottish Home and Health Department.

Simpson Memorial Maternity Pavilion

The building of the Simpson Memorial Maternity Pavilion and the transfer to it, in 1939, of patients from the former Simpson Memorial Maternity Hospital were described earlier. At that time the Managers of the Royal Infirmary confidently declared their new maternity accommodation to be 'as up-to-date as medical science can make it and there is not a better equipped building in the world'. In 1946, the authors of the Department of Health's Scottish Hospitals Survey so far supported that claim as to describe the pavilion as 'the best laid out and best equipped institution of its kind we have had the opportunity of inspecting'. The total bed complement, they reported, was 140 grouped in wards taking from three to twelve beds and in 19 two-bedded and 23 single-bedded rooms. The top floor was reserved for patients who had to be isolated and was reached by a separate lift so that it could be completely cut off from the rest of the building. They added, 'there is liberal provision of labour rooms and spacious operating theatres and accommodation for healthy, for premature and for sick infants is provided in air-conditioned rooms'. They also praised the facilities provided for the teaching of medical students and midwives. The authors' only reservation concerned the ante-natal, post-natal and child welfare clinics on the ground floor of the two-storey, northern part of the building, the space for which they thought was 'perhaps hardly sufficient as the patients attend in greater numbers than was anticipated'. 'The hospital', they added, 'has its own matron and trained nursing staff and being a recognised training school has 96 pupil midwives on its staff . . . The visiting staff are all specialist obstetricians who serve in an honorary capacity. They are assisted by specialists in training and by house surgeons . . .'

As a matter of policy, the Managers of the Infirmary had decided that the affairs of their new Maternity Pavilion should be administered separately from those of the main hospital and they appointed a special committee of their members for that purpose. For the remaining years of the voluntary hospital system the finances of the Pavilion were a constant source of concern to that Committee and to the Managers. In September 1940, the Managers reported that in the first full year of operation the accounts of the Pavilion had revealed:

a deficit of over £13,500 on the year's working and, as the capital funds [transferred from the old hospital] are practically exhausted, it means that this special unit is a very heavy drain on the resources of the Infirmary generally . . . It is obvious that this state of affairs cannot continue and that new sources of revenue must be obtained, otherwise the present service cannot be maintained. The latter alternative seems unthinkable . . .

The concern expressed by the Managers was fully justified by events. No major new sources of revenue appeared; but, to their great credit, they never allowed the 'unthinkable' to happen. For their remaining seven years in office they met the Simpson Pavilion's increasing deficits annually from the general funds of the Infirmary. During those years the 'Simpson' was receiving income from four main sources:

   (i) payments by patients (including maternity benefits from Insurance
       Societies) charged under the powers contained in the old Maternity
       Hospital's Act of 1932;
  (ii) payments by Edinburgh Town Council in respect of statutory ante-natal
       and domiciliary midwifery services provided on the Council's behalf;
 (iii) payments by medical students for 'hospital tickets'; and
  (iv) fees paid by pupil midwives including, latterly, government training
       grants paid on their behalf.

Small amounts, never totalling more than £4,000 in any year, came from legacies and gifts.

Between 1940 and 1946 the annual ordinary expenditure in respect of the Maternity Pavilion rose from £29,000 to £66,000 and the deficit to be met annually from the Infirmary's general funds varied between £12,000 and £21,000. These 'subsidies' from the parent hospital enabled the maternity service to be satisfactorily maintained until the advent of the National Health Service in 1948.

An inescapable problem in hospital planning arises from the extent to which changes occur both in medical knowledge and practice and in social demands. The Simpson Pavilion had been designed to meet the requirements of the 1930s which, in fact, differed little from those of the 1920s. In the years that followed there were many changes which had to be met by adaptations to the building and re-organisation within it. Already, before 1948, difficulty had been caused by the growing numbers of women seeking to book accommodation. The Simpson Pavilion Committee's report for 1945 recorded that 'the shortage of maternity beds in the city continues to be an acute problem and it is significant to note that, in the course of the year, 715 patients who had applied for bookings had to be refused'. The report added that fifty of those were refused 'on the ground that their financial circumstances did not warrant their admission'. In other words, the pressure was so great that those who appeared able to afford to book at a private maternity home or nursing home with maternity beds were urged to do so. At that time there were about sixteen such homes in the city; ten years later there were only eight and by 1970 none was registered.

As the years passed it was, fortunately, found possible to accommodate increasing numbers of women in the Simpson Pavilion, partly because adaptations to the building (including the incorporation of open balconies into the adjoining wards) enabled the bed complement to be increased from 140 to 208 and partly because the average length of stay was reduced from 10-14 days in the early years, to 5 or 6 days. Though not formally adopted as policy, it was the practice after 1968 to allow some mothers and babies, in straightforward cases, to leave hospital after 48 hours provided their home conditions were suitable and in the knowledge that they would receive regular visits at home by members of the midwifery staff.

The increasing demand for bookings was not due to a rising birth-rate for, except in the immediate post-war years and briefly in the early sixties, the birth-rate remained fairly steady until it began to fall in the later sixties. The trend was largely due to a growing preference by women to have their babies in hospital, where every facility would be available in case of need, rather than at home. The following table of figures for selected dates shows the growing number of admissions to the Pavilion and the diminishing number of home confinements.

Year	Birth-rate (Scot.) (per 1,000 pop.)	Confinements attended by S.M.M.P. staff	
		in hospital	at home
1947	22·3	3,349	1,371
1948	19·7	3,188	831
1955	18·1	3,375	213
1960	19·6	3,912	311
1965	19·3	4,711	241
1970	16·8	4,902	39
1975	13·1	4,309	0
1976	12·5	4,227	0
1977	12·0	4,083	1
1978	12·4	4,275	1
1979	13·2	4,887	3

The figures given above for home confinements show the number of such cases in the district allocated to staff from the Simpson Pavilion under the local authority domiciliary midwifery arrangements. In 1975 and 1976 there were no such cases and in later years the number has not been higher than four. Though the demand had almost vanished the statutory requirement to provide the service if required remained and so trained staff had to be available. Such staff were not idle, however, for they were increasingly engaged in post-natal visits, including the all-important visits to those mothers and babies who had been able to return early to their homes.

The near disappearance of home confinements, combined with increasing availability and effectiveness of ante-natal care, also reduced demands on an emergency service which had been introduced in February 1948 and had saved the lives of many mothers and infants. This was the Edinburgh Flying Squad, based on the Simpson Pavilion and serving the whole of south-east Scotland. Within minutes of receiving a call from a doctor or midwife in any part of that area, sometimes from as far as sixty miles away, a team of obstetrician, anaesthetist and sister or staff midwife could be on the way, by ambulance, to take their skilled help to the patient and, if necessary, bring her back to hospital. In the first ten years of the service an average of forty such calls were answered each year. In 1966 a peak of 66 calls was reached but, by 1974, the number had fallen to 23. In later years there were only one or occasionally two calls monthly, the reduction being largely due to the earlier identification of potential dangers, enabling the patient at risk to be brought to hospital before any emergency has arisen.

Comparable to the service given by the flying squad was that provided by a vehicle presented to the Simpson Pavilion in 1972 by the Variety Club of Great Britain. This was an ambulance specifically designed and equipped to carry premature or other new-born infants at risk to the hospital, often from another hospital which did not have the sophisticated equipment or highly specialised skills available at the 'Simpson'. It was the second such ambulance in Scotland and proved of value where speed, combined with the use of special equipment during the journey, was necessary. By 1979, however, use of the special ambulance had been almost wholly superseded as a result of the development of a new type of transport incubator which could provide the environment necessary for the baby and could be carried in any ambulance.

Yet another social trend, or changing fashion, twice had an effect on the work of the Simpson Pavilion. This was the attitude of mothers to breast-feeding. In the 1930s breast-feeding was normal practice for almost all mothers who were able to adopt it. So the Simpson Pavilion contained ward kitchens in which, it was assumed, milk for just a few babies' bottles would have to be prepared by ward staff, and there was no fully-equipped central milk-kitchen. For a decade and more this was not seen as a serious lack. But in the later 1950s and early sixties breast-feeding became increasingly unfashionable until, at one stage, only about 20% of mothers practised it. With an average of ten new babies arriving daily, the problem of preparing so many bottle-feeds with the facilities available began to be a serious one. So space was found in which to construct a well-equipped milk kitchen in which babies' feeds could be prepared in sterile conditions, under the supervision of a Sister-in-charge. In 1964, after a trial period of several months the milk-kitchen was brought into full use. Besides relieving ward staffs of a time-consuming task its up-to-date equipment and skilled supervision ensured the safe condition of the feeds and their suitability for the needs of individual infants. Not many years elapsed, however, before a reverse trend began. Perhaps under the influence of the view that 'nature knows best', breast-feeding began to come back into fashion and by the late 1970s more than 80% of the mothers in the Simpson Pavilion were breast-feeding their babies. The provision of the milk-kitchen, however, had not been in vain for it remained equally important to ensure safe and scientific facilities for the preparation of feeds for the minority of babies requiring that service, however small that minority might become and for the storage of breast-milk, particularly for babies in special care.

'Rooming-in' began to be adopted experimentally in the late 1950s and before long became the normal procedure, except where medical or other circumstances prevented it. That was the name given to the practice of allowing babies, instead of being segregated in a nursery, to stay in the wards beside their mothers thus enabling mother and baby to become thoroughly accustomed to one another before leaving hospital. Other changes in practice led to the need for adaptations to the building, among them the coming of 'early rising' whereby mothers were encouraged to be up and about in the wards as soon as possible after the birth of their babies. That required the provision of additional toilet facilities and day-rooms which had been lacking before, all of which had to be constructed by conversion of whatever space could be made available. Despite the difficulties it was reported in 1963 that 'toilet facilities, baths, showers, basins etc., have been more than doubled in number'.

Such piece-meal alterations, however useful, are no substitute for a complete internal reconstruction of the building to bring it into line with modern requirements. In the early 1960s, authority was obtained from the Scottish Home and Health Department for a sum of one million pounds to be set aside for the purpose and a scheme was devised under which the work was to be done in four stages. Supervening financial crises and changing ideas, however, resulted in the work of only two stages being undertaken. These provided a special-care baby unit, opened in 1968, and an improved and enlarged labour ward suite, completed in 1972.

The special-care baby unit is of particular interest because its opening marked a culminating point in a development which had been going on for a very long time. Already, in the earliest years of the Simpson Pavilion there had been a close link between its work and that of the child welfare service provided by the local authority whose Child Welfare Medical Officer held a hospital appointment as associate paediatrician. Yet, in 1947, when Professor Charles McNeil of the Chair of Child Life and Health at Edinburgh and Paediatrician to the Infirmary, reported to the Managers on his work, there was still apparent a division between the concern of obstetrician, and that of paediatrician, for the babies' welfare. The new-born infant was still, in a sense, the 'property' of the obstetrician. Gradually, in the years that followed, the two interests began to merge, as he had urged, until eventually, the paediatrician became concerned with the well-being of the infant

even before birth, a concern aided from 1973 by the use of ultra-sound to produce
a 'picture' of the baby while still in the mother's womb. As such techniques
developed, as new treatment and monitoring equipment became available and as
the need for highly specialised nursing skills became increasingly apparent the
wisdom of concentrating the expertise and equipment in one specialist unit was
obvious. The special-care unit was opened in 1968 in part of the former isolation
block on the top floor of the Pavilion. This was possible because the need to use the
area for potentially infected cases was much diminished, the number of emergency
admissions having decreased steadily over the years as the proportion of women
booking in advance and receiving adequate ante-natal care had grown; and also
because of the availability of antibiotics. The new unit contained thirty cots in
four nurseries, one for respiratory problems, one for premature babies (later
known as 'light-for-date babies'), one for metabolic problems and one for infected infants. Conveniently beside the unit a paediatric research laboratory was
constructed.

The up-grading of the labour ward suite in 1972 was probably the most
Besides having its own specialists and highly-trained nurses, the unit benefited
from the ready co-operation of experts in cardiology, haematology, anaesthesia
and other branches of medicine. Their co-operation, of course, had been available
before but could now be given more effectively because of the facilities provided
in the new unit. All had to adapt their expertise to meet the requirements of the
smallest of infants. When it is noted that some light-for-date babies may be little
more than 12 inches long and that only 10 millilitres of blood given to such an
infant may be the equivalent of a transfusion of more than a pint to an adult, the
skill and precision necessary in their treatment can be appreciated. During the first
year's operation of the special-care unit, 765 infants were admitted to it, representing 16.3% of all those born in the Pavilion.

The up-grading of the labour ward suite in 1972 was probably the most
important event of that year in terms of long-term benefit to the Simpson
Pavilion. It was not, however, the year's most remarkable event. That description
must surely belong to the successful delivery, by Caesarean section, in February
1972, of a baby girl whose mother, having suffered for many years from renal
disease, had received a kidney transplant in 1966. The annual clinical report of the
Simpson Pavilion for 1972 refers to two almost similar cases in America, but adds:
'This is probably the first case reported from this country in which there has been
a non-twin cadaver kidney homotransplant and a successful pregnancy and outcome'. Ante-natal care of the mother had been given in the out-patient clinic of the
Simpson Pavilion but the operation was carried out, by a Consultant from the
Simpson, in the Nuffield transplantation unit at the Western General Hospital.
The infant was immediately transferred, in the Variety Club Ambulance, to the
special care baby Unit, thereby achieving for herself two 'firsts'—first baby born
in the Nuffield unit and first baby carried in the new vehicle. Her mother was able
to leave hospital twelve days later and both made normal progress afterwards.

So far, the changes that have been noted have all been concerned with mothers
and their babies. The fathers have seen changes too. When the Simpson Pavilion
was opened, and until about 1958, fathers were allowed to visit their wives and
new sons or daughters for only half-an-hour each evening. A daily sight in

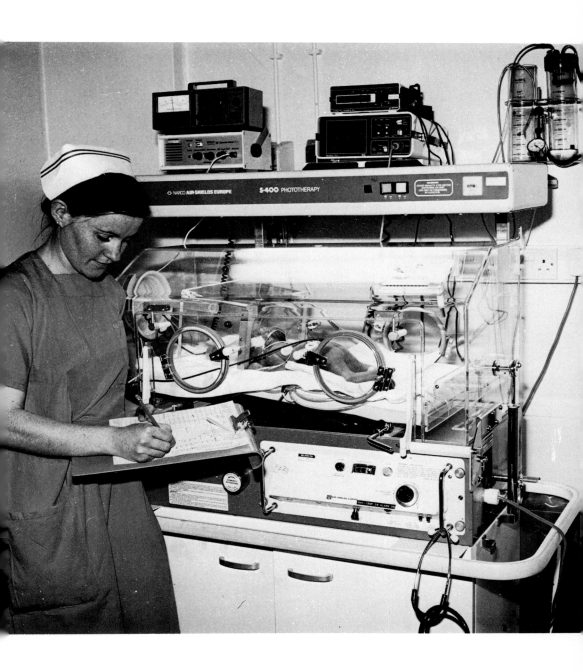

**Plate 29   Simpson Memorial Maternity Pavilion —
Special Care Baby Unit, opened 1968**

Progress of an infant at risk is checked, within the unit

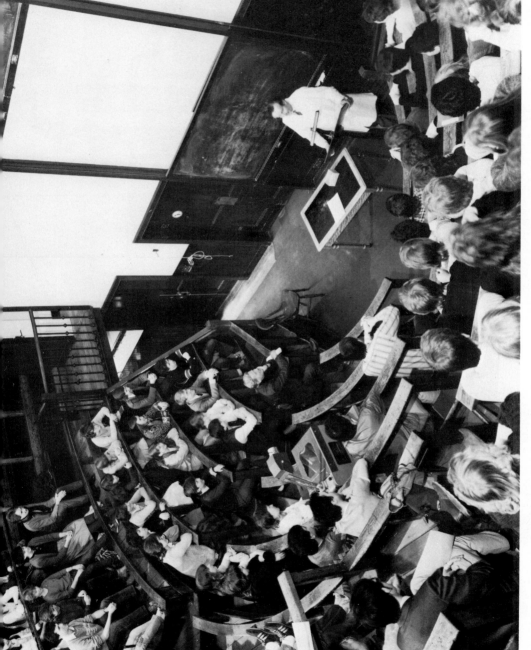

Plate 30 West Medical Lecture Theatre

Standard pattern in 1879; still occasionally used in 1983

Lauriston Place was the queue of fathers impatiently waiting outside the west gate of the Infirmary; then, as the gate was opened at precisely 7.15 p.m., a race began down the west entrance drive, everyone bent on seeing that none of the thirty minutes would be wasted. Visiting times were later extended and, since 1974, visiting by fathers has been unrestricted; but a trial (in response to public demand) of unlimited visiting by other relatives was quickly vetoed by the mothers themselves, asking for more peace and quiet. Fathers first attended at births in 1968 and by 1974 that practice had become officially recognised as a routine one.

For 35 years (1939 to 1974) the beds in the Simpson Pavilion were organised in three units, one on each of the first, second and third floors, each with an obstetrician/gynaecologist in charge who also had responsibility for the care of patients in a gynaecological ward in the Jubilee Pavilion. From 1939 until 1946 the obstetricians in charge of the units were three who had held honorary posts in the old Simpson Memorial Hospital. They were Professor R. W. Johnstone, Dr. W. F. T. Haultain and Dr. Douglas Miller, all recognised as men of distinction in medical and midwifery circles in pre-National Health Service Edinburgh. In 1946 Professor Johnstone and Dr. Haultain retired and were succeeded, respectively, by Professor R. J. Kellar and by Dr. E. C. Fahmy who had been an Assistant Obstetrician in both the old and new hospitals.

When Dr. Douglas Miller and Dr. Fahmy retired in 1958, Dr. John Sturrock and Dr. Clifford Kennedy became obstetricians in administrative charge of two of the units. They had been associated since their student days in the Infirmary in the 1920s. Both had been on the staff of the 'old' Simpson and their careers continued to run in parallel until they both retired on the same day in September 1966.

The two were succeeded in administrative charge of their units by Dr. Douglas Matthew and Dr. W. D. A. Callam. In 1974, however, in which year both Professor Kellar and Dr. Matthew retired and were succeeded by Professor M. G. Kerr and Dr. K. Boddy, the organisation of clinical work within the Pavilion was changed. The traditional 'unit' system was discontinued and each obstetrician (of whom there were then ten) undertook full responsibility for patients admitted to his care. Under the clinical Divisional organisation previously described the medical staff of the Simpson Pavilion became members of the Obstetric and Gynaecology Division, with representation on the South Lothian District Medical Committee responsible for advising the District Executive Group. When the Queen Mary Maternity Home annexe to the Simpson (in which general practitioners attended their own patients) was closed in 1976 the practice of enabling general practitioners to care for patients was introduced to the Simpson Pavilion and those participating in that scheme were then also represented in the Obstetrics and Gynaecology Division.

Miss J. P. Ferlie, OBE who, as Matron, had directed midwifery procedures at the Simpson Memorial Hospital and the Simpson Pavilion for a combined total of 24 years, retired in 1958. Her early training had been in the Royal Infirmary School of Nursing and in the 'old' Simpson where she qualified as a midwife in 1924 and to which she returned as Matron in 1934. The intervening years had been spent in England, including five years in Newcastle-upon-Tyne as one of the youngest Matrons ever appointed to a maternity hospital. Her professional skill

P

was matched by skill in administration and she possessed perhaps the most important quality for leadership in any walk of life, the ability to combine discipline
with understanding and compassion. After her retiral she served for ten years as
Honorary Secretary of the Scottish Council of the Royal College of Midwives and
from 1960 till 1963 she was President of that College—the first Scottish midwife
to be so honoured. She died in 1974. At the Simpson Pavilion she was succeeded as
Matron by Miss M. J. W. Taylor who had earlier been her Deputy but had been
for some years in England.

Miss Taylor continued in office until her retiral in 1968. The Annual Report
for that year records that she had successfully organised many changes for the
benefit of the patients; and she had taken an active part in the planning of the
paediatric special-care unit. Miss Taylor, in her turn, was followed by her Deputy,
Miss M. G. Auld who, as Matron, became responsible for developing special
training for the nurses staffing that unit and for the organisation of their work. On
the introduction of the 'Salmon' senior nursing staff structure in 1972 Miss Auld
was re-designated Principal Nursing Officer (Midwifery). Following the re-
organisation of 1974, she was appointed by the Borders Health Board as their first
Chief Area Nursing Officer and in 1976 she was appointed to the Scottish Home
and Health Department as Chief Nursing Officer for Scotland. Her place at the
Simpson Pavilion, since 1974 designated Divisional Nursing Officer (Midwifery),
was filled by the appointment of Miss B. Jamieson, present holder of that post.

From the first year of its opening the Simpson Pavilion began to acquire its
reputation as a leading centre for the training of midwives—a reputation which
soon became world-wide. For the rapid achievement of that position credit must
go to Miss Ferlie, ably and enthusiastically aided by Mrs. M. F. Myles (affectionately known as 'Maggie Myles') who was the first Principal Midwifery Tutor
at the Simpson Pavilion, a position she held from 1939 till she retired in 1952.
Important as was her contribution in that capacity it was afterwards overshadowed
by her world-wide reputation as author of a comprehensive, standard text-book of
midwifery published in 1953. By 1981 it had reached its ninth edition, each revised
and updated by the author, with world sales of half a million copies. Also after her
retiral Mrs. Myles achieved wide recognition as a lecturer on midwifery. She
undertook extensive and exhausting lecture tours in Canada, America, New
Zealand and many African countries, especially those where new hospitals and
new nurse-training schools were being established. The global fame of the Simpson
Pavilion as a school of midwifery owes much to the work of the many highly
qualified midwives who have gone out from it to practise their skill in this country
and across the world; it also owes a great deal to the remarkable energy of 'Maggie'
Myles and her wide acclaim as author and lecturer.

Not only have many qualified midwives from the Simpson gone to practise
overseas but many student midwives have come to it from Commonwealth and
other countries to learn and gain experience. By the late 1970s, however, the
numbers doing so tended to be fewer. Partly, no doubt, this was due to the growing
number of training schools in other countries, but it was related also to altered
training requirements and other organisational changes. In April 1976 administrative and nursing management of the Simpson Pavilion were joined with those of

the Elsie Inglis Memorial Maternity Hospital (82 beds) on the east side of the City, with a combined student midwife establishment of 130, of whom about 80 might be in post at the Simpson at any one time. In December of the same year their combined School of Midwifery was joined with the Royal Infirmary School of Nursing to become part of the South Lothian College of Nursing and Midwifery. A senior tutor from the staff of the College then became responsible for midwifery training of students who obtained practical experience both at the Simpson Pavilion and at the Elsie Inglis Hospital.

Following the examples set by the nurses who had qualified in the Infirmary School of Nursing, midwives who had trained in the Simpson Pavilion decided in 1967 that a distinctive badge should be awarded to each student midwife on successful completion of her training; and in 1968, they formed a Simpson Midwives League. The central motif chosen for the badge was a butterfly, derived from the butterfly carved on the headstone above Sir James Y. Simpson's family burial place in Warriston Cemetery, Edinburgh. The badge also bore the words 'Victo Dolore' (Victory over Pain), the motto adopted by Sir James when he received his baronetcy. The badge, however, had a life of only ten years. In 1977 it was superseded by the official badge of the South Lothian College of Nursing and Midwifery.

During the 1970s the Simpson Memorial Maternity Pavilion began to take part in a field of research which those who planned and built it almost certainly never envisaged. The approach of this new role was signalled in June 1972 when the Medical Research Council announced their decision to set up, in the University of Edinburgh, a Reproductive Biology Unit whose research team would work in close association with consultants and laboratory experts in the Simpson Pavilion. The Unit, it was explained, would be the first of its kind in Britain and one among only a few in the world. Edinburgh had been selected for the work in preference to all other British medical schools because it already had a strong contingent of research workers in related disciplines. The Unit began to operate in August 1972 with, as its Director, Dr. Roger V. Short, until then Reader in Reproductive Biology at Cambridge University who was appointed an Honorary Professor at Edinburgh in 1975. As Deputy Director Dr. David T. Baird was appointed. He was then a Consultant in the Simpson Pavilion and Senior Lecturer in Obstetrics and Gynaecology in the University and became Professor in that Chair in 1977.

Within a year of the setting up of the Unit the Ford Foundation intimated their intention to make a grant of more than £250,000 towards building and equipping a Centre for Reproductive Biology, to be sited near the Simpson Pavilion, in which the Unit's research team could work and could exchange ideas with other scientists and physicians concerned with problems such as those posed by the rapid growth of world populations, the control of fertility and means of improving the quality of human life. While the research was getting under way, a site was provided to the west of the Simpson Pavilion by the demolition of houses (including the former residence of the Lady Superintendent of Nurses) at the south end of Chalmers Street. There the new Centre—a joint University—Medical Research Council—Health Service venture—was built. It was formally opened on 12 July 1980 by Madame Simone Veil, President of the European Parliament, and formerly France's Minister of Health and Family Affairs. On the same day, the University conferred on her the Degree of Doctor *honoris causa*. To the new building had been transferred the University Department of Obstetrics and Gynaecology, the laboratories of the Reproductive Biology Unit and endocrinology, hormone and clinical laboratories from the Simpson Pavilion to which it was linked by a bridge at second floor level. Thus the Pavilion, designed forty years earlier to be the main centre serving the maternity hospital needs of south-east Scotland, now also plays an important part in a research and teaching project of world-wide significance.

Pathology and Bacteriology

If the ages of these two branches of scientific study in Edinburgh are counted only from the dates of foundation of their University Chairs, then pathology is by far the older. John Thomson, the first Professor of Pathology was appointed in 1831 and James Ritchie, first Bacteriology professor, not until 1913.

Pathology

By 1929, at which point this history of the Infirmary began, the fifth Professor of Pathology had been in the Chair for seventeen years. He was James Lorrain Smith. During his tenure of the Chair an effort was made to clarify the relationship between the University and the Infirmary in the provision of pathological services. The Infirmary had its own pathology laboratories near the mortuary, just beyond the west gate. The University's pathology laboratory was in their medical building at Teviot Place. In 1930 the Managers of the Infirmary (apparently re-affirming an earlier agreement) resolved that the Professor of Pathology should be in close and continuous touch with their laboratory 'and be responsible to the Board for its general supervision and direction'. They added that 'the discharge of these duties is quite consistent with the delegation to competent pathologists of the daily work of the department and in particular the post-mortem work in the theatre'. It was decided therefore that the Professor should be Honorary Pathologist to the Infirmary. A post of senior pathologist was created to take charge of the laboratory and the holders of that post, though usually lecturers or senior lecturers in the University, tended to regard themselves as head of the Infirmary department, independent of the University hierarchy.

At this point it may be convenient to distinguish between two branches of the pathologist's work—autopsies, or post-mortem examinations, which tend to loom large in the mind of the layman, and biopsies, which involve examination of tissue taken from the living body and which are therefore of more direct concern to the patient. The situation in the 1930s and 1940s was complicated by the fact that some clinicians themselves dealt with gynaecological, ophthalmological and dermatological biopsy specimens in laboratories attached to their own departments. There was also the laboratory in Forrest Road maintained by the Royal College of Physicians of Edinburgh which was sometimes used by members of staff. It operated on a fee-for-service basis and it ceased to function soon after the advent of the National Health Service.

In 1931 Professor Lorrain Smith had been succeeded in the Chair and as

Honorary Pathologist to the Infirmary by Professor Alexander Murray Drennan. He continued until 1954 when Professor George L. Montgomery was appointed. Professor Montgomery was designated 'Pathologist-in-Charge to the Royal Infirmary' and he played an important, leading part in bringing the pathological work of University and hospital together until in 1965, the two departments were united in new laboratories within the University Medical School buildings.

Professor Montgomery was succeeded in 1972 by Professor (since 1979 Sir), Alastair Currie who extended the 'single laboratory' concept; moving forward from the idea of two laboratories working together to the principle of the whole being regarded as one laboratory serving hospital and University equally. Meanwhile areas of specialised interest within pathology had been developing steadily, each no doubt now benefiting from closer contact with the others. Edinburgh had been among the first to introduce neuro-pathology as a sub-discipline. That branch of work continued in the Infirmary until the early 1970s when it was transferred, though still within the ambit of the Pathology Department, to the Western General Hospital. Other pathologists developed particular interests in the kidney, the lung, the breast and the lymphoreticular system and performed pioneering work in those fields.

Hand in hand with these areas of study the use of new techniques steadily developed. The electron microscope came to be used almost routinely in the examination of biopsies, particularly from the kidneys and from tumours. The introduction of such aids and other new techniques led naturally to a need for more advanced scientific training of laboratory technical staffs—a trend which progressed over the years in many fields of hospital laboratory work besides pathology until the highly qualified Medical Laboratory Scientific Officer (MLSO) of today bears no resemblance at all to the 'Lab boy' of fifty years ago.

In addition to the pathologists' usual services, a 'frozen section' service was introduced to the Infirmary in the early 1960s. Provision was then made for a pathologist and a technician to work within easy reach of the main operating theatres in a room equipped with up-to-date facilities for freezing, preparing and examining specimens of tissue so that an immediate diagnostic opinion could be offered to the surgeon in course of an operation enabling him to make 'on the spot' decisions as to whether to proceed as planned, to vary his procedure or to postpone the operation.

Alongside these and other changes the volume of work undertaken by the pathology laboratory steadily increased. As an indication of that growth the following figures from a statement supplied by the Pathology Department speak for themselves: Taking, as examples, the years 1929, 1949 and 1959, the numbers of biopsy specimens processed in the Royal Infirmary laboratory were, respectively, 840, 2,620 and 2,940. In 1971, about six years after the Infirmary and University laboratories were united, a total of 11,265 biopsy specimens were processed. Of these, 3,765 were from other hospitals and 7,500 from the Infirmary (frozen sections—1,260; others—6,240). By the year 1979, the overall annual total was nearly 17,200 specimens.

For the other aspect of the pathologists' work—the carrying out of autopsies— conditions were immensely improved in 1981 when Phase 1 of the Infirmary

re-building project was completed. Until then autopsies were still performed in
the 1879 mortuary block beside the west gate. Although it had been improved and
up-graded within the confined limits of the old building it was still far from
satisfactory. In the new building, in addition to normal facilities of the most up-to-
date kind, the post-mortem suite contains a specially designed 'high risk' area in
which to undertake examinations involving the possibility of more than ordinary
exposure to risks of infection. The whole suite must surely be one of the most
advanced and best equipped in any hospital in the country.

Bacteriology

In 1929 Professor Thomas J. Mackie was Bacteriologist to the Royal Infirmary.
He had been appointed to the Robert Irvine Chair of Bacteriology (of which he
was the second incumbent) and to the Infirmary in 1923 and he continued in both
these appointments until his death in 1955. He was a pioneer in the teaching of
medical bacteriology and is remembered for the high quality of his lectures in the
era of 200 students to a class. He was much more than a theorist, however, for he
was an indefatigable worker at the laboratory bench until quite late in his career
when the demands of administration and committees made it impossible for him
to continue such work except in a supervisory and guiding capacity. In 1928 he
wrote a 'Report on an Inquiry into post-operative tetanus'. He had conducted the
Inquiry on behalf of the Scottish Board of Health and it was based largely on his
work in the Infirmary. The Report was highly praised and its publication led to
the introduction, nationally, of new standards for the production and sterilisation
of catgut used for surgical sutures.

In 1930, as for pathology, the Infirmary Managers sought to clarify the connection between the University and the hospital in the field of bacteriology. They
considered that the nature of the work of that department 'does not call for the
same close touch and supervision of the work as in the case of the Pathological
Department' and continued, 'The Bacteriologist will, however, consult with the
Professor as the official head of the Department in regard to any matters of
importance . . . and the senior assistant to the Professor of Bacteriology for the time
being will be attached as a member of the staff with the title of Extra Bacteriologist'
—a title which continued until 1946. Thus, although the link between the hospital
and University was already a close one, their laboratories remained separate—
beside the Infirmary west gate and in Teviot Place, respectively, until very
recently.

Professor Mackie was succeeded, in 1958, by Professor Robert Cruickshank.
In contrast to his predecessor's intense interest in work at the bench, the new
Professor was more concerned with a wide epidemiological approach to his
subject. His period in office coincided with years of immense increase in the work
of his department for the Infirmary. In 1958, 61,000 specimens were received,
involving nearly 290,000 investigations; by 1968 these numbers had grown,
respectively, to 112,000 and over one million. Yet the staff had not increased
proportionately and they frequently had to work under great pressure. The
increase was largely caused by the setting-up and expansion of several special units.
Already in the year 1961-62 the Department's Report referred to 'the relatively

enormous number of specimens taken daily in connection with seriously ill patients under treatment in the artificial kidney unit, the assisted respiration unit and elsewhere in the hospital . . . [In these units] specimens are taken from the patient, from those in attendance and from the environment in order to isolate and identify the probable causative organisms—even before clinical signs and symptoms of infection become manifest. For a single patient, this may entail the examination of more than 100 specimens a day.'

Professor Cruickshank retired in 1966. He was followed, in 1968, by Professor Barrie P. Marmion who brought a third kind of interest and ability to the Department. Besides his expertise as bacteriologist and virologist he was a skilful planner and administrator and he was the instigator of improvements in the University and hospital laboratories, both in their physical equipment and lay-out and by the revision of management methods. At the same time he did much to bring the work of the two departments closer together.

Professor Marmion's attributes were of prime importance during and after the outbreak of serum hepatitis in 1970. He was then, undoubtedly, the right man in the right place at the right time. As Chairman of the Advisory Committee appointed by the Board he not only brought his special knowledge to bear in guiding the Committee but also took charge, for a period of about three months, of the precautionary measures adopted to give effect to the Committee's recommendations; the handling of that alarming situation by all concerned, under Professor Marmion's leadership, was internationally applauded. From that episode there came into being a busy hepatitis reference laboratory, doing research and development in Edinburgh, and other important virological studies began.

Virology had for many years been one of Professor Marmion's special interests and in August 1978 he resigned from his posts in Edinburgh to take up appointments as Director of Virology at the Institute of Medical and Veterinary Science in Adelaide and as Clinical Professor of Virology at the University there.

He was succeeded in 1978 by Professor J. G. Collee who has continued and extended much of his predecessors' work. In particular, he brought to fruition two developments. These were the merging of hospital and University laboratories by transfer of the work formerly done in the building beside the Infirmary west gate to an enlarged laboratory in the Teviot Place Medical School building and the transfer of the hepatitis reference laboratory to the clinical virology section of the Department. Also at Teviot Place, a 'Category A' laboratory was constructed which was specially designed to enable highly infective material to be examined with safety. It is reserved for use in cases or suspected cases of exotic and dangerous diseases of rare occurrence in this country but less so in some other countries. In this era of mass foreign travel it is reassuring to know that such essential facilities are within immediate reach of the Infirmary if the need arises.

So far, this account has dealt with the branch of hospital bacteriological work directed to the search for and identification of harmful bacteria. A different but closely related aspect of the bacteriologists' work which has figured prominently in the story of the Infirmary in the post-war period has been their contribution to the planning of premises, the design and installation of sterilising equipment and the devising of safe working conditions and practices—all aimed at the maintenance of aseptic conditions and the prevention of infection. During the 1960s much work was done in the Infirmary along these lines, under the guidance of Dr. John Bowie, Senior Bacteriologist, who had a knowledge also of engineering principles involved in the design and operation of high pressure autoclaves and other types of equipment. Examples of that aspect of bacteriological work have been given in describing the construction of the medical renal unit and the development of the theatre service centre; it will be mentioned again in relation to the Infirmary Pharmacy. In fact there has scarcely been any project in the past thirty years or so in which the expertise of the bacteriologist has not been called upon to enhance the protection of patients and staff against infection.

The Pharmacy

Until 1949, the Royal Infirmary Chemical Laboratory was at the east end of the Medical House with a dispensary and store-room opposite, across the lower end of the east entrance roadway. In that year the dispensary and store were altered and extended to accommodate the whole department which then became known as the Pharmacy. It was responsible not only for preparing and issuing medicines, ointments and pills but also for the purchase and supply of medical gases and for buying bandages, surgical dressings and surgical instruments. To ensure that the instruments were maintained in perfect condition for use there had long been a skilled cutler, with a workshop, on the Pharmacy staff. The department was directed by Mr. Gordon Perrins, PhC, MPS, FCS who had been appointed in 1926 with the title of 'Dispenser' and who was one of the first qualified pharmaceutical chemists in Scotland to hold such a hospital post. In 1946 his designation was changed to 'Pharmacist' and, later, to 'Chief Pharmacist'. He continued in the post until his retiral in 1958.

The drugs supplied from the Pharmacy in the 1930s, compared with those of today, were few in number, simple and relatively cheap. Among them would be digitalis, organic arsenicals and chemical disinfectants. There would be iron for anaemia, salicylates for rheumatic fever, bromides, chloral, paraldehyde and opium derivatives for sedation. Liver extract, thyroid extract and insulin would be in demand—the forerunners of a wide range of laboratory-made endocrine substances to follow. The total cost of drugs, dressings and surgical supplies in 1939 was almost the same as the cost of provisions for the hospital; in 1979 it was seven times as much.

Having presided for some twenty years over the preparation and issue of that time-honoured assortment of mainly herbal drug extracts and other pills and potions, Gordon Perrins became involved, during the last twelve years of his service in the Infirmary in helping to bring about the transformation of his department to meet the different, more sophisticated demands of the new era of penicillin and the sulphonamide drugs. It was a transformation in which he took much interest and in 1951 the University of Edinburgh conferred on him the Degree of Doctor of Philosophy in the Faculty of Science for his thesis on 'The Solubility of Sulphanilamide Derivatives'.

The new era also saw a growing appreciation of the paramount need, in many branches of the department's work, to maintain strictly sterile conditions if the dangers of cross infection were to be successfully combatted. Even as late as 1958, among the first features that met the eye in the basement of the Pharmacy were two 100-gallon wooden casks, with tops open to the air, from one of which boric acid lotion, and from the other, carbolic acid lotion were by ancient custom dispensed daily by re-filling stock lotion bottles for ward and theatre use. Soon afterwards that practice was replaced by a system of pre-packing all solutions as soon as they were prepared. The use of corks in bottles was thereafter prohibited and all bottles returned from wards were sterilised before re-use.

During the 1950s it had become clear that facilities in the Pharmacy would have to be radically changed to meet the needs of the new era. At first a complete re-building of the Pharmacy was contemplated but that scheme was abandoned in 1959 because it was then believed that within ten years a new Royal Infirmary, which would include a fully up-to-date pharmacy, would have risen on the site of the old. So the Board of Management and the Pharmacy staff had to be content with an internal adaptation and re-arrangement of the premises.

On Dr. Perrins' retiral in 1958 he was succeeded by Mr. John A. Myers, BPharm, FPS, LLB who, since 1946, had been Chief Pharmacist at Bradford Royal Infirmary. He was immediately faced with the task of organising a modernised pharmaceutical service in the adapted premises and in the next few years the department pioneered the use of several new items of scientific equipment. For example, the demand for sterile water for use in intravenous injections and in other treatments was rapidly growing and the Pharmacy was greatly helped in meeting that demand by the installation, in 1960, of a thermo-compressor still which was said to be the first equipment of its kind in any hospital in Britain. The new still was capable of producing 60 litres of distilled water every hour and, because several safety devices and warning signals were incorporated in its mechanism, it could be left to operate, unattended, for 24 hours a day.

Two years later it was reported that two quick-cooling autoclaves for high pressure steam sterilisation had been provided and that they, too, were the first of their kind in a British hospital. Their quick-cooling facility, it was explained, enabled a full load of bottles to be sterilised, cooled and removed in $1\frac{1}{2}$ hours compared with the four hours required by older types of autoclave which cooled slowly, by radiation. Other pieces of equipment installed within the next few years to enable the Pharmacy to keep pace with the demands made on it were an automatic bottle-washing machine and an electronic tablet counter. That these modern aids had been provided none too soon was evident from the Chief Pharmacist's statement in 1962 that, although the work of his department had more than doubled in three years and was steadily growing, his staff had not appreciably increased. He drew attention also to the fact that almost seventy per cent of the valuable drugs then in use had been introduced to medicine during only the previous ten years—a rapid increase calling for constant up-dating of knowledge and expertise on the part of his staff.

A small sterile solutions room had been built on to the Pharmacy in 1949 in which infusion fluids and other sterile solutions were regularly prepared, sometimes to a formula particularly specified by a surgeon undertaking a new or unusually complex operation. The development of haemodialysis for patients suffering from renal disease led, during the 1960s, to a rapid growth in the demand for concentrated haemodialysis solution. In 1966, in conjunction with a commercial company, the Pharmacy staff devised an ultra-sonic machine which much increased the speed with which the solution could be prepared. In the same year a quality-control laboratory was brought into use, its items of advanced technology including an atomic absorption spectrophotometer for routine control checks of calcium, potassium and magnesium in various solutions. By this time the Pharmacy was well on the way to becoming a centralised pharmaceutical centre not only for the Royal Infirmary Group but also for hospitals throughout the south-eastern region which had neither the equipment nor the staff required to produce the kinds of sterile bottled fluids and other new items being demanded by medical staffs.

The adaptation of the Pharmacy had been completed by 1964. Its accommodation then included, on the top floor, an aseptic suite designed, with advice from the Bacteriology Department, to eliminate, so far as humanly possible, the harbouring of harmful germs which might contaminate fluids and materials being prepared there. The room was supplied with sterile, filtered air and there was a shower at the entrance and an air-lock through which staff entering the room must pass. The aseptic suite—which is still in use—was claimed as another 'first' in a hospital pharmacy.

Meanwhile other changes had been taking place. Hypodermic needles and syringes for very many years had been issued by the Pharmacy to wards and theatres and kept there, to be disinfected by the ward and theatre staffs after every use. Inevitably the effectiveness of disinfection under such a system was variable. So, in 1958 a central syringe service organised by a ward sister and the Chief Pharmacist had been set up in a laboratory in part of the skin department. There a small staff were trained in the techniques of servicing and disinfecting syringes and issuing them to the wards, each to be used once and returned for treatment before re-issue. In 1961 it was reported that the output of sterile syringes from the centre had risen, in one year, from 19,000 to 29,000. By 1963 the output was often 2,000 sterile syringes and tubes daily. As may well be imagined, it was a service much appreciated by the doctors and nurses; and, doubtless, also by patients since the servicing staff, by seeing that the hypodermic needles were always sharp, ensured that the pain of injections would be minimal. At its peak the service required a staff of about twelve, working hard to keep pace with demand. By 1968 demand had so diminished that only three or four people were needed. Several of these no longer required were useful recruits to the developing theatre service centre where their experience stood them in good stead.

The trend which led to this and other changes in the work of the Pharmacy—and also of nurses—was the rapid growth in the use of 'disposables', articles of many kinds, including syringes, which having been used once could be sent to the incinerator, thereby ensuring beyond any shadow of doubt that they could not carry infection from one patient to another. In 1961 the Pharmacy had co-operated with 33 commercial firms in organising, in the Florence Nightingale Nurses Home, an exhibition of sterile 'disposables' which aroused much interest among members of the medical, nursing and pharmaceutical professions who came from many parts of Scotland to inspect the items on display. The paper industry exhibited disposable face-masks, operating theatre drapes, ointment containers, bedpan covers and urinals, to list only a few. The plastic and rubber industries displayed disposable sterile syringes, kidney coils, tubing for various uses, surgeons' gloves and other items which had formerly had to be laboriously washed and disinfected for re-use; even items wholly or partly of metal were available in sterile packs to be used once and then discarded.

Between 1962 and 1967 the Department's expenditure on 'disposables' rose from £12,000 to £55,000. Although part of the increase could be attributed to the general increase of prices and part could be set off against the saving that resulted from elimination of labour costs of cleaning and disinfecting former non-disposable items, the increase was alarming. Yet the use of disposables, if they are properly handled, spells freedom from the dangers of cross-infection from articles used twice or more—and how can the value of that be measured?

In January 1967 the Regional Hospital Board approved of the addition to the Pharmacy staff of a Research Pharmacist and urged the Board of Management to give high priority to the appointment. The statement of duties of the post included: 'to investigate the use and suitability of drugs, dressings and equipment in hospital wards and departments and to undertake such other research as is appropriate, the services of the appointment to be made available to other hospitals in the Region if requested'. That final phrase is an indication that, by then, the Royal Infirmary Pharmacy was serving more than the Infirmary group of hospitals. For some time, in fact, it had been giving help and advice to hospitals throughout the South-Eastern Region, thus anticipating its post-1974 function as district pharmacy for the South Lothian District.

In line with these developments the Royal Infirmary Group Pharmacist became District Pharmaceutical Officer for South Lothian. In 1972, Mr. J. A. Myers had been promoted to the position of Regional Pharmacist and after 1974 he became the Chief Administrative Pharmaceutical Officer of the Lothian Health Board. He had been succeeded at the Infirmary by Mr. T. M. Furber, BPhar, MPS who became the South Lothian District Officer in 1974. When he left in 1976 to take up another appointment he was replaced by Mr. Peter Jones, BPharm, MSc. Under their direction the department's programme of modernisation continued to develop.

Among the important advances after re-organisation was the introduction of ward pharmacists each attached to a group of wards and departments. There they were made available to consult with clinicians and nurses about the prescribing and administration of drugs for individual patients; they could help to renew ward stocks of medicines and appliances; they could often save the time of ward staffs in communicating with the Pharmacy and sometimes prevent or correct errors. Their arrival on the wards, following the trend already noted in other fields, demonstrated the value of close co-operation among personnel trained and experienced in different disciplines, all concerned to work as a team in providing the best possible service to the patients.

An impression of the growth of the work of the Royal Infirmary Pharmacy in the twenty years between 1959 and 1979 can be quickly gained by comparing the staff in 1959 (three qualified pharmacists, four technicians and about seven others) with the numbers of staff shown in the following statement:

Pharmacy Staff in 1979	Serving Infirmary	Serving District	Total
Pharmacists	20	15	35
Technicians	12	7	19
Pharmacy Assistants	10	4	14
Others	43	11	54
	85	37	122

It may seem surprising that such an increase in numbers could take place in premises only slightly extended since 1959. The answer lay partly in the adaptations made in the early 1960s, partly in the deployment of staff to wards and other departments and partly in the 'out-housing' of several branches of work. The central syringe service, for example, had been accommodated since its inception in the dermatology pavilion; the cutler's workshop was housed in separate premises in Lauriston Place; and, after 1972, the sterile fluids unit operated in the former laundry premises which had been vacated when arrangements were made for the Infirmary's laundry work (along with that of several other hospitals) to be done at the Western General Hospital.

Despite the inconvenience naturally resulting from such out-housing the work undertaken by the Pharmacy as it evolved during the 1970s was astonishing in its volume and variety. Its range was well summarised in the Royal Infirmary's 250th Anniversary Booklet issued in 1979, in the following words:

The Pharmacy spends some £2,500,000 of the Infirmary's budget. It has special facilities for the manufacture of sterile products that are not available from commercial sources and produces in the region of 180,000 items annually; these are supplied to all the hospitals in the South Lothian District. In addition 100,000 non-sterile items are produced annually for use in the Royal Infirmary together with 4,000 kilograms of creams and ointments, 40,000 litres of dialysis fluid and the pre-packing of three million tablets. In conjunction with the Department of Medical Physics and Medical Engineering the Pharmacy also produces every year 11,000 doses of radiopharmaceuticals. The quality control laboratories provide the Quality Controller, who is responsible for the overall quality of all manufactured products, with analytical facilities for testing items during their production and before final release and administration to the patient. . . . Several members of staff are involved with the teaching of medical students and nursing staff and the department is currently engaged in research into the formulation and shelf-life of ophthalmic preparations, and the micro-biological attributes of non-sterile production, especially creams and ointments.

The Para-medical Professions

It comes as something of a surprise to find that the para-medical professions whose practitioners now play such indispensable roles in hospital work did not begin to appear among the staff of the Royal Infirmary until the 1920s and some not till much later. An account was given earlier of the emergence in Wards 25 and 26, during that decade, of dietitians as pioneers in their profession. The coming, in 1924, of the first official Infirmary almoners and their eventual metamorphosis into hospital social workers will be described later. Here, let us look at five other para-medical groups, each with special knowledge and skills, who help in the cure and rehabilitation of patients—the radiographers, the physiotherapists, speech therapists and occupational therapists and the chiropodists.

Radiographers

In the Royal Infirmary radiography began with William Law. As Dr. Dawson Turner and Dr. Hope Fowler were developing the use of X-rays for diagnosis and treatment William Law, as an apprentice electrician, became involved in the maintenance of their early X-ray equipment and his interest in that branch of electrical work led him to acquire an expert knowledge of it and its uses. When the new X-ray department was built beside the 'duodenum' in 1926 he became superintendent radiographer there, with a staff of four. In that capacity he was responsible for the operation of the department's equipment, much of which was of entirely new design. Law retired in the 1930s. He died a few years later, his death, like those of the two pioneer radiologists for whom he worked having been hastened by over-exposure to radiation in the days before the new department with its safety components had been built or codes of safe-working fully evolved.

Law's successor as Radiographer-in-Charge was Neil Longden whose father, Richard Longden, senior electrical engineer for many years in the Works Department, was responsible for adapting and inventing several ingenious devices including, in the 1950s, those in the Oral Surgery Department. Son seems to have inherited father's ingenuity and during his long service in the Radiology Department, Neil Longden collaborated with many medical experts in the Infirmary in adapting and developing new ideas for equipment and methods which later became standard. He was well-known throughout Britain and abroad for his important contributions to techniques in the fields of arterial, cardiac and brain investigation and was awarded the MBE for services to radio-diagnostic and X-ray work. He retired in 1972 after a career of more than forty years in the Infirmary and was succeeded as Superintendent Radiographer by Miss Jean Brown DSRD.

When the X-ray department opened in 1926 it had no official school of radiography attached to it. There was only a 'demonstration room' in the basement where some lectures were given to students who worked as dark-room technicians while studying independently for examinations of the Society of Radiographers which had been founded in 1920. In 1936 the department was recognised by the Society for teaching purposes. Under the direction of Dr. John P. McGibbon systematic lectures were then given on anatomy, physiology, photography and radiographic techniques. At first, a single diploma was awarded but after 1948 there were separate diplomas for radio-diagnosis and radiotherapy. After 1955, when the main radiotherapy work was transferred to the Western General Hospital, the school was also divided but first year students of both branches continued to attend lectures at the Infirmary on subjects common to the two courses.

In the twelve years from 1946 to 1958 the number of X-ray investigations at the Infirmary rose steadily from about 50,000 to nearly 80,000 annually. During that time the demonstration room had to be brought into use for the daily work of the department and lectures were then delivered in borrowed classrooms elsewhere in the hospital.

Re-arrangement after 1958 enabled some space for teaching again to be made available in the department but it was not until 1972 that it was possible to provide fully satisfactory premises for the School. This was done by adapting part of the old Simpson Memorial Maternity Hospital in Lauriston Place which had been vacated by the National Health Service Supplies Division of the Scottish Home and Health Department who had occupied it for several years. There, in former wards and hospital rooms, completely re-furbished, the South-East Scotland School of Radiography was established under the management of the Royal Infirmary Board, with Miss I. R. West, FSR, TE, formerly head of the Infirmary's own School, as Principal. It was opened in November 1972 by Sir John Brotherston, then Chief Medical Officer of the Scottish Home and Health Department and its accommodation and facilities were described at the time as being 'among the most impressive in the United Kingdom'. After the Health Service re-organisation of 1974 the two divisions of teaching were separated and given distinctive titles as The Edinburgh School of Radiotherapy whose students received their practical training at the Western General Hospital and the Edinburgh School of Diagnostic Radiography whose students were attached for practical experience to the Royal Infirmary. As Principal of the Diagnostic School, Mr. M. S. Pitt, FSR, TE, succeeded Miss West, who had died in 1973.

By the mid-1970s, the annual numbers of new students enrolling for the two-year courses were 25 for radio-diagnosis and 6 for radiotherapy, the wide difference in numbers being inherent in the fact that many hospitals and hospital departments require the services of trained diagnostic radiographers but only a few highly specialised hospitals are equipped for radiotherapy. By 1978 it had been found that, for both groups of radiographers, supply had overtaken demand and so the annual 'intake' figures for the two schools were reduced to 15 and 5 respectively.

That satisfactory teaching facilities at last existed away from the department was fortunate, the volume of radio-diagnostic work undertaken annually having increased tenfold, from about 13,000 examinations in 1926 to 130,000 in 1972, leaving no spare space within the department for teaching and study. Afterwards, the volume of work continued to grow, reaching (in 1981) 185,000 examinations including those undertaken in other departments and in the Simpson Pavilion. With the introduction of each new radiological procedure and technique, the range of teaching had to be expanded and new skills in the handling of increasingly complex, expensive and, in some cases, potentially dangerous equipment had to be acquired. They are skills, too, which have to be acquired without diminishing the radiographer's equally valuable ability to put each patient at ease in the presence of machines which, to the patient, may have a forbidding aspect.

Physiotherapists

In the Royal Infirmary, the Physiotherapy Department traces its origin back to 1922 when a 'massage department' was set up in a small room in the Surgical Out-patient Department. Two years later the massage department was 'expanded' if that word may be applied to its transfer with two part-time staff to a hut provided for the purpose near the SOPD.

It is more realistic, perhaps, to regard the Physiotherapy Department as dating from 1926. That was the year in which the Radiological Department was opened in its new building beside the 'duodenum'. The upper floor of the building was (and still is) occupied by the Physiotherapy Department, then known as the Massage and Electrical Department. In a booklet issued in 1926 it was described as follows:

> One room is equipped with remedial exercise and gymnastic apparatus.
> Adjoining the gymnasium are two large rooms for male and female
> electrical treatment. Each is equipped with wall-type treatment
> boards . . . supplied by the 80-volt motor generator in the basement. A
> Schnee bath with unbreakable receptacles for the arms and legs is
> installed in each room, together with many other appliances, including
> diathermy and high-frequency apparatus. Massage couches are placed
> around the walls of each room. . . . Two rooms are also provided for
> treatment by ultra-violet rays. Both carbon-arc and mercury vapour-lamps
> have been installed.

Massage was still a predominant part of the work of physiotherapists and it was not until 1943 that the name of their professional body was changed from 'The Chartered Society of Massage and Medical Gymnastics' to 'The Chartered Society of Physiotherapists' so as to embrace all the varied forms of treatment practised by their members.

When the new Department opened in 1926, Miss M. I. V. Mann, from Guy's Hospital, London, became its first Superintendent Physiotherapist with a staff of eight. With the object of encouraging the highest standards of work she was anxious to form a training school in the hospital but, for a variety of reasons, was unable to do so until 1941. War-time restrictions had, by then, made it even less likely that a school could be started in the near future, but it was, in fact, war time conditions that led to its opening. Because of the disruption caused by air-raids on London and other southern cities the establishment of a physiotherapy school in Edinburgh was encouraged by the authorities and the Royal Infirmary Managers gave the idea their blessing. On 1 April 1941, the School was inaugurated and Miss Mann's dream of fifteen years became a reality.

Physiotherapy being of great value in the treatment of orthopaedic patients it was natural for Mr. (later Sir) Walter Mercer to become the first Director of the School and the rapid growth of its reputation owed much to his enthusiastic guidance and support. Miss Mann became the School's first Principal. The course provided was one of two-and-a-half years (later, three years) and the subjects covered were those required for membership of the Chartered Society including anatomy, physiology, medical gymnastics, medical electricity, light and electrotherapy. Miss Mann continued as Principal until her retiral in 1961. Her successor was Miss E. A. Shaw, MCSP, who had joined the staff in 1947. In an article about the development of the School which she wrote in 1966, Miss Shaw said:

> No school of physiotherapy can function as a separate entity. Its success depends in no small measure upon the co-operation of all members of hospital staff. Due especially to the enthusiasm, co-operation and encouragement given by the Medical Consultants in the early days (and which we enjoy to this day) this school was very quickly integrated into the hospital service in Edinburgh and its reputation as a successful establishment had spread far and wide before I came in 1947. The fact that many of the well-known medical staff in the Royal Infirmary from the orthopaedic, surgical and medical sections gave up a considerable amount of their time to visit the department weekly, not only to review patients sent for treatment but also to give clinical teaching to our students was, and still is, the envy of many other training centres.

Miss Shaw died in 1970. She was succeeded as Principal of the School by Miss C. M. Murray, MCSP, TCSP, who transferred to Queen Margaret College, Edinburgh in 1977 when that College undertook responsibility for the training of physiotherapists. Miss Shaw's successor as Superintendent Physiotherapist in the Infirmary was Miss Joan C. Tait, MCSP, who remained in that post until 1981. The students of the College, after 1977, continued to obtain their clinical and practical experience in the Infirmary which thus still plays a vital role in the training of new members of the profession.

In 1979 the staff of the Physiotherapy Department numbered 22, in addition to the Superintendent and there were 10 students in training. During its existence of rather more than half a century, the Department had experienced many changes. From the patients' point of view there had been, since the early 1960s, trends away from group exercises in ward classes towards treatments geared more specifically to individual needs; and away from mechanical exercises towards various other mobilisation techniques. For the physiotherapist there had been an almost opposite trend from acting largely in isolation towards becoming a member of a multi-disciplinary team, including doctors, nurses and colleagues in the other para-medical professions, jointly aiming to provide a comprehensive rehabilitation programme for each patient. Along with that development, a growing recognition of their professional skills had led to physiotherapists, instead of being expected mainly to carry out prescribed procedures, being encouraged to ascertain each patient's needs and themselves assess the nature and extent of treatments most likely to meet those needs.

The conditions treated by physiotherapists had increased in number during the same period and ranged through acute and chronic chest disease, orthopaedic trauma, neurological disorders, head and spinal injuries and many others, including soft tissue injuries, met with among patients in the Accident and Emergency

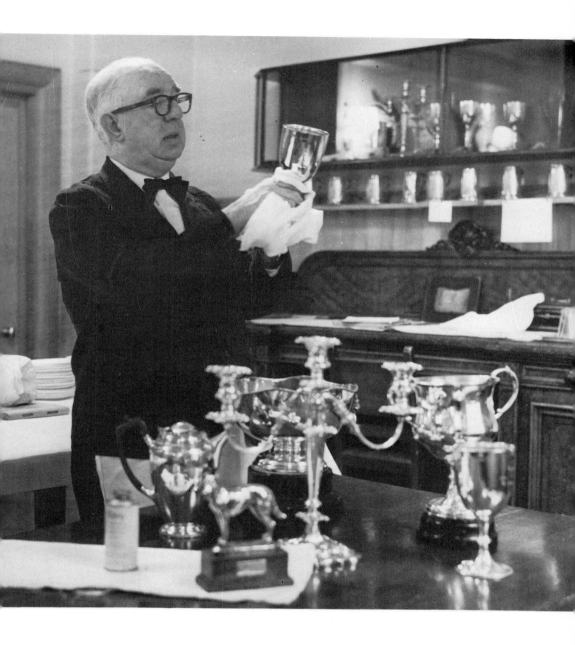

Plate 31   House Officers' Residency

Mr. Bob Morris, The Residency Butler in 1966, polishes the silver
belonging to the Residency Mess

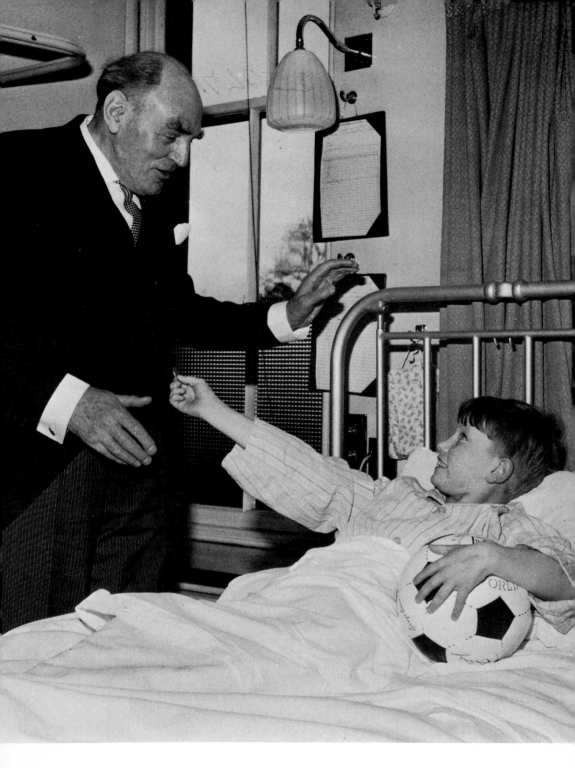

Plate 32   Lord Reith, visiting in 1967 as Lord High Commissioner to the General Assembly of the Church of Scotland

The young patient is showing him a two-shilling coin which he had accidentally swallowed and which had been retrieved by operation

Department. With the introduction of the geriatric unit in 1963 new demands came to be made on the department as they were called upon, if not to cure, at least to ease some of the painful conditions that accompany old age.

While these changes were taking place more scientific aids to treatment were becoming available. As these were developed, active exercises were increasingly preceded by the application of heat, through short-wave diathermy or infra-red irradiation; by the application of intense cold (cryo-therapy); or by ultra-sound. By the use of such methods the physiotherapy department, still based in its original premises had sought to keep abreast of the latest advances in its field and the skills of the staff had greatly widened; but their basic concern to help in the fullest possible rehabilitation of each patient remained unchanged.

Speech Therapists

In Britain the profession of speech therapy—the assessment and treatment of disorders of communication—is about fifty years old. It began to be organised in the 1930s, the first school of speech therapy having been opened in London in 1929 and the first in Scotland, in Glasgow in 1935. Two professional organisations founded at about that time merged, in 1945, to become the College of Speech Therapists, the profession's controlling body.

The first annual report of the Royal Infirmary Board of Management to contain a section describing the work of their speech therapy department was that for 1972-73 (the Board's last report); but that does not mean that speech therapy had not been practised earlier in the Infirmary—it had. The insertion, then, of a separate section dealing with it was prompted, as the report itself records, by 'the recent publication of the Government enquiry into speech therapy services and the subsequent upsurge of interest in the profession'. The government report to which that was a reference was the *Quirk Report* issued in 1972 by a committee under the chairmanship of Professor Randolph Quirk, Professor of Linguistics (later Vice-Chancellor) of the University of London, who had been appointed to consider for England, Wales and Scotland the need for and role of speech therapy in the fields of education and medicine.

Two sentences in that report which may well have caught the interest of the Board of Management were the following, under the heading of 'Wartime Developments': 'Professor Norman Dott, neuro-surgeon at the Royal Infirmary, Edinburgh established an effective rehabilitation team for neurosurgical cases at the Bangour Head Injuries Unit, near Edinburgh. The speech therapist appointed to this team was the first full-time speech therapist in the hospital service.' After the war, the speech therapist in that team continued to work with Norman Dott, thus becoming the first full-time speech therapist in the Infirmary. For about twenty years the Infirmary's speech therapist continued to be based in Ward 20, dealing mainly with patients whose powers of speech had been impaired by brain injury or other neurological defects. So far as time permitted, she was available also to work with patients from other Infirmary departments.

In the mid-1960s the speech therapist became much involved in the work of the Ear, Nose and Throat Department where Dr. Malcolm Farquharson, in collaboration with the University Linguistics Department, was engaged in research

Q

into the causes of certain speech defects. A second speech therapist was appointed and the Board's Report for 1972-73 described their work as it had then developed as follows:

> Despite its origins in the Department of Surgical Neurology and the very great interest shown by them in it, the Speech Therapy Department is now housed in the Voice and Speech Disorders Clinic in the Department of Otolaryngology, with two full-time therapists assessing and treating in-patients and out-patients suffering from any type of disorder of communication. Patients are referred from the surgical neurology department, the medical neurology department, from medical wards and from ear, nose and throat out-patient and in-patient departments as well as from general practitioners. The volume of work is increasing enormously as more emphasis is being laid on rehabilitation and as the wide scope of speech therapy is being slowly recognised to include all aspects of disorders of communication.

By then, the speech therapy unit had become an autonomous department, no longer incorporated in either the surgical neurology or the ear, nose and throat departments. After re-organisation in 1974, the department, consisting of senior therapist and one other qualified therapist became a branch of the co-ordinated speech therapy service of the Lothian area. None too soon, if one may judge from the description of their work quoted above, the staff was increased, in 1976, from two to four. It then became possible for them to undertake regular work for the oral surgery department, bringing help to patients whose jaws, palate and other organs used in speaking had been damaged by injury or disease.

The Senior Speech Therapist who had been appointed in 1971 (Mrs. M. McIntosh) and who is the present holder of the post, became responsible also for work at the Western General Hospital. As part of their out-patient work the speech therapists in the Infirmary became participants in lively and effective 'stammering groups' designed to help those afflicted in that way to overcome their impediment. Increasingly, as in so many other branches of the Infirmary's work, co-ordination and joint action became normal procedure, with valuable results. The speech therapists co-operated with their other para-medical colleagues, especially the physiotherapists and occupational therapists; they collaborated with fellow speech therapists of the community health service and in the educational field, with general practitioners and with social workers. They also joined in multi-disciplinary assessment and monitoring teams, helping to provide, in the words of the Quirk Report, 'not only a diagnosis of the basic disability but also a complete picture of the patient's problems and potential, together with a co-ordinated plan for treatment'.

Occupational Therapists

The Royal Infirmary, being primarily a short-stay hospital, formerly saw little need to employ occupational therapists. Patients, after the acute stages of their illnesses had passed, did not usually remain long enough to benefit from courses of occupational therapy. It was accepted that assessment of ability to manage at home or in other residential accommodation could be done by medical and nursing staff.

When necessary patients could be, and often were, referred to the Astley Ainslie Hospital's rehabilitation clinic. There had been a time, in the late 1940s and early 1950s, when an occupational therapist was employed in the surgical neurology unit, but their employment elsewhere in the Infirmary did not begin until about twenty years later.

It was the introduction in 1970 of special provision for geriatric patients, that brought an occupational therapist back on to the Infirmary scene. Then, in 1977, a small but well-equipped unit was provided on the ground floor of the former ear, nose and throat pavilion. There a senior therapist, three qualified assistants and a part-time helper were installed to assess and treat patients. Three of the therapists undertook responsibility for four medical wards each and also assessed the abilities of elderly patients in surgical wards awaiting discharge. The other therapist and the helper attended to the geriatric wards' patients.

Accommodation within the unit included an 'activities room' to which patients could come to practise occupations designed to improve the use of limbs and fingers and to help those who had suffered strokes to regain co-ordination between brain and limb. Another room was fitted out to simulate living conditions at home, with sink unit, cooker, bed, bath and other appliances. Using them, patients could be encouraged to practise normal household activities, watched and guided by a therapist who could assess whether or not they were able to be discharged from hospital to their homes, to a longer-stay hospital or to a residential home.

The occupational therapists co-operate regularly with their other para-medical colleagues and also participate in multi-disciplinary meetings, including weekly case conferences with geriatricians to consider the abilities of patients more than 65 years old anywhere in the hospital. As with so many innovations, it soon became difficult to understand how the hospital had been able to manage for so many years without the kind of help that occupational therapists are equipped to give.

Chiropodists

This summary of work of para-medical professions in the Infirmary is completed with the chiropodists. Their story starts with the Edinburgh Foot Clinic and School of Chiropody in Newington Road, Edinburgh, the first such clinic and school in Scotland, which was begun by a voluntary organisation in 1924. From the outset it had links with the Infirmary, several of its office-bearers, consultants and teachers being members of the Infirmary's honorary medical staff. From 1948 until 1970, the clinic and school were administered by the Edinburgh Central Hospitals Board of Management, from then until 1974 by the Regional Hospital Board and thereafter by the South Lothian District of the Lothian Health Board. Throughout that Board's area there were by then some 90 chiropodists, most working in the community, in clinics and residential homes and only a few in hospitals.

The chiropody clinic in the Infirmary was started in 1958 with the object of ensuring that skilled foot care appropriate to their special needs would be given to patients suffering from diabetes and peripheral vascular disease for whom, if such care is not given, the danger of gangrene developing is increased. For that reason the clinic was accommodated within the diabetic out-patient department. It was staffed by one chiropodist, Mr. R. S. Paterson, MChS, SRCh, who was then 'on loan' from the Edinburgh Foot Clinic. In the first year of operation of the new clinic he gave 3,288 treatments to 396 patients of whom 266 were sufferers from diabetes. In 1963, he was joined by a second chiropodist, also on loan from the Foot Clinic, and by 1965 the number of treatments had risen to 5,000. Four years later both chiropodists were transferred to the staff of the Infirmary and eventually a third chiropodist was engaged, the three being responsible (in 1982) for about 6,500 treatments annually.

By the nature of their work chiropodists tend to have less need than their other para-medical colleagues for mutual consultation but they work in close association with medical staff concerned not only with diabetes and patients suffering from peripheral vascular disease but also with sufferers from haemophilia and patients in the renal dialysis unit. The clinic was not intended, and is not staffed, to provide a general ward service. Its staff are few in number but, as their work has developed over the years, the help they have given to the departments they serve and the comfort and freedom from serious complications they have brought to patients have been of great value.

Ancillary Services

The staff of the Royal Infirmary and of other hospitals are often described as a 'family'; in this case a very large family with about 1,100 members in 1929 and some 4,000 in 1979. It is scarcely possible to think of any other organisation whose members are so diverse in knowledge, skills and activities as those of a hospital. From surgeon to domestic, from physician to porter, from accountant to catering assistant, administrator to engineer, the range and variety are immense. Each is a link in a chain with the common purpose of serving the patients and if one link weakens, the whole chain may be affected. The contributions to the common cause made by medical, nursing and other professionals have already been described. This section deals with the work of some other groups of staff as it changed during the fifty years covered by this history; and, first, the work of the domestics.

Domestic Services

If anyone should ask why the domestic staff are placed first in this group, the answer is that in the former voluntary hospital days it was judicially declared that the only undertaking required of a hospital board of managers was that they would provide, first (in a striking if inelegant phrase), 'a clean, wholesome sick-house' and, second, a competent staff. Though, after 1948, the managements' legal responsibilities became much wider, the provision of a clean, wholesome hospital continued to be, and remains, one of their prime duties. Only through a well-organised domestic staff fully understanding the importance of their work can management meet that requirement. More, perhaps, than any other section of staff, the domestic workers penetrate into every nook and cranny and any extension to any unit in the hospital brings added work for them.

According to regulations made by the old Board of Managers as published in 1897, it was a duty of the Lady Superintendent of Nurses, as 'Mistress of the Household', to see that the hospital was kept scrupulously clean and, with that end in view, 'to hire, promote, suspend and dismiss the Female Servants'. (The nurses, she could only 'engage, promote and suspend'.) She had at her disposal an 'army' of domestics, many of whom might be seen daily scrubbing and polishing on hands and knees throughout the hospital. Until the 1950s almost all ward floors were still of wood with no other covering and corridors, except the main surgical one, still had their original bare stone floors. The toil involved in constantly cleaning these, without modern aids, was immense.

In the 1930s the number of domestics was about 220. Many of them had spent years in the service of the hospital. So, in some cases, had their mothers and grandmothers, because several families cherished a long tradition of work in the Infirmary. A high proportion of the domestic staff, then, were resident—some in attic rooms above wards, others in part of the Red Home and, later, some in the former Simpson Memorial Maternity Hospital. Their welfare and their conduct, on duty and off, were carefully watched over, something deemed necessary when many of the younger wardmaids were far from their homes in the Highlands and other country districts, experiencing their first taste of city life.

The trend towards employment of non-resident staff which accelerated during the 1950s and 1960s meant that such close supervision was relaxed. Although some space was still needed to provide non-resident staff with changing-rooms and lockers, the trend also brought a valuable bonus to the hospital as former residential accommodation became available for use as offices or laboratories and for other purposes.

Until 1971 there was one section of domestic staff who formed a distinct and close-knit group and, if one judges aright, they were proud of that distinction. They were the laundry workers, some fifty in all. The laundry building, near the west entrance gate, had been rebuilt in the 1890s and it extended over part of Lauriston Lane; in 1936 it was again extended and modernised to cope with a growing volume of work. On an upper floor living accommodation was provided for thirty laundry maids, with their own dining-room; and their comings and goings were strictly scrutinised by a Laundry Mistress acting on behalf of the Lady Superintendent. About 1939, however, the employment of resident laundry staff was discontinued. Then, in 1947, a new era opened with the appointment of a male Laundry Manager, experienced in the maintenance of the increasingly mechanised plant as well as in laundry management.

Four years later a Department of Health survey gave 'top marks' to the Infirmary laundry for general efficiency as evinced by its output and the quality of its finished articles. In the years that followed, the need to reduce the heavy labour of laundry work called for the introduction of still more sophisticated and expensive machinery. That led the South-Eastern Regional Hospital Board and other hospital authorities to seek ways of re-organising laundry arrangements by concentrating the work in a smaller number of larger laundries whose through-put would justify the high cost of installing the most modern equipment. As a result, the Royal Infirmary laundry was closed in 1971 by stages and its work, along with that of some other hospitals, was transferred to the Western General Hospital where a new laundry was capable of processing eventually more than six million articles annually, about three million of them for the Royal Infirmary. The transfer, besides achieving a rationalisation of the laundry service, brought to the Infirmary (hard-pressed as ever for space) the added benefit of a large vacant building which was quickly re-occupied for much-needed storage and other purposes. Most important of these was the housing of apparatus for the production, in sterile conditions, of dialysis fluid, the demand for which was growing rapidly.

Meanwhile, in other fields of domestic work, modernisation and mechanisation were taking place. In 1960 supervision of the general domestic work had been allocated to a Domestic Superintendent, at first on the staff of the Lady Superintendent of Nurses, some eight years later directly responsible to the Secretary and Treasurer and after the re-organisation of 1974 responsible to the South Lothian District Domestic Manager. Under the District Manager's control three Domestic Managers organised the provision of domestic services in the Infirmary covering fifteen hours daily (from 7.00 am to 10.00 pm) in three areas—the main buildings, the Simpson Pavilion and the Nurses' Homes. To achieve this a staff of about 700 came to be employed but, as many worked part-time, that figure represents a whole-time equivalent of about 420.

The new district organisation enlarged the opportunity for new standards to be established and the status of domestic work to be raised. Supervisors of the several sections of domestic workers in the Infirmary were encouraged to attend training courses and, through them, staff were made aware of technical aspects of their work to which they may have given little thought before. They learned to understand how their work contributes to the safety of patients by removing possible sources of infection and how best to meet the need for scrupulous cleanliness in areas of highest risk. The introduction of equipment such as heavy-duty vacuum cleaners, scrubbing and polishing machines made day-to-day work lighter but called for a new understanding of the use and maintenance of such machines and also of the kinds of treatment appropriate for the different types of floor-covering and furnishings that were being introduced.

These steps were all designed to increase efficiency and reduce drudgery; but there was at least one long-serving member of staff who distrusted them and continued to scrub and polish her section of the main surgical corridor by her own well-tried 'hands and knees' method. Wisely, her superiors allowed her to do so for the few remaining years until her retiral.

In 1977 a new kind of 'hybrid' appointment was introduced to the Royal Infirmary and other hospitals, designed to help nurses, domestic supervisors and, above all, patients. This was the post of housekeeper/receptionist in wards or groups of wards. The duties were (and are) to receive and welcome patients, putting them at their ease and explaining ward routine. They relieve the nurses by completing any necessary admission documents and with other non-medical, non-nursing tasks; they help patients by distributing and collecting menu-slips, assisting in the service of meals and in other ways; and they co-operate with the domestic supervisors by seeing that stocks of non-medical equipment are maintained for ward use and kept in good order. When it is remembered that, previously, almost all those duties had to be undertaken by nurses in intervals snatched from their main duties, the value of these new functions of the domestic service department is obvious.

House Steward's Department

For four-fifths of the period covered by this history a key figure in the Infirmary was the House Steward, of whom there were three in that time. They were Andrew Whyte (1920-44), Adam S. Thomson (1944-55) and Colin W. Henderson who, having joined the Steward's department as provisions clerk in 1925, was House Steward from 1955 until he retired in 1969, having thus given 44 years service to the department. After his retiral the post of house steward was discontinued and the work transferred to the administrative department and dealt with by a Principal Administrative Officer (Supplies).

An important function of the House Steward was to ensure that every kind of article required in the hospital (with only a few exceptions) would be available when wanted. Some of the articles required changed with changing times and arrangements for obtaining them also changed but the basic requirement to keep the hospital properly supplied and equipped remained the same.

In 1932 a correspondent of a daily paper who had visited the Infirmary wrote: 'Every Scottish woman will envy Mr. Andrew Whyte, for he is a "housekeeper" with a housekeeping allowance of £1,000 a week. . . . Here are some of the things he buys annually for his family of nearly 2,000 people.' There then followed a long list of commodities (including 223,900 lbs of bread, 41,664 lbs of butter and margarine and 37,500 lbs of oatmeal) but what is perhaps of greater interest, now, is the correspondent's reference to gifts which, in those voluntary hospital days, helped to supplement the purchases. 'Mr. Whyte', he continued, 'receives many useful gifts. . . . Women's rural institutes throughout the lowlands and even from as far north as Perth, regularly collect boxes of eggs from farmers and send them along to the Infirmary and last year, in addition, he received in common with other institutions in Edinburgh, a share of all the eggs laid on Sundays by hens on one of Scotland's largest poultry farms.' Very occasionally large gifts came unexpectedly. In November 1947, the Managers' minutes record that the Infirmary was about to receive nearly 12,000 cans of pears, pineapples and chopped carrots, its share of some 1,200,000 cans given to the British Hospitals Association by Mr. H. J. Heinz for distribution to voluntary hospitals, in proportion to their bed-complements— the hospitals to pay the cost of carriage only.

The purchase (or acceptance) of provisions, however, was not the only function of the House Steward—far from it. To give a quick idea of the extent of his duties in the 1930s, here is a paragraph from a paper written in 1935 by Mr. Colin Henderson when he was a clerk in the Steward's office and now quoted with his permission:

> The Steward's Department deals with goods of a very comprehensive
> nature, namely; provisions, furniture, furnishings, beds, bedding,
> bed-linen; napery, uniform, clothing; house coal; cleaning articles;
> stationery, etc . . . The Steward also has charge of the general porters,
> attendants, storemen . . . the upholsterers' shop and, in conjunction with

the Lady Superintendent of Nurses has also to deal with the kitchens and
laundry . . . The total expenditure of the Department, per annum, is
£42,000 or roughly one quarter of the total expenditure of our large
Institution . . . On provisions alone, the annual expenditure is £26,000.
Among the items quoted, one finally disappeared from the shopping list about
1955. It was 'house coal'.

Contracts were placed, on the authority of the Managers, for annual, six-
monthly or shorter periods and an important part of the Steward's duty was to
check deliveries for quantity and quality. He was also expected to check usage and
discourage waste.

So much for pre-National Health Service days. After 1948, with the Infirmary
no longer an independent hospital, a different system was evolved. Joint Committees were formed, to be responsible for placing contracts at regional, area and
board of management levels. Some highly specialised requirements were obtained
under contracts placed nationally by the Department of Health for Scotland.
Some were bought through regional contracts; others, for which local purchasing
was likely to be advantageous, were placed on an 'area' basis to supply several
boards of management. Some items were bought at board of management level
and a very few continued to be obtained by hospitals individually. These arrangements, designed to give the advantage of lower prices for larger purchases, still left
the House Steward with the important responsibilities of ordering goods at the
right time, checking quality and supervising their issue and usage. He also had to
collaborate in preparing specifications for several items; and in the period of many
extensions, adaptations and improvements that filled the years between 1950 and
1970 he and his staff were kept constantly busy in ensuring that furniture and
equipment for the new and extended departments would be on the spot at the right
time; the largest single commitment in that period being the furnishing and
equipping of the Princess Alexandra Eye Pavilion.

Porters

When the Principal Administrative Officer (Supplies) took over the Steward's
functions in 1969, these functions still included overall responsibility for the Porters.
In 1975 that responsibility was brought within the ambit of general administration.
Hospital Porters have many duties to perform, some of which have changed from
time to time but many of which are basic tasks, as essential today as they were half
a century ago. The number of staff required to cover these duties throughout the
Infirmary has varied surprisingly little, remaining around 110 for many years.
This is no doubt because progress, having removed the need for time-consuming
tasks such as coal carrying and disposal of ashes from ward and office fires has also
brought new duties in its wake. An ever growing dependence on scientific tests,
for example, has steadily increased the need for conveyance of specimens, sometimes urgently, from ward to laboratory; and each new department opened has
brought its own requirements for additional portering services.

While on the establishment of the House Steward's department and, since
1969, attached to the deparment of administration, the portering staff have always
formed a distinct unit with a Chief Porter (later designated Head Porter) in

charge. Since 1929, five have held that position. Alexander Strathdee who had been appointed Chief Porter in 1920 retired in 1942 after 42 years service on the portering staff. He was followed by Andrew Johnstone (1942 to 1961), Peter Anderson (1961 to 1972), Charles Moodie (1972 to 1975) and the present Head Porter, Mr. Robert Munro.

An instruction sheet, issued in 1935, contained a list of duties to be done by the Chief Porter or by his Deputy, who was then known as Sergeant Porter, a title appropriate to the tendency towards military style discipline prevailing in those days. The duties listed included, among others:

Attendance at main entrance hall—the main (central) entrance being used then almost exclusively by senior honorary medical staff, by Board members attending meetings and by senior officers;

Attending the Superintendent's and Secretary and Treasurer's private bells—as a kind of major-domo to those officers;

Seeing that the Boardroom is prepared for meetings—this function then included making arrangements for tea to be served, the water for which was boiled on an open fire in the Chief Porter's office;

Keeping roll of patients—this enabled him to direct visitors to the appropriate ward, a service now provided elsewhere.

For these and his other duties the Chief Porter then received 64 shillings (£3.20) weekly with free house (the gate lodge) coal and uniform. As several of his duties were transferred elsewhere, the Head Porter's function became predominantly a supervisory one with responsibility for allocating staff either geographically among wards and the growing number of departments or functionally according to duties—conveyance of linen and other goods to and from wards, taking patients on trolleys, or escorting patients, between ward and X-ray room; taking food trolleys from kitchen to ward and back; and all the other varied and essential functions, pleasant and unpleasant, that fill a porter's days. Until the 1950s these would include for some the making of soft soap for use in wards and the daily filling of lotion bottles from the two large open casks in the basement of the pharmacy.

Members of the portering staff still man the kiosks at the east and west entrances but attendance as 'gate-men' to open the gates at visiting times and on the approach of ambulances and authorised cars became unnecessary when the gates were removed in 1962. That function, however, was soon replaced by the new need for porters to act as car-park attendants supervising the use by permit holders of the severely limited space within the hospital grounds.

Traditionally porters helped to control 'unruly' patients in the Surgical Out-Patient Department, especially on Saturday nights when the treatment of those who indulge unwisely during the evening has always been a matter of regular routine. Sadly, that problem increased during the 1970s, exacerbated by the presence of patients under the influence of drugs and unable to control their own behaviour. In helping to restrain such patients, protecting both patient and staff, the porters allocated to the Accident and Emergency Department continue to play a difficult but necessary role.

For many patients arriving in the Infirmary the porter who pushes their trolley or otherwise lends a helping hand may be the first hospital employee they meet. Then, or later, many an apprehensive patient must have had confidence restored or boosted simply by the cheerful, friendly manner of the portering staff. That is a part of their service to the hospital, no less valuable because it is intangible.

Catering

Little imagination is needed to recognise the size of the problem of catering daily for the Infirmary's populations of about 2,000 (in the 1930s) and nearly 5,000 (in the 1970s)—numbers equalled by the guest and staff lists of very few of the largest hotels. In hospital, too, there are problems with which a hotel does not have to cope. Most of the hospital 'guests' have to be given their meals in bed, some are on special diets, a few have to be spoon-fed; many staff are on night duty and have to have meals at unorthodox hours.

The Infirmary main kitchens from which almost all these needs have to be met are in the old George Watson's Hospital building, immediately below the doctors' residency. Though perhaps not the most desirable position from the residents' point of view, they are just about as centrally placed as they could be which is important when food has to be delivered to wards as quickly as possible by trolley.

In the 1930s the kitchens produced what was accurately described as good plain food. For the main meal of the day changes were rung on a limited repertoire of dishes and it was probably possible to tell the day of the week by the content of the main course. The resultant monotony mattered little to short-stay patients but must have begun to pall for those whose stay was longer, as in the medical wards where the *average* stay was then 25 days. In certain wards in those days some items of food might be brought for patients by their visitors, to be cooked in the ward kitchen by the nurses who might also have to prepare light puddings and 'fish custards' for those with gastric complaints. War-time and early post-war rationing restrictions brought additional complications.

Traditionally, the Royal Infirmary was noted for the quality of its breakfast porridge; but, as elsewhere, the taste for that diminished as packaged breakfast cereals appeared on the market in increasing varieties. One statistical comparison will demonstrate the change. In an article in *The Pelican* in 1946 it was stated that the hospital 'porridge pot' each morning contained 112 lbs of oatmeal and 90 gallons of water. The catering department, in 1982, reported that the comparable figures then were: '20 lbs of pinhead oatmeal and 20 gallons of water'.

Towards the end of the first ten years of the National Health Service the Infirmary's kitchens were described as having been well-maintained and to be in no need of any large modification. For patients and staff, it was said, about 2,750,000 meals (not counting teas) were being served annually. But the impression was growing that the whole system should be reviewed and brought more into line with current large-scale catering trends. The Board of Management therefore sought and were successful in obtaining the services of the King Edward's Hospital Fund Catering Advisory Service to survey and report on the arrangements. It was the first time that Service had undertaken such a survey beyond the London area.

Their report, 90 pages long, was received early in 1960. Its comments and main recommendations were summarised in a foreword from which the following points are taken: The standard of feeding for patients was 'below that usually found in teaching hospitals in England'; 'the old-style discipline and service arrangements for staff' and the large number of staff feeding-points (eleven) were noted; the therapeutic diet arrangements were described as 'poor'.

The Report went on to recommend that 'much could be done to improve the position if a well-experienced caterer were appointed to co-ordinate the whole of the catering activities instead of the responsibilities being divided among the "catering officer", the Matron and the Steward' and that 'a good communal restaurant should be provided for all staff, supported by a well-appointed service counter'.

The Board of Management accepted the Report and set about remedying the shortcomings to which it had drawn attention. By 1962 an experienced Catering Officer, Miss E. W. B. Coneghan (afterwards Mrs. Lennon) had been appointed. She was later designated Group Catering Manager and after 1974 she became South Lothian District Catering Manager. In the intervening years many improvements were made in the catering arrangements at the Infirmary. Kitchen equipment was modernised and the catering staff grew, both in ability and number, to meet the rising expectations of patients and staff who were becoming increasingly accustomed to more varied meals in their homes and in hotels at home and abroad.

As explained earlier the Board had long been aware of the need for a new diet kitchen and it was at last provided in 1966. For most patients, almost certainly, the most popular advance was the introduction of menu-slips on which they could show beforehand their preferences as between choices offered for main meals—a welcome improvement on the 'take it or leave it' system of old. The new system was begun in 1962 in the Simpson Pavilion and the reconstructed Corstorphine Hospital; its adoption generally had to be done by stages and everywhere, as it appeared, it was greeted with expressions of pleasure. By 1971 choice was available in every ward of the Infirmary.

Welcome improvements were made in staff dining facilities. Instead of retaining the eleven separate 'staff feeding points' mentioned in the Report it was decided to move away from the old segregated arrangements towards the provision of one central diningroom; and, instead of the traditional system of fixed 'sittings' for meals, to introduce a cafeteria system. The change had to be made by stages. With difficulty and by the exercise of much ingenuity the nurses' diningroom in the central administrative area was altered and enlarged. By 1969 it had been converted into a cafeteria restaurant, comfortably furnished, brightly decorated and capable of serving more than 1,000 people during the main meal period. It soon proved popular and came to be patronised by members of every group and grade of staff.

Welfare Services

For anyone who is ill or injured, expert medical and nursing care however essential, are not the only requirements. Comfort, peace of mind and freedom from worry are also important; in some circumstances they may be even more important.

There is a sense in which all members of the hospital staff, not just the doctors and nurses, may contribute to a patient's well-being simply by the way in which they go about their duties and by showing a cheerful interest in the patients they meet whenever opportunity offers. That is the unofficial informal approach to patient welfare. Its value must be immense but it is unchronicled and impossible to estimate.

There are, however, at least three officially sponsored channels through which the hospital seeks to ensure the patients' welfare and whose activities are recorded. Of longest standing—and that by many years—is the Infirmary Chaplain whose office was created in 1756 when the Infirmary itself was less than thirty years old. Next in length of service are the voluntary organisations among whom the oldest are the Edinburgh Royal Infirmary Samaritan Society who began their benevolent work in 1879, the year in which the present main Infirmary building was first occupied; and the Royal Infirmary Volunteers who, as the Women's Maintenance Council, came into being in 1938 but can legitimately claim descent from the Ladies' Extension Appeal Committee formed in 1929.

The third channel of help to patients and their relatives is that provided by the social workers whose profession has experienced several changes since the Board of Managers, in 1924, first appointed an Almoner to the Infirmary staff. All these groups, despite their different origins and the varying aims and emphases of their work, continue to collaborate in the common purpose of service to the patient. Their histories deserve to be looked at more closely.

The Chaplain

Correctly one should write 'The Chaplains' because, in addition to the Church of Scotland Minister appointed as whole-time Infirmary Chaplain and his whole-time Assistant (first appointed in 1976) there have been, since 1948, a Roman Catholic Chaplain and, since 1960, an Episcopal Chaplain each acting on a paid part-time basis. Previously the pastoral care of Roman Catholics had been under-taken, from 1886, by a succession of Priests from their three City Parishes; and the care of Episcopalians, from 1958, by Chaplains appointed successively from Episcopal Churches in the city. The three Chaplains are helped by voluntary workers in the Chaplaincy office and in the visiting of patients. The Infirmary Chaplain, besides ministering to those who have stated a connection with the Church of Scotland, has responsibility for offering, or arranging for others to offer, pastoral visits to those of religious persuasions not represented in the chaplaincy, or of none.

In the half-century since 1929 there have been five Infirmary Chaplains. The Rev. Thomas C. Macaulay, MA died in 1934 after ten years service. He was succeeded by The Rev. Peter Lockhart, MA (1934-46), The Rev. William B. Taylor, BD (1947-52), The Rev. William Anderson, MA (1953-70) and, since 1970, The Rev. T. Stewart McGregor, MA, BD. Throughout forty of those years the duties and activities of the Chaplains varied little from what had become a pattern of long standing. They visited wards on a regular weekly basis and on other occasions when asked to do so; they saw to it that patients' own ministers, if known, were notified; they arranged Sunday services in the Infirmary Chapel and conducted monthly services there for nurses and, after 1966, also for other members of staff. They organised concerts of sacred music in wards and, occasionally, in a lecture theatre; each Christmas they conducted special services and they took part in other seasonal events. Until 1969 the hospital library came under their wing. Deaconesses of the Church of Scotland helped the Chaplains in their pastoral work and voluntary lady visitors also co-operated by visiting patients, especially on days when wards were not open to other visitors.

It was with a sense of satisfaction that the Chaplains reported, at the end of each year, that they had visited every ward in the Infirmary every week. Their visits gave support and comfort to many of the patients and doubtless each successive Chaplain helped many patients and members of staff in other ways and at other times that are not recorded. Nevertheless, it may be doubted whether an automatic weekly visit to every ward is the best way of using the Chaplain's time and the general impression that is gained from the annual reports is of an unchanging and unchangeable routine.

In 1970, however, things did change. From then on the impression of the Chaplaincy that emerges is of a department taking a full and active part in the life of the hospital. What happened was in keeping with the theme which, as we have seen, ran through the whole story of the nineteen-sixties; the theme of fuller and closer collaboration among departments and with the University—but, this time, with the University Faculty of Divinity. The new Chaplain, The Rev. T. Stewart McGregor, inducted in April 1970, was also appointed to a part-time lectureship in the University.

There was thus added to the Chaplain's duties the responsibility, in consultation with other hospital staff, for arranging and supervising practical experience in hospital pastoral work for students of divinity. From this he gained the benefit that senior students were sometimes able to act as his assistants by visiting some patients on his behalf. The additional functions of the Chaplain did not stop there. Arrangements were also made for him—and his colleagues—to take part in the teaching of student nurses by giving lectures and conducting seminars on religious, moral and ethical questions relevant to their work. He began also to participate in programmes of teaching for medical students and in the training of hospital social workers and to arrange inter-disciplinary discussions among members of different professions within the hospital.

Besides these new activities it was essential that the old duties of the Chaplain should continue. Because of the time occupied by the Chaplain's new duties a system of priorities had to be adopted. Instead of making a routine visit to every ward every week it was decided that the Chaplain would visit as a priority (i) those patients who, either on admission or later, asked to see him and (ii) those whom he was asked to visit either by a member of the ward staff or hospital social worker or by the patient's own minister or a relative. In the time available after these priorities had been met, wards would be visited, priority among such visits being given to the geriatric wards where visits are specially appreciated and to some of the special care units. To speed response to requests the Chaplain was provided with a pocket 'bleep'.

For the new system to be effective, co-operation by other groups of hospital staff was all important. Attention to requests to see the Chaplain made by patients at the time of admission was speeded up after 1975 when computer 'print-outs' began to be delivered every morning to the Chaplain's office. These give particulars of every patient admitted during the previous day, including the ward to which each was allocated and the answer given to the question whether a visit by the Chaplain is desired—one way in which the 'impersonal' computer can help to provide a very personal service.

The Edinburgh Royal Infirmary Samaritan Society

The work of this Society, 'the Infirmary Samaritans' who reached their centenary year in 1979, grew out of social conditions very different from those of today. Help for people in need, other than those receiving parish relief or small payments from Friendly Societies, depended wholly on friends and neighbours, often as poor as themselves, and charity organisations. Yet today, the Society find that they still have a role to play, working closely with official social workers.

The Society's work grew out of the benevolence of an Edinburgh lady, Mrs. Elizabeth Cleghorn, widow of Thomas Cleghorn, Sheriff of Argyll who died in 1874. After his death, Mrs. Cleghorn began to take an interest in helping destitute patients in the medical wards of the Infirmary, in Infirmary Street. She visited the wards, distributing clothing and sometimes money to those she described as 'the more needy'. When the burden of her self-imposed task became too great for one individual she wrote to her friends and acquaintances appealing for help 'either in the form of money or readymade clothing'. So many responded to that appeal that, in January 1879, it was decided to create a formal organisation and thus the Edinburgh Royal Infirmary Samaritan Society was born. Its objects were stated as being: 'to assist the families and dependents of patients being breadwinners, to give clothing, travelling expenses or other needful help to patients on leaving the Infirmary, to endeavour to procure work for them and generally to befriend and be of use to them as much as possible'.

As time passed the Society's range was extended, enabling help to be given to patients in any wards instead of medical wards only, and in some other hospitals. Further extensions were made in later years. By 1979 the Objects of the Society, as formally stated, covered help to patients in any Edinburgh hospital, and their families, by giving money, food or clothing, by contributing towards the cost of special diets and extra expenses of convalescence and by assisting in many other ways. The statement still included the words 'and generally to befriend patients and their families'. Despite the extension of the Society's concern to other hospitals their work has always been largely with patients of the Infirmary and so their title has remained unchanged. (The designation 'Royal Infirmary' also helps to distinguish the Society from the 'Telephone Samaritans', the nationwide organisation devoted to helping people who are in despair.)

The Royal Infirmary Samaritans' funds come from subscriptions, gifts, proceeds of appeals, sales and other activities and also from legacies. Soon after the Society was formed they appointed a Lady Superintendent to advise their Committee and ensure that prompt effect was given to their decisions. An almoner was also appointed to visit the wards of the Infirmary and, in consultation with the ward sisters, to identify patients who were in need of help or were likely to need help after returning home. Later, other almoners were appointed and their duties included regular visiting of patients' homes to distribute cash (in the early 1930s the sum given might be five shillings (25p) or seven shillings and sixpence (37½p) weekly for a few weeks) or to arrange other kinds of help.

Guidance, as well as cash, was given to help patients to obtain medical appliances, special foods and medicines prescribed by the hospital doctors. That was of great value, and often essential, in enabling diabetic patients and others receiving dietetic advice to follow the instructions given. Besides providing immediate help, a regular part of the Samaritans' work was to direct patients to other organisations, official and voluntary, to which they or their families might apply for longer-term aid.

A leading light in all this effort was Miss R. Wharton Duff, the Society's principal almoner from 1923 till 1939 and, thereafter, Superintendent of Clothing until her death in 1961. She rarely took a holiday and then only for less than a week, so that she would never miss the regular meetings of the Samaritans' Committee! She was a familiar figure, cycling about Edinburgh on the Society's business 'with her skirt hitched up and attached to her boots in a completely individual way'—according to the Society's centenary booklet, issued in 1979.

Another office-bearer who favoured the bicycle as a means of transport was Mr. W. J. ('Pussy') Stuart, Surgeon-in-Ordinary from 1923 till 1937 and thereafter Consulting Surgeon, a much-loved figure in the Infirmary and also among the Samaritans whom he served, as Vice-Chairman and Chairman, for sixteen years until his death in 1959. Long service has been an attribute of the Society's office-bearers. Sir Robert Maconochie, a distinguished lawyer, joined their Committee in 1921 and served in several capacities, retiring as President, after forty years, in 1961. Even that record, however, was bettered by Mr. Alexander Morrison, CA, who was the Society's Treasurer for 57 years—from 1898 to 1955.

As we have seen, the almoners of the Samaritan Society concerned themselves with in-patients and their welfare after leaving hospital. As will shortly be explained, the Managers of the Infirmary in 1923 began to employ their own almoners to work on behalf of out-patients. The two groups worked thus in parallel for twenty-four years. Then, in 1947, the Samaritans who were employing two qualified almoners (and one unqualified lady who left about this time) began to find that the almoners' nationally-negotiated salaries were taking too high a proportion of the Society's income. They therefore asked whether the Infirmary Board would relieve them of payment of these salaries.

For some time the Infirmary's Head Almoner had been advocating, unsuccessfully, the merging of the two agencies of social work if only to remove the anomaly whereby the social service support of an in-patient who became an out-patient (and vice-versa) had to be transferred from one group to the other. So, after some negotiation, it was decided that in January 1948 the Society's two almoners would be transferred to work as senior almoners for the benefit of both in-patients and out-patients with the Head Almoner and her two assistants on the Infirmary's social service staff. The Samaritan Society would go on collecting clothing and making monetary grants to necessitous patients, at the request of the almoners.

When, six months later, the National Health Service came into being the Samaritans continued as a voluntary organisation administering their own funds. They still do so, their Committee of Management meeting regularly with the hospital social work staff in consultation with whom they make grants for the benefit of patients and their families to tide them over the time-lag that often occurs before official help can be given, and sometimes to provide for their welfare in ways not covered by statutory rules and regulations.

Infirmary Social Work Service

As we have seen, organised social work for the benefit of Infirmary in-patients was begun by the voluntary Samaritan Society in 1879. That was sixteen years before the Royal Free Hospital in London appointed the first official hospital almoner in Britain. Twenty-nine years after that, in 1924, the Royal Infirmary Managers decided to establish their own Social Service Department. The initiative which led them to do so had come from another voluntary organisation, the University of Edinburgh Settlement Association, whose objects include the promotion, especially among University students and staff, of interest in social problems and in educational and social work in the community.

In 1923 permission was given to the University Settlement to commence, through their lady visitors, social service work among the medical out-patients by following up necessitous cases at their homes, providing them where necessary with medicine or special nourishment, securing their admission to convalescent or rest homes or improving from the health point of view the conditions under which they were living. This work proved to be so beneficial and was so much appreciated by the members of the Honorary Staff that the Managers of the Infirmary adopted a scheme to be linked with that of the Samaritans which involved the appointment by the Infirmary of a Principal Lady Almoner with a staff of assistants, at an annual expenditure of £500.

The Principal Lady Almoner first appointed, Miss E. A. Callender, remained for only a few years. Her successor, Miss H. Y. Watt who was appointed in 1930, continued in office for thirty years. She began with a staff of two fully-trained almoners, one assistant and a part-time worker attached to the mental health clinic. Already the Department had begun to participate in training, with students from the University School of Social Study and from the Institute of Hospital Almoners in London working in the Infirmary as part of their study programme.

In her report for the year 1930-31, Miss Watt recorded that 2,500 patients had been referred to her Department. With some help from voluntary workers nearly 2,300 home visits had been made and there had been 7,700 interviews in the almoners' office. (In the same year the Samaritans dealt with 956 patients and made 596 visits.) The Department had no funds of their own and much of their work consisted of identifying needs and then seeking help from, or referring patients to, organisations able to supply these needs.

The report included reference to a new development during the year which had added to the almoners' duties and must also have changed their image in the

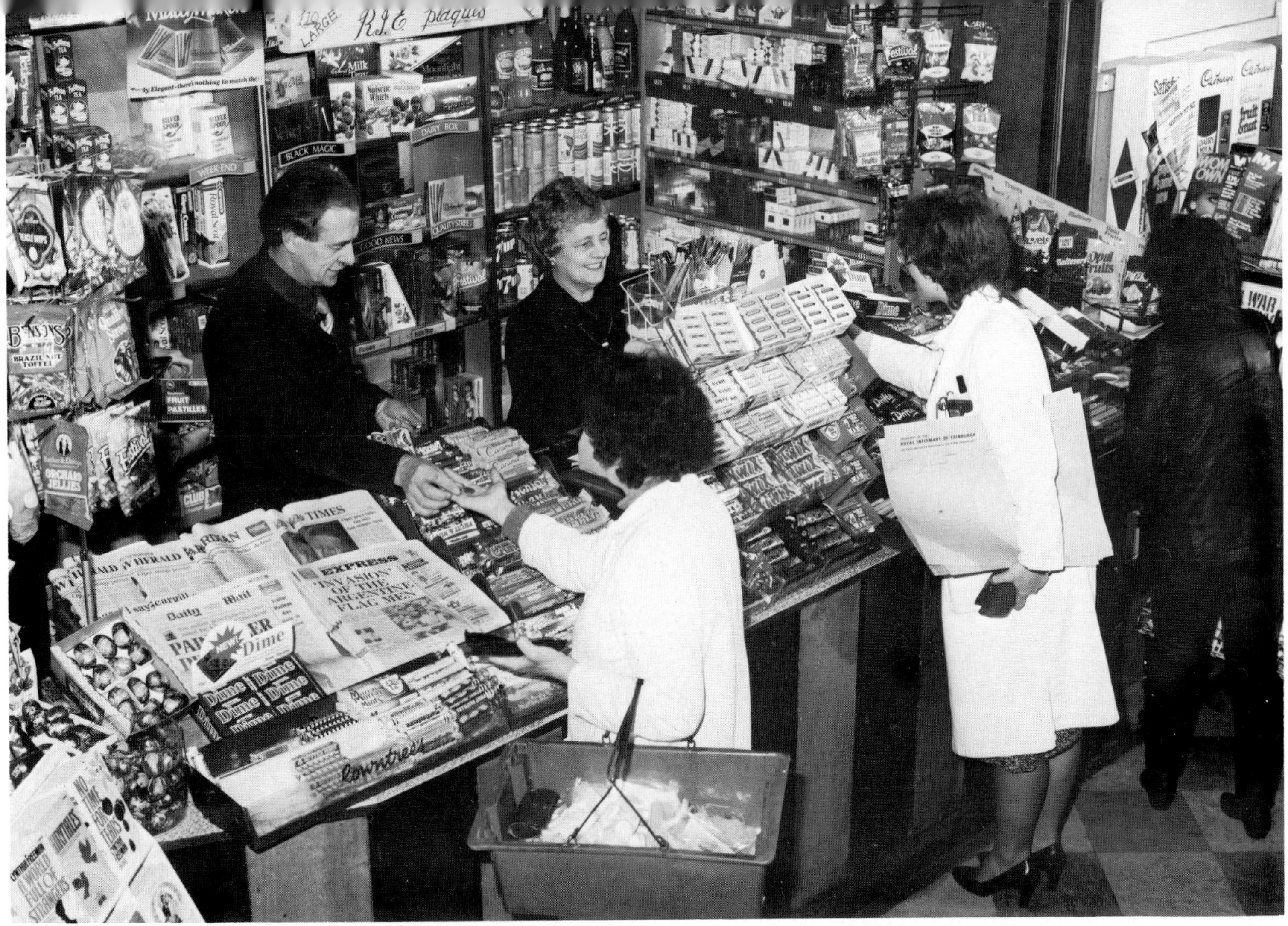

Plate 33   The Royal Infirmary Shop in the lower surgical corridor, opened in 1959

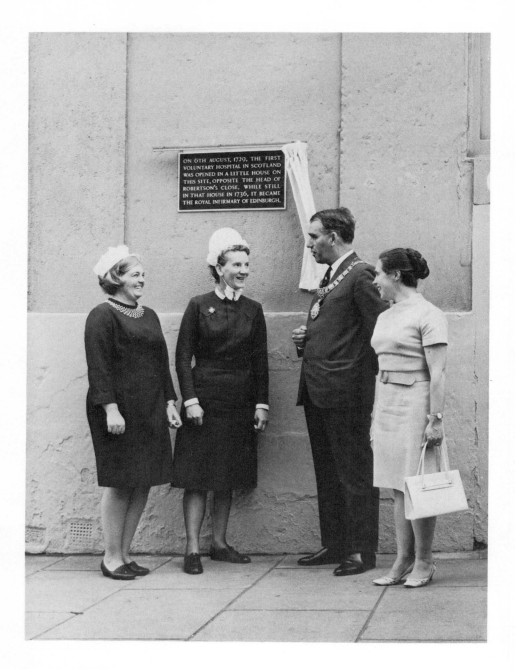

Plate 34   Identifying the site of 'The Little House', the first Royal Infirmary of Edinburgh, 1729

The plaque has just been unveiled by the Rt. Hon. James McKay, Lord Provost of Edinburgh on 12 August, 1969. With him are (left to right) Miss Margaret G. Auld, Matron, Simpson Memorial Maternity Pavilion (afterwards Chief Nursing Officer, Scotland), Miss Muriel F. Cullen, Lady Superintendent of Nurses and Mrs. Patricia Eaves-Walton, Royal Infirmary Archivist.

eyes of some patients. It arose from a decision by the Board of Managers that, as well as seeking to help patients and relieve them from worry during illness and convalescence, the almoners should try to recover from patients who were able to pay, or from a charitable fund, all or part of the cost of items supplied by the Infirmary for their use at home. The report added that adoption of the practice had already resulted in a 'fair sum' being recovered. The amounts collected in this way were not recorded in the reports till 1938 when the sum was £159, a 'considerable increase' over the previous year, and 1939 when £250 was obtained. At that time the Almoners were also expected to encourage patients whose circumstances might enable them to do so, to make donations, however small, to the funds of the Infirmary. The dual role of the almoner as bringer of help with one hand and assessor and collector of payments with the other, though new in the Infirmary was not new elsewhere, especially in hospitals in which fees were charged subject to abatement in necessitous cases. They were roles which the almoners' profession had had to master together from the outset. Most played the two parts with skill and discretion until 1948 when the National Health Service left them free to concentrate on their primary purpose of seeking to promote the patients' welfare.

When the Simpson Memorial Maternity Pavilion was opened in the Spring of 1939, there was statutory authority to charge fees there subject to abatement when necessary. To deal with these and generally look after the patients' welfare, an additional almoner was appointed by the Infirmary and allocated to the Pavilion. Before the end of her first year's work it was recorded that assessment and collection of fees took up the greater part of her time and that she had been able to do only a 'certain amount' of social work. Much, it was said, needed to be done to develop that work and, a year later, a second almoner was appointed to the Maternity Pavilion.

Wartime conditions produced some interesting results from the point of view of the hospital's Social Service Department. In 1942 the almoners reported that, while previously most patients referred to them had been unemployed before becoming ill, it was now unusual for a patient to have been out of work and, in 1944, 'speaking generally, patients are much better off than in pre-war times and in many cases advice is all that is necessary'. A year later they reported 'The general health of patients has greatly improved. It is now rare to find the type of patient, all too common in the pre-war days of mass unemployment, suffering from malnutrition and who, while not requiring active hospital treatment, were in great need of a long period in a convalescent home . . .' The need still existed, however, for convalescence as a follow-up to active treatment and for homes to which aged and chronic sick patients could be moved. Several such homes had closed and almoners were finding it increasingly difficult to obtain places in those that remained. As a result, hospital beds needed for acute cases were blocked and waiting-lists grew.

One problem which dominated almoners' reports for years after the war was the housing shortage. Because of overcrowding and insanitary conditions many patients who could otherwise have gone home to recuperate had to remain in hospital while almoners spent much time trying to persuade housing authorities to allocate suitable houses to patients or their families; but there were simply not

R

enough houses. The shortage greatly exacerbated the already serious problem facing the almoners of the Simpson Pavilion during the post-war 'bulge' in the birth rate. The head almoner there reported in 1947 that, except for emergency admissions, the available accommodation was usually booked six months ahead, that during 1946, 1,518 applications had had to be refused compared with 715 the year before and that these figures took no account of the many women who, knowing the position, made no application. It had even been necessary to refuse admission to patients whose home circumstances were appalling. After quoting examples of some of the worst conditions she had found (including three couples and two children living in one room) she wrote: 'Even although a woman may be admitted to hospital for her confinement, it is terrible to have to send new-born babies back to such conditions, but many cases only slightly better have had to be refused a hospital booking even for the confinement'.

Practical training of student almoners at the Infirmary had come to an end after 1939 and it was not resumed after the war, except in the Simpson Pavilion, partly because the former division of work between Infirmary and Samaritan almoners had been thought not to be conducive to comprehensive training. In 1954 it was noted that the Institute of Hospital Almoners had decided to leave the selection, teaching and supervision of such students in Edinburgh to the University who proposed to arrange practical training only at the Western General Hospital and the Simpson Pavilion. This did not please the Infirmary Board of Management who thought it 'strange and a matter for enquiry that a great teaching hospital like the Infirmary which can train doctors, nurses, physiotherapists, radiographers etc., should be unable to train hospital almoners'. So, after some negotiation, it was agreed that the practical training of students should be resumed in the main hospital. Accommodation for the Social Services Department had had to be moved from time to time and had always been inadequate. As an essential requirement for training, it was decided to form a students' unit by converting one of two former air-raid shelters on the Lauriston Place boundary of the hospital. It was opened in October 1956 when four students began their training.

In 1960 Miss Watt retired as Head Almoner and her place was taken by Miss M. R. P. Andrews, AMIA. During the 1950s there had been a shortage of trained almoners but by this time the position had improved and, during 1961, the establishment was increased to ten almoners, although this was still regarded as insufficient, especially as the Department had to serve other hospitals in the Group. Referrals to the Department, mostly from Ward Sisters, were being received at an average rate of 230 each month, a total of 2,770 in the year. Many required only brief interviews, for advice and answers to questions. Many were helped by arranging for the supply of appliances, for the attendance of District Nurses or for the provision by the local authority of meals-on-wheels or home helps to enable them to return to their own homes. Aid to others, involving help in making domestic arrangements or resolving family or financial difficulties, could be much more time-consuming. In 1963 it was reported that some seventy per cent of the problems met with were emotional or environmental in origin and that in twenty-five per cent of cases contact with the patient had to be maintained for at least six months.

Although some grants of money were (and are) still made, the almoner's time was increasingly spent in counselling and other forms of social work. As their professional skills had developed over the years to embrace a widening knowledge of human behaviour and reaction to stress they had come, gradually, to be accepted as members of a team, with medical, nursing and other staff, in the overall care of the patient. They were concerned, now, not only with the poorest patients, but with any patient for whom help with a personal or other problem might contribute to recovery or to general well-being. This was a trend throughout the country and it was formally recognised in 1965 when the out-dated name 'almoners' was changed to 'medical social workers' and their professional body became the Institute of Medical Social Workers.

In 1966 training facilities for medical social workers in the Infirmary were increased by the conversion for that purpose of the second former air-raid shelter beside Lauriston Place. By 1968 there were 25 students in training. Not all were prospective medical social workers though all wished to have experience of work in hospital. That was the year in which the Social Work (Scotland) Act required the three separate branches of social work—welfare, child care and probation work (but not yet hospital social workers)—to be combined in one co-ordinated social work department, an arrangement which came into effect late in 1969.

The Infirmary Report for 1968-69 recorded that there had been a fall of 300 (from 4,080 to 3,780) in the number of patients referred by doctors and others to the medical social workers during the year. The reduction was attributed in part to the fact that many more local authority social workers were following up those of their 'clients' who became hospital patients by visiting them in hospital, thereby avoiding duplication of interviewing and time-consuming transfers of information from medical to community social worker. This trend provided a welcome lessening of pressure on the medical social workers although the demand on their services still continued to be greater than could be fully met by the available staff. It reflected a growing awareness, to which the Infirmary Board drew attention in their report for 1971-72, that a hospital patient should be seen as part of a family network and not just as an individual.

It was a trend, also, that foreshadowed an important organisational change introduced in May 1975 when hospital social workers were transferred to local authorities, the Infirmary's medical social workers becoming members of staff of the Lothian Regional Council's Social Work Department. That Department then became responsible for providing social services for patients in the Infirmary and all other hospitals in the Region. This enabled the medical social workers based in the Infirmary to have direct and immediate access to all the resources of the Social Work Department, including advice from experts in special fields, provision of care for single-parent children while the parent was in hospital and of accommodation (when available) for old people not requiring continuing hospital care.

In 1976, twelve social workers (increased to eighteen by 1979) were attached to the Royal Infirmary, with responsibility also for the Simpson Pavilion, Chalmers Hospital and the Elsie Inglis Memorial Maternity Hospital. The Lothian Health Board continued to be responsible for their accommodation and office services, managerial control remaining with the Principal Social Worker in the

Infirmary, under the Regional Director of Social Work. Within the Infirmary some social workers were thereafter attached to particular units, enabling them to participate with doctors, nurses and others as regular members of unit teams and to attend ward meetings. Their concern, in co-operation with their colleagues working in the community, was, as before, to relieve the patient of worry that might retard recovery and to assist patient and family to re-adjust to normal life— or, in some cases, to adjust to a changed pattern of life.

Royal Infirmary Volunteers

Today there are about 200 names on the roll of Royal Infirmary Volunteers who give their services freely in a variety of ways to provide amenities for patients and their visitors and to help in promoting the patients' welfare and the smooth running of several branches of the hospital's work. Almost all the volunteers are women and the majority are middle-aged or older. This is partly because they are the group most available during normal working hours and partly because of the kind of voluntary work they are mainly called upon to do. But it also has roots in the origin and history of the Volunteers.

In 1929 when the appeal for funds for extension of the Infirmary was about to be launched, a Ladies' Extension Appeal Committee was formed and for the next ten years they helped in many ways to raise money for the extension fund. When the Simpson Pavilion and the Florence Nightingale Nurses Home were nearing completion in 1938, the fund was closed but members of the Ladies' Extension Committee were reluctant to end their work for the Infirmary. So, on the invitation of the Board, a new organisation was formed 'to continue to work for the maintenance of the Infirmary'. It was named 'The Women's Maintenance Council'. Many members of the former Committee joined the Council and the Countess of Minto, who had been Chairman of the Committee since 1937, was again appointed Chairman, an office she continued to hold until 1971. Mrs. A. D. Stewart, wife of the Superintendent, became Hon. Secretary.

The objects of the new Council were: 'to interest women in the work of the Royal Infirmary and the Simpson Memorial Maternity Pavilion; to further that interest by organising workers willing to give personal service; and to provide garments and linen for use in the wards and theatres'. The five types of membership, and the annual subscriptions then were: Honorary Member 10/- (50p); Member 5/- (25p) and a gift of one garment; Guild Member 2/6d (12½p) and a gift of one garment; Associate Member 1/- (5p); Sewing Member (no subscription). An urgent task at the outset was to help to equip the new Simpson Pavilion with 'literally hundreds of babies' vests' and, to this end, it appears that members were at first asked to give two vests instead of the prescribed 'one garment'.

A workroom was established in the semi-basement under Ward 34 in the Jubilee Pavilion and there a large group of members and their friends met daily from 10 a.m. till 5 p.m., on three nights weekly till 9 p.m. and on Sunday afternoons, sorting and cutting and sewing to make and repair garments and linen articles for use in wards and theatres. With the prospect and then the actuality of war, there developed an urgent demand for dressings and bandages and the workroom ladies turned their hands to producing these in great numbers. The extent of this work is described in the Council's Report issued at the end of 1940, which also contains a reference to the use of a commodity unlikely to be in demand for surgical dressings today:

> During the ten months to September 1940, 9,050 garments and articles for Theatre use have been made and 149,772 swabs and dressings. Owing to the difficulty of procuring plaster bandages and their increased cost, these are now being made in the work-room; at present about forty dozen of these are made and used every week. In the last three months of the year the following materials were used for swabs, dressings and plaster bandages: 25,050 yards of gauze, 4,180 yards of plaster muslin (this making about 25,080 yards of bandage) and one ton of Plaster of Paris.
>
> Sphagnum Moss is being largely used to save cotton wool and an average of about fifty dozen pads of this material are made and used daily in the Royal Infirmary and Simpson Maternity Pavilion. The moss has been sent in from all parts of the country; one parcel even coming all the way from Canada . . .

The work-room long continued to be the Maintenance Council's principal source of help to the hospital. Then, gradually, as the availability of pre-packed goods increased, the demand for the work-room's products diminished. This was perhaps fortunate because, over the same period, volunteers willing to spend many hours with a sewing machine were becoming fewer. To-day a smaller band of workers continue making, mending, folding and otherwise preparing various articles for use in wards and theatres, providing a service that is still of value.

When the National Health Service began in 1948 there was some brief doubt as to whether the Council's work should continue or whether such voluntary work might be frowned upon by the authorities who had set their face against the new Service making appeals for money. It was quickly agreed, however, that this was different and that even in a fully organised State service there would still be room for the kind of personal touches and helping hands that voluntary workers could contribute. So the Women's Maintenance Council continued and went from strength to strength. In November 1959 the Council celebrated their 21st birthday with a tea-party attended by about 200 people at which HRH The Duchess of Gloucester congratulated the Volunteers on the work they were doing and then ceremoniously cut their birthday cake.

During those 21 years the most important activity of the Council, apart from that of the work-room, had been the running of a canteen. That began in 1943 when they took over responsibility for a small buffet, in an alcove off the main surgical corridor known as 'the hole in the wall', on the withdrawal of the commercial bakery firm who had previously run it. There they began to serve light meals to out-patients and their friends. Three years later the canteen was moved to rather more spacious accommodation, still in the surgical house. Finally, in 1958, it was transferred to the red-brick building near the foot of the west entrance road which had recently been vacated by the nurses' training unit. The building was converted into a well-equipped cafeteria with seats for 70 customers. Associated with the canteen, a 'tea-trolley service' to out-patient departments was begun; it still continues, with each trolley manned by two volunteers paying daily visits to out-patient departments and other units.

In November 1959, at the request of the Board of Management, the Women's Maintenance Council opened a shop in the lower surgical corridor for the sale of newspapers, books, confectionery, soft drinks and other items. A few years earlier the demand by patients for such facilities had led to the provision by the Maintenance Council, of trolleys with items for sale which were taken from ward to ward by volunteers. This service continued, the trolleys becoming mobile branches of the main shop.

The shop is not far from the hospital's branch Post Office, opened by the GPO in 1959 and the Royal Infirmary Branch of the Royal Bank of Scotland. The Bank was opened, also in 1959, at the request of the Board, primarily to facilitate payment by banker's order of salaries of nurses and other staff but it soon began to provide general banking services. The trio—Post Office, Bank and Hospital Shop— with their steady stream of customers, give almost a town shopping centre atmosphere to that part of the surgical house. They are a reminder that the Infirmary's population of staff and patients is nearly 5,000 and larger than that of many a small town.

The success of the first shop was such that, in 1966, another was opened, this time in the Simpson Pavilion. In 1969 a cafeteria was provided in the newly opened Eye Pavilion. These activities—shops and cafeterias—are run on business lines, by professional managers and paid staff, with some help from volunteers. In most years they have been able to hand over a surplus to add to the Women's Maintenance Council's and Volunteers' funds.

From these funds, in 1969, a gift of £2,000 was made to the Board of Management towards the cost of building a children's playroom close to the Simpson Pavilion. The playroom, for which furniture and toys were given by members of the public, is staffed by volunteers in whose care young children can play in safety while their mothers attend clinics.

Since 1970, the volunteers have been organised from an office in the former chief porter's lodge at the central entrance gate in Lauriston Place. Long out of use as a dwelling-house, the lodge had been used for storage and for a variety of other purposes before being made available to the Women's Maintenance Council. From that office, a full-time organiser, in consultation with honorary group conveners, recruits persons willing to give service to the hospital and allocates them to groups undertaking the kind of work for which they have expressed a preference or may have shown a special aptitude. Besides the members who provide the services already described, there are others who:

> —staff the enquiry office established in 1970 in the surgical house and the
> enquiry office in the Princess Alexandra Eye Pavilion;
> —give clerical assistance in a few departments including the office of the
> Chaplain;
> —provide some non-nursing help in wards—a service, however for which
> the need diminished as ward secretaries came to be appointed after 1973;
> —undertake various duties for which a temporary need may have arisen.

A welcome trend was recorded in the Council's report for 1970-71. In it they noted 'this year has been especially noteworthy for the contribution made by young people. Three schools seconded pupils for voluntary service. Very many gave voluntarily of their holiday time to work in hospital, 36 girls being particularly helpful with holiday relief during the summer vacation.' Since then, young people have continued to supplement the work of the regular volunteers. Throughout the years only a few men ever enrolled for voluntary work among the ranks of the Women's Maintenance Council. With the advent of the young volunteers and, possibly, in the hope that more men might be encouraged to join, it was decided in 1976 to change the name of the Council to 'The Royal Infirmary of Edinburgh Volunteers'.

The Hospital Library

The provision of books and magazines for patients has long been recognised as a worth-while welfare service and one that may often have a therapeutic value. Traditionally the library service in the Infirmary was provided by the Chaplain's Department, being looked after mainly by a lady assistant. For the year 1929-30 the Chaplain reported: 'The library is well-stocked with books, but gifts of new and popular books, magazines, children's papers, gramophone records etc. are always acceptable . . . The Scottish *Monthly Visitor* Tract Society is thanked most heartily for their ever welcome monthly gift of Tracts.' His reference to gramophone records is a reminder that, before the arrival of radio in the wards in 1934, some had a gramophone to provide occasional entertainment; the fact that the stock of reading-matter depended almost entirely on gifts meant that the librarian had little control over the subject-matter or quality of the books available; and the Chaplain's final sentence reflects the idea that often prevailed that literature of an 'improving' nature was particularly suitable for invalids.

The last of the Chaplain's librarians, Miss E. Campbell, served the library devotedly and well for 39 years—from 1930 until her retiral in 1969. By that time there were 10,000 books in stock and the number issued to patients or placed in ward bookcases by her during the year was reported as being 12,000. Maintaining these arrangements with very little help must have been a formidable task made even more so in the 1960s by the fact that, to make room for alterations and reorganisation of other departments, the library, with its 10,000 books had more than once to be moved from one location to another.

By 1970 there was a growing awareness of the value of a hospital library service and of the need for professional management if its full value was to be achieved. So the Chaplain was relieved of responsibility for the Infirmary Library which became a separate department of the hospital under the charge of a professionally qualified Librarian with, later, a qualified assistant.

The Librarian's first task was then to 'weed' the library stock, removing books in poor condition, those which had been only of ephemeral interest and those which, because of changing tastes, were unlikely to be in demand. Eventually the stock was reduced to under 6,000 volumes; they were classified and arranged in accordance with modern library practice and the library premises were attractively set out and furnished to encourage ambulant patients to visit and select books from its shelves—in itself a valuable therapeutic exercise.

For many years grants had been made from the hospital's Comforts Fund to enable some books to be bought. After 1970, annual grants were made by the Board of Management (later, by the Lothian Health Board). These increased from £150 in the first year to £1,700 in 1980—a welcome increase but, in real terms, much smaller than it seems.

In the work of re-organisation the Librarian had the help of Volunteers. Since then, a group of up to 20 Volunteers have manned the Library trolleys, each trolley carrying some 80 books, which they take twice weekly to every ward in the main hospital and once weekly to the Simpson Pavilion.

8

History Remembered

Research and Celebration

Among members of the Royal Infirmary staff, in whatever profession or capacity they may serve, and among Edinburgh people generally, pride in their famous hospital is often expressed through the interest they take in its long history. During the 1960s that interest was quickened by the knowledge that plans were afoot to demolish the old, familiar buildings and replace them by a new hospital in modern form which would be unlikely to arouse any similar aura of interest and affection until, perhaps, a generation had passed. It was also recognised that the buildings were certain to contain, in wards, offices, store-rooms and cupboards, valuable records in the form of reports and correspondence of medical personalities and about incidents which, whether important in themselves or not, are the stuff of which social history and medical history are made. It was well known that successive Lady Superintendents of Nurses had carefully preserved letters which Florence Nightingale had written to her 'dear nurses of the Infirmary'. There might well be other interesting documents, less well cared for or even unnoticed which could disappear for ever in the clearance preceding demolition.

Infirmary Archivist

It was, therefore, proposed to appoint an official Archivist under whose guidance such records and memorabilia could be collected, recorded and preserved. Not everyone was convinced of the need for such an officer but, eventually, authority was given for the appointment of a qualified Archivist, on a part-time basis, whose salary would be met from endowment funds.

The Infirmary's first Archivist took up her appointment in September 1967 and was provided with an office and limited storage accommodation at No. 43 Chalmers Street (later transferred to No. 23). She was Mrs. Patricia Eaves-Walton, an honours graduate in history of Edinburgh University, who had worked for the Scots Ancestry Research Society and had specialised in the tracing, translation and interpretation of documents.

The appointment quickly proved its worth. Within a year it was reported that 'the majority of the administrative records of the Infirmary earlier in date than 1900 which, with very few exceptions, have survived in good condition are now being kept in the record room and others are being traced . . . Approximately 580 accessions have been noted so far and over 600 volumes of records after 1900, previously kept in unsuitable conditions, have been brought over. Progress has been made in listing and classifying, and a programme of binding and repairs to the volumes has been started.' (These records, of course, did not include clinical records which were, and are, the concern of the Medical Records Officer.) The report also expressed the Board's appreciation of gifts received of books, photographs and other articles of historic interest related to the Infirmary.

Between August and October 1968 an exhibition of over 100 items selected from the collection was held in the National Library of Scotland and was seen by more than 5,000 visitors. The items on view ranged from a Treasurer's account book of 1729 showing the names of all who had contributed to the first £2,000 raised for the Infirmary to 19th and early 20th century photographs of wards and operating theatres and of doctors, nurses, porters and other staff of those days.

It soon became clear that the newly-appointed Archivist's interest in the Infirmary and in medical history went beyond the collection, preservation and display of documents and other items. She undertook original research into aspects of the Infirmary's past and gave valuable help to others preparing lectures or learned papers on the development of their departments or specialties; and she became widely sought after as a lecturer on hospital history to Edinburgh organisations of many kinds who soon discovered that her illustrated talks on the founding and growth of the Infirmary were models of accuracy and clarity.

With the coming of administrative reorganisation in 1974, the Archivist's duties, though continuing to be concerned primarily with the Royal Infirmary, were enlarged to include the history of other hospitals in the Lothian Area but, with only such clerical help at her disposal as could be provided by members of the Royal Infirmary Volunteers, her ability to cover that extended field was limited.

In September 1981 Mrs. Eaves-Walton died, after a short illness. Only a few months earlier, her department had been transferred to premises belonging to the University in the historic precincts of old Surgeons' Hall. There, a new phase of her work as Health Board Archivist had just begun, in a partnership with the University's History of Medicine and Science Unit—a partnership since continued and developed by her successor, Mrs. Rosemary Gibson, MA; demonstrating yet again the close relationship between the Royal Infirmary and the University of Edinburgh.

Identifying the 'Little House'

An early piece of research undertaken by Mrs. Eaves-Walton concerned the location of the 'Little House' in which the Infirmary had first opened its door in 1729. Dr. Logan Turner, in his history, had said that uncertainty remained about its position although he appeared to favour a site on the west side of Robertson's Close, part of which still exists, running uphill from the Cowgate to Infirmary Street. His statement, and the frequent reproduction in books and articles about the Infirmary of a drawing dated 1854 by James Drummond, R.S.A. showing old houses in a continuous row on one side of the Close, had led to the widely-held assumption that the work of the Infirmary had begun in one such house.

Having examined the evidence, Mrs. Eaves-Walton pointed out that the house was variously described in contemporary documents as being, not in the

Close itself, but 'in Robertson's Close head', 'at the head of Robertson's Close' and 'opposite to the head of Robertson's Close'. She had noticed that the last of these descriptions corresponded with three houses shown within the College Garden on William Edgar's map of 1742 when the 'little house' was still leased to the Infirmary Managers although their great new building nearby, from which Infirmary Street later took its name, was by then nearing completion.

From other sources it appeared that in 1729 and the following years the east-most of the three houses was occupied by the Professor of Divinity and that the westmost one was used as a laboratory by the Professors of Medicine who grew medicinal herbs in the College garden. She concluded, therefore, that the central house must have been the one occupied as the Infirmary.

The research leading to that information had been begun in response to a wish expressed by the Board of Management that the site of the original Infirmary should be marked by a commemorative plaque. The three houses had been demolished in the 1780s to make way for the construction of the South Bridge and of the building now occupied by James Thin's bookshop. So, in Infirmary Street, on a side wall of the bookshop 'opposite to the head of Robertson's Close' a plaque was unveiled on 12 August 1969, 240 years and six days after the Infirmary's first patient, Miss Elizabeth Sinclair from Caithness, had been admitted. The plaque was unveiled by the Lord Provost, The Rt. Hon. James W. McKay, on the invitation of Sir John Bruce, Professor of Clinical Surgery and Surgeon in Administrative Charge of Wards 7 and 8 in the Infirmary. It bears the following inscription:

> On 6th August 1729 the first Voluntary Hospital in Scotland was opened
> in a little house on this site, opposite the head of Robertson's Close.
> While still in that house, in 1736, it became The Royal Infirmary of
> Edinburgh.

Foundation Stone Centenary and a Loyal Address

The next historic celebration to which the Board of Management turned their attention was the centenary of the laying of the foundation stone of the Lauriston Place buildings which had been done with much pomp and ceremony on 13 October 1870. As October 1970 approached all were agreed that some formal commemoration of the occasion should be organised but, again, there arose a question of place. Where, beneath David Bryce's huge complex of buildings, did the foundation stone lie? Though an answer to that question was not essential to the holding of a ceremony, it would be desirable and certainly interesting to know exactly where the stone that was the object of the commemoration had been laid.

It was known that the stone-laying ceremony had been held somewhere in the north-east corner of the grounds of George Watson's Hospital which then had very recently been acquired by the Infirmary Managers and, among the archives, was a lithograph showing the scene at the ceremony in great detail. The drawing, however, contained no clue to the exact point at which it had taken place. So a search for the stone was begun. This involved much creeping and probing in the labyrinth of tunnels and ducts beneath the massive buildings until, at last, on 18 September 1970 the stone was found in a position approached only with difficulty. It was underneath the original casualty ward which, in 1967, had been modernised as part of the Accident and Emergency Department, near the East Gate.

On 13 October 1870, which had been declared a public holiday in the city, the stone had been laid by HRH The Prince of Wales (later King Edward VII) accompanied by Princess Alexandra. It was the Prince's first official engagement since he had become Patron of the Freemasons of Scotland and the ceremony which was attended by 4,000 Freemasons from all over Scotland, by representatives of many public bodies and by a crowd of other spectators, was conducted with full masonic ritual and symbolism.

After that 19th-century ceremony and symbolism it was sad that the stone had disappeared from view for 100 years; and it was fitting that the 20th-century Board of Management, while making no attempt to vie with the splendour of the first occasion, decided to mark its centenary with a modest ceremony of their own. On 13 October 1970, before a small company of invited guests, Professor G. J. Romanes, Chairman of the Board, unveiled a plaque on the outside wall of the Accident and Emergency Department, bearing the following inscription:

> The Royal Infirmary of Edinburgh. This plaque was unveiled on 13th October 1970 to mark the site of the original Foundation Stone laid by HRH Albert Edward, Prince of Wales, exactly one hundred years ago.
> The stone lies six feet six inches directly under this plaque.

Tea was then provided in the Board Room for the invited guests and in the evening a Centenary Board Dinner was held in the Florence Nightingale Nurses Home. On the following Sunday a Joint Service of Thanksgiving took place in the Kirk of the Greyfriars to mark both the 350th Anniversary of the dedication of the Kirk and the Royal Infirmary's centenary occasion.

Commemorative events continued, including the display of a selection of relevant records in the main entrance hall of the Infirmary; and the programme was concluded by a reception given by the Lord Provost, Magistrates and Council, on 29 October, in the Assembly Rooms in George Street, in recognition of the good work done by the Infirmary for the citizens of Edinburgh and the fame which the Infirmary had brought to the city.

Unpretentious though the Board of Management's celebrations were, the research and preparation for them had heightened the Board's appreciation of the importance of the Royal occasion which they were commemorating. Two years earlier Her Majesty The Queen had graciously agreed to become Patron of the Infirmary, thus continuing the long connection of members of the Royal Family with the hospital and following the example of her grandmother, Queen Mary, who had become a Patron in 1937, having previously been Patron of the Simpson Memorial Hospital. This centenary occasion, the Board decided, would be an appropriate one on which to send a loyal message to their Royal Patron. So a Loyal Address was sent to The Queen in the following terms:

> In this year of the celebration of the centenary of the laying of the foundation stone of the present hospital of the Royal Infirmary by Your Majesty's illustrious great-grandfather, H.M. King Edward the Seventh, then Prince of Wales, the Board of Management for the Royal Infirmary

of Edinburgh and Associated Hospitals, with humble duty, wishes to record this assurance of its gratitude for the continued gracious patronage of Your Majesty and its loyalty to the Crown.

To that Address, Her Majesty sent the following reply, received on the centenary day:

Please convey my warm thanks to the Board of Management for the Royal Infirmary of Edinburgh and Associated Hospitals for their kind and loyal message of devotion which they have sent on the occasion of the celebration of the centenary of the laying of the foundation stone of the present Royal Infirmary.

As Patron, I greatly appreciate their message of greetings and I send my very best wishes for the successful continuation of the valuable work carried out by the Royal Infirmary and its Associated Hospitals.

Three Anniversaries

Celebration of the anniversary of a great event may be important for several reasons. One is the opportunity it gives to express pride in past achievement; another, the chance it brings to show gratitude to those whose foresight and effort established great institutions which still benefit the community but which might otherwise be taken for granted; and a third is the inspiration such an occasion may provide. If, for any or all of these reasons, one anniversary makes a year an important one, then in the story of the Royal Infirmary of Edinburgh, the year 1979 was of triple importance. It saw the celebration of one 250th anniversary and of two centenaries.

In 1979—

Monday 6 August was the 250th anniversary of the admission, in 1729, of the Infirmary's first patient, the event commemorated ten years earlier by the erection of the plaque in Infirmary Street and celebrated now for its full significance as the base from which every aspect of the Infirmary's two and a half centuries of development had grown;

Tuesday 1 May was the centenary of the opening in 1879 by Dr. Alexander Peddie, President of the Royal College of Surgeons, of the Edinburgh Royal Maternity and Simpson Memorial Hospital which, sixty years later, had handed on its work, its tradition of service to the community and, in part, its name to the Infirmary's Simpson Memorial Maternity Pavilion.

Monday 29 October was the centenary of the day in 1879 on which the Lord Provost, The Rt. Hon. Thomas Jamieson Boyd had formally declared open the Infirmary's new building in Lauriston Place and, in the afternoon and evening of which nearly 40,000 members of the public had accepted the Managers' invitation to walk through its corridors and wards admiring what they saw.

The Lothian Health Board, having accepted a suggestion by members of the staff of the Infirmary and the Simpson Pavilion that these three occasions should be officially commemorated, an organising committee was formed with the Chairman of the Board, Dr. Rina Nealon, as committee chairman. Other members included representatives of the University of Edinburgh, the Royal Colleges of Physicians and of Surgeons of Edinburgh, the Royal College of Obstetricians and Gynaecologists, the Lothian Regional Council and the City of Edinburgh District Council. Medical, nursing and administrative staffs were also represented. Mr. Donald McIntosh, FRCSE, then recently retired as the Senior Consultant Surgeon in the Infirmary was appointed as Organising Secretary; to work with him Mr. John Laidlaw, FCIS, FHA also recently retired, after a career in hospital adminis-tration which had begun in the Infirmary almost fifty years before, was appointed Administrative Secretary. Celebration of the year of anniversaries, the Committee decided at an early stage, should take many forms so as to appeal to people of widely differing interests.

In January 1979 the Committee learned with the greatest of pleasure that the events they were planning were all to be outshone by one Royal occasion.

They were told that a letter had been received from the Private Secretary to Her Majesty intimating that 'The Queen and the Duke of Edinburgh would be delighted to visit the Royal Infirmary of Edinburgh on the occasion of the 250th anniversary of its foundation and the centenary of the foundation of the Simpson Memorial Maternity Pavilion' and adding that Her Majesty would like the visit to take place on Monday 2nd July, if convenient.

So it was arranged. The Royal visit, demonstrating Her Majesty's interest in and affection for the hospital of which she is Patron, cast a lustre over the whole programme of events. Though it took place early in the programme, it seems fitting to describe it last of all, as being truly the zenith of the Infirmary's year of anniversary celebrations.

Simpson Memorial Hospital Centenary

The other events began modestly with a simple ceremony held on 1 May 1979. Although it took place in Princes Street, it was related to the opening on 1 May 1879, of the Edinburgh Royal Maternity and Simpson Memorial Hospital at 79 Lauriston Place. That hospital, however, had been effectively commemorated in October 1970—on the day of the Infirmary foundation stone centenary. Then, a plaque had been placed beside the doorway of the building which for sixty years had been the Maternity Hospital and which since April 1939 has been used for a variety of hospital purposes, ranging from Infirmary maids' home to school of radiography and district medical records office. That plaque was unveiled in 1970 by Mr. J. R. Cameron, President of the Royal College of Surgeons of Edinburgh and great-grand-nephew of Sir J. Y. Simpson. He was accompanied by Professor R. J. Kellar. The plaque carries the following inscription:

> On this site was erected The Edinburgh Royal Maternity and Simpson
> Memorial Hospital, opened 1st May 1879. The first purpose-built
> maternity hospital in Edinburgh, it was erected in memory of Sir James
> Young Simpson (1811-1870), discoverer of chloroform anaesthesia.

The former Maternity Hospital itself having thus been sufficiently com-memorated already, attention turned, on its centenary day, to the great man in whose memory it had been founded, Sir James Young Simpson, Bart. It was for that reason that the 1979 ceremony took place near the west end of Princes Street, beside the statue of Simpson by William Brodie, which had been placed there in 1877. There Simpson sits, a benign yet impressive figure in his academic robes, sculpted in bronze, above a stone plinth; and there, against the plinth, a wreath was placed on 1 May 1979 by Miss B. Jamieson, Divisional Nursing Officer and Dr. M. G. Pearson, Consultant Physician, both from the Simpson Pavilion. The Chairman of the Lothian Health Board, Dr. Rina Nealon, officiated and a small representative group attended, including Miss Margaret Auld, Chief Nursing Officer of the Scottish Home and Health Department (a former Matron of the Simpson Pavilion), Miss Anne Grant, Central Midwives Board, representing the Simpson Midwives League and Professor David T. Baird on behalf of the Faculty of Medicine.

Service of Thanksgiving and Celebration

Fittingly, the first major event of this commemoration year was the Service of Thanksgiving and Celebration held in the High Kirk of St. Giles on the afternoon of 1 July 1979. It was conducted by the Rev. Gilleasbuig Macmillan, Minister of St. Giles, assisted by The Rev. T. S. McGregor, Chaplain of the Infirmary. The Service was ecumenical in character, the other participating Clergy being—

The Rev. Dr. John Gray, Moderator of the Presbytery of Edinburgh of the Church of Scotland.

The Rt. Rev. Monsignor Patrick Grady, Vicar General of the Archdiocese of St. Andrews and Edinburgh, of the Roman Catholic Church.

The Most Rev. Alastair I. M. Haggart, Bishop of Edinburgh, Primus of the Episcopal Church in Scotland and

The Rt. Rev. Professor Robin A. S. Barbour, Moderator of the General Assembly of the Church of Scotland, who preached the sermon.

The importance of the Royal Infirmary and the respect and affection in which it is held by all sections of the community was symbolised by the formal procession into the Church of representatives (wearing robes of office where appropriate) of organisations which had participated in the founding of the Infirmary or had later become entitled to make nominations to its Board of Managers; followed by representatives of other public and professional bodies and of the many groups that go to make up the staff of the Infirmary. The number of individuals in the formal procession totalled about 250—one for each year of the Infirmary's life, though that was by coincidence not design. Many members of the St. Giles' congregation and of the general public had also come to give thanks for the Infirmary's two and a half centuries of service, with the result that the great church was filled to capacity.

So that the Service might be seen in perspective it was preceded by the reading of a historical narrative and extracts from early documents relating to the founding of the Infirmary, by Tom Fleming, distinguished equally as actor and as radio and television commentator. To reflect the present-day context in which the Service was being held, it included two Statements of Affirmation and Dedication. The first, on behalf of Health Service Staff, was read by Dr. John D. Matthews, Consultant Physician in the Infirmary. The second, on behalf of members of the public, was read by Robin Cook, then Member of Parliament for

Central Edinburgh, the constituency in which the Royal Infirmary is situated. Together, these two Statements summarised in simple yet impressive words the ideals of the Infirmary and the Health Service and of the community they serve and on whose support they depend.

Professor Barbour had adopted for his sermon a similar theme of inter-dependence likening hospital staff, patients and general public to one great family. 'This is a family celebration', he said, 'Birth, life and death all find their meaning within a community which is what, despite their size and complexity, the Royal and the Simpson can surely claim to be; and for that we can praise God.'

Along with the general desire to give thanks for the Royal Infirmary's years of service, a wish had been expressed to honour the memory of one who had done more than any other individual to ensure the success of the campaign for its founding. He was George Drummond, six times Lord Provost of Edinburgh who had died, aged 80, in 1766 and had been buried with full public honours in Canongate Kirkyard. So, immediately after the Thanksgiving Service, a small group from the congregation made their way down the Royal Mile to the kirk-yard. There a wreath was laid on Drummond's grave by Dr. Haldane P. Tait, President of the Scottish Society of the History of Medicine, in a ceremony which, though simple and brief, fittingly acknowledged George Drummond's importance in the Infirmary story.

Three Exhibitions

The Thanksgiving Service had recognised the worth of the Infirmary's work and its growth from simple beginnings to all the complexities of modern medicine. To show the extent of these complexities and the variety of skills, technical expertise and equipment available to help the patient of today, a comprehensive exhibition was arranged in the recreation hall of the Florence Nightingale Nurses Home. Entitled 'The Royal and the Simpson Today' and 'manned' by a rota of Royal Infirmary Volunteers, it was open daily from July till October. It was an exhibition which, by its varied and clear displays, must have opened the eyes of many to the resources of the Infirmary that could come to their aid in time of need.

Two smaller exhibitions were also held during the celebration period. Under the title 'Open to All', the Royal Scottish Museum in Chambers Street displayed documents, pictures and other items, drawn from their own collections as well as from the hospital archives, which summarised the history of the Infirmary and the Simpson Pavilion, thus bringing their anniversaries to wider public notice. At Surgeons Hall, the Royal College of Surgeons of Edinburgh exhibited surgical instruments and related items to show how they had developed over many years.

Lectures

The triple anniversary year seemed a suitable opportunity to arrange lectures and discussions on three levels of interest—for those experienced in medical, nursing and administrative matters to exchange ideas; for members of the public who might like to learn more about the Royal Infirmary and its place in Edinburgh's

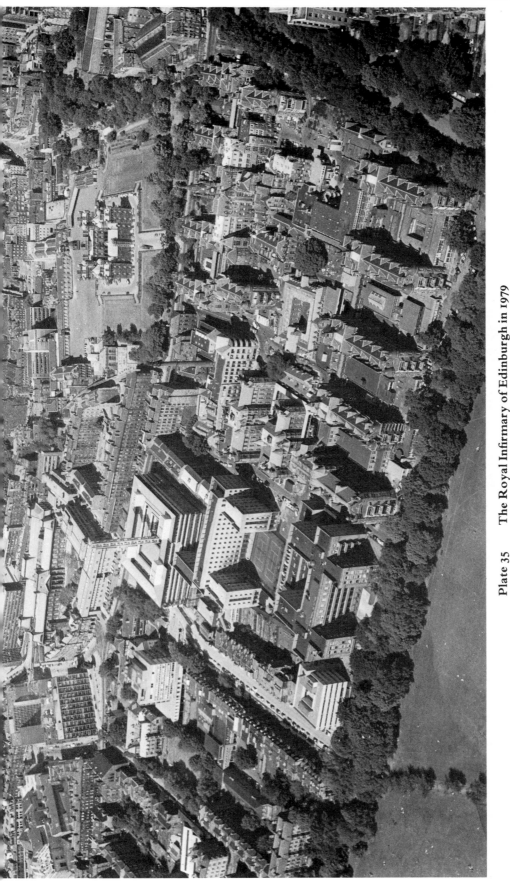

Plate 35   The Royal Infirmary of Edinburgh in 1979

All available open spaces are built upon; and three important new buildings are seen — 1: Princess Alexandra Eye Pavilion, West of Chalmers Street. 2: 'Phase 1' building, first stage of the new Infirmary, between Florence Nightingale Home and Lauriston Place and 3: Reproductive Biology Unit, West of Simpson Pavilion.

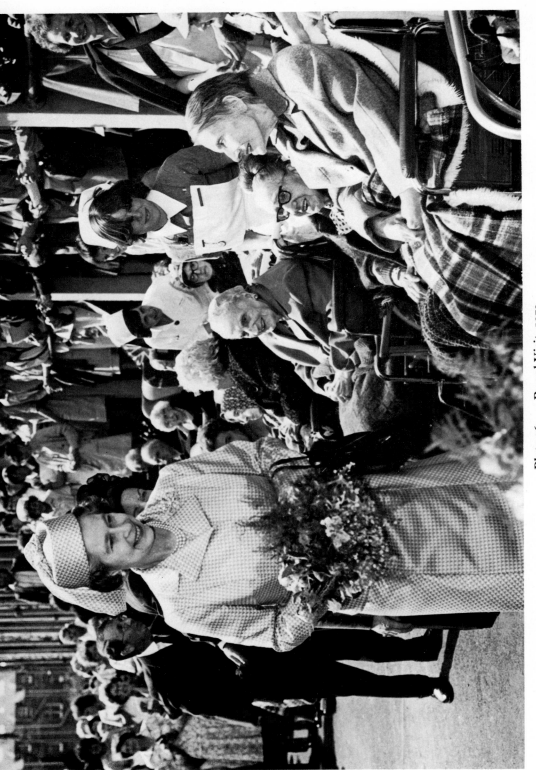

Plate 36   Royal Visit, 1979

H.M. The Queen exchanges greetings with elderly patients and their nurses medical history; and for a younger group interested in aspects of health care who might perhaps be encouraged to seek careers in medicine, nursing or some related profession. Three lecture series were therefore arranged.

Chief among these was a Symposium held in the Hall of the Royal College of Surgeons of Edinburgh on three mornings in September 1979. At these meetings papers were read by distinguished figures in medicine, nursing and hospital administration from McGill University and the Royal Victoria Hospital, Montreal. Their contributions were matched by others from more familiar but no less distinguished figures in similar fields of work in Edinburgh, and useful discussions followed. There had long been a friendly rapport with the Canadian Royal Victoria Hospital even, as mentioned in an earlier chapter, to the extent that the plans of that hospital, built in the 1890s had been modelled on David Bryce's plans for the Royal Infirmary of 1879.

In association with the Symposium six academic lectures were held in the afternoons in the surgical lecture theatre in the Infirmary. These had been arranged by three founder bodies of the Royal Infirmary—the Faculty of Medicine, the Royal College of Physicians and the Royal College of Surgeons. They were all memorial lectures, commemorating prominent medical men. Five of them were given by speakers from the Medical School of McGill University.

For a more general audience a one-day programme of ten lectures, organised by the Scottish Society of the History of Medicine under the title of 'Edinburgh's Infirmary' was held in the University's George Square Theatre on 27 October 1979. The other lectures were given in the Infirmary's surgical lecture theatre on several evenings between July and September. They were delivered by senior members of the medical and nursing staffs of the Infirmary and the South Lothian School of Nursing and Midwifery and were aimed at the younger generation.

Exhibitions and lectures were not the only means adopted for spreading knowledge of the Infirmary and the Simpson Pavilion. A finely produced and well illustrated brochure was published describing the history and current work of the hospitals; and Dr. Logan Turner's admirable book—*Story of a Great Hospital—The Royal Infirmary of Edinburgh, 1729 to 1929*, first published in 1937, was reprinted by James Thin, the Mercat Press, Edinburgh. Souvenirs, including prints, plaques and photo-engravings on copper of past and present Infirmary buildings were on sale in the hospital shops and elsewhere. On 6 August 1979, anniversary of the first patient's admission, every patient in the Infirmary and the Simpson Pavilion was given a leaflet outlining the hospitals' history.

One last note on the subject of 'publication', though in a different sense, may not come amiss. For fifty years or so, the façade of the Infirmary had 'published', high above the main entrance doorway, to be seen by all who entered or passed by, two dates: '1730', presumably intended as the Infirmary's year of origin and '1870', the foundation-stone year. They had been carved there, at the expense of a benefactor, in the 1920s. That the first date was wrong had been noticed soon after it appeared but to make the correction then, it was thought, would be discourteous to the donor and it was allowed to remain. In the anniversary year of 1979, however, it would have been quite inappropriate to allow the stonework to continue to publish its misleading message to the world. So, during restoration

s

work on the masonry, the opportunity was taken for '1730' to be removed and '1729' substituted.

Social Occasions

No anniversary celebration would be complete without a social occasion. For this triple celebration, to ensure that as many as possible could enjoy a sense of participation, the organising committee arranged two such events in July for members of staff of every profession and occupation, retired staff and others connected with the Infirmary. The first, an evening reception, was held in the concourse of the University's Appleton Tower, beside George Square. The concourse was filled to capacity by some 1,700 guests. The other was an afternoon garden party in the spacious garden of George Heriot's School enjoyed in pleasant sunshine by nearly 2,000. With the 100-year-old Infirmary to the south, the three centuries old Renaissance-style Heriot's School to the north and the mediaeval castle rising behind it, the garden was an impressive setting for the occasion. In such surroundings it was impossible not to see the story of the Infirmary in its context as part of the city's history.

Royal Visit 1979

As has been said, the celebrations for the Royal Infirmary's year of anniversaries reached their zenith early with the visit of Her Majesty The Queen and His Royal Highness the Duke of Edinburgh on the afternoon of Monday 2 July, the day after the main series of events had begun with the Service of Thanksgiving in St. Giles. Such timing was admirable, for the Queen and the Duke brought with them a happy atmosphere of interest and goodwill which pervaded all the events that followed.

Within the fifty years covered by this history members of the Royal Family had visited the Infirmary on several occasions, some of which have already been described, the latest being the opening of the new Eye Pavilion by Princess Alexandra in 1969. Within the one hundred years life of the Lauriston Place buildings there were four occasions on which the reigning sovereign had honoured the hospital with an official visit:

In August 1881, Her Majesty Queen Victoria, accompanied by Princess Beatrice and Prince Arthur visited the hospital and The Queen then gave the names 'Victoria' and 'Albert' to Wards 11 and 24 respectively;

In July 1911, Their Majesties King George V and Queen Mary visited and graciously agreed that Wards 7 and 30, respectively, should be named after them;

In June 1916, King George visited wounded servicemen from the Battle of Jutland; and

In July 1920, King George and Queen Mary made a return visit to the hospital, accompanied by HRH Princess Mary, The Princess Royal.

None of those Royal visits, however, can have been conducted in a more friendly manner or have left happier memories with patients and staff than that on 2 July 1979. It was the first visit in a week-long royal tour of Scotland and it took place immediately after the Royal Party's arrival in the city. Having driven direct from the airport, the Queen and the Duke went first to the Nurses' Home to see the exhibition—'The Royal and the Simpson Today'. From it they were conducted by the Chairman of the Lothian Health Board, Dr. Rina T. Nealon and Mr. Donald McIntosh across the courtyard to the Simpson Pavilion where their visits to the wards began and where both Queen and Duke showed much interest in the mothers and babies. From there they were conducted to the main building, happily greeted on the way by elderly patients seated in the warm sunshine along their route. The tour of the main building included visits to the Coronary Care Unit in Ward 31, the Physiotherapy Department and two Surgical Wards, at all of which members of staff were formally presented to Her Majesty and at each of which she and the Duke spoke informally to patients and staff. In the Board Room the Visitors' Book was signed and more presentations were made. Her Majesty and the Duke then left for the Palace of Holyroodhouse, there to receive from the Lord Provost, in time-honoured fashion, the Keys of the City of Edinburgh.

The Royal tour of the hospital, involving a walk of almost three quarters of a mile and lasting nearly two hours, was said at the time to have been one of the longest 'walkabouts' the Queen had undertaken. The mood of the occasion was well caught next day in a press report beginning: 'The Queen showed a sparkling bedside manner and gave patients at the Royal Infirmary, Edinburgh, a real tonic when she made visiting time a Royal occasion yesterday'.

There could have been no better way of marking the Infirmary's two and a half centuries of service to the community.

s*

Appendices

compiled by

Donald McIntosh

I: Comparative Statistics—Royal Infirmary of Edinburgh, 1729-1978.

II: Lists of Medical and Surgical Officers, Senior Nursing and Senior Administrative Officers, of the Royal Infirmary of Edinburgh, 1929-1979.

APPENDIX I

Comparative Statistics—Royal Infirmary of Edinburgh 1729-1978

	1729-30	1836-37	1935-36	1939	1947	1978
Total patients discharged	30	3,829	20,612	21,341	22,233	37,124★
Available beds	4/5	373	1,117	1,161	1,450★	1,202★
Average stay medical (days)	35·8	c. 35	26·04	22·75	22·82	15·85
Average stay surgical (days)	40·2	c. 43	13·87	13·67	15·07	9·1
Medical & surgical officers	2	13★★	82★★	c. 100	207	495
Nursing staff (W.T.E.)	1	50	460	499	712★	1,614★
Annual ord. expenditure	£97. 19. 7¾	£6,727	£169,694	£195,225	£350,108	£M17
Average cost/day/patient	10¾d (4·5p)	1/- (5p)	9/7¼ (48p)	11/3 (56p)	18/1 (90½p)	£42

★ Includes SMMP   ★★ Does not include residents

APPENDIX II

MEDICAL AND SURGICAL OFFICERS

From 1930 the Managers continued the practice of appointing and reappointing for set periods (2 or 5 years) assistant physicians and surgeons, the most senior of whom became a physician or surgeon 'in ordinary' as a vacancy arose through resignation, retiral or death. Appointment to the latter posts was for a period of fifteen years or until the age of 65, whichever was the earlier.

Associate appointments were made in certain specialties or to holders of certain senior university appointments.

From the inception of the National Health Service in 1948 appointments were as consultant physicians or surgeons who initially might, on application and after interview, be appointed physician or surgeon 'in charge', as a vacancy arose. From 1955 seniority again governed this appointment, subject to the recommendation of the Board of Management who consulted the relevant section of the staff. From 1960 the post was designated 'physician/surgeon in administrative charge' and appointments to such posts ceased with the re-organisation in 1974, when 'Divisions' with elected chairmen were formed. The last remnant of the Scottish hierarchical system thus disappeared although it is fair to say that within divisions a unit or charge system tended to persist. Associate status disappeared in 1948 and was shortly replaced in the case of professors and senior lecturers by honorary consultant status arising from and for the duration of the university appointment. This status is marked ★ throughout the appendix. The names of those who held an appointment 'in charge' before 1974 are marked ᶜ when their initial appointment was post 1948.

MEDICAL DEPARTMENT

	Assistant Physicians	Ordinary Physicians	Retired or Resigned, Died
Douglas Chalmers Watson	1907	1919	1934
Edwin Matthew†	1909	1921	1934
John Eason	1912	1923	1938
John Dixon Comrie	1913	1927	1939, died
Alexander Goodall	1913	1928	1941, died
George Douglas Mathewson	1919	1934	1935, died
Andrew Fergus Hewat	1920	1934	1949
Herbert Lindesay Watson-Wemyss	1921	...	1933, died
Charles George Lambie	1922	...	1930
William Douglas Denton Small, CBE	1923	1935	1954
Andrew Rutherford	1924	...	1930, died
William Alister Alexander	1927	1936	1955
Leybourne Stanley Patrick Davidson	1928	...	1930
Andrew Rae Gilchrist, CBE	1930	1939	1964
Thomas Robert Rushton Todd	1930	1941	1961
James Kirkwood Slater	1932	1949	1964
Sir James Davidson Stuart Cameron, CBE	1932	1954	1965
Sir Derrick Melville Dunlop†	1934	1936	1962
William Ritchie Russell	1934	...	1939

† See Professors of Medicine

	Assistant Physicians	Ordinary Physicians	Retired or Resigned, Died
Ranald Malcolm Murray Lyon	1936	1956	1969, died
William Lindsay Lamb	1936	1961	1969
Sir Leybourne Stanley Patrick Davidson†	1938	1938	1959
Sir Ian George William Hill, CBE	1938	...	1950
James Gilbert Murdoch Hamilton	1939	1964	1972, died
Sir William Melville Arnott	1946	...	1946
Charles Kelman Robertson	1946	...	1966
Sir John Halliday Croom	1946	1965	1974
Donald Marcus Fielding Batty	1946	1969	1974

	Consultant Physicians	
James Innes^c	1949	1974
Henry Johnston Scott Matthew^c	1950	1974
Ronald Haxton Girdwood^c†	1951	1982
Alastair Gould Macgregor★	1952	1959
Robert Macfie Marquis, MBE^c	1955	1979
John Duncan Matthews^c	1956	...
Kenneth William Donald, DSC★†^c	1959	1975
James Scott Robson★†	1959	...
Samuel Howard Davies, Haematology^c	1961	1979
Leslie James Patrick Duncan	1962	...
Michael Francis Oliver†	1963	...
John Richmond★	1963	1973
Andrew Doig	1963	...
Desmond Gareth Julian	1964	1974
Clifford Mawdsley ★	1966	...
William James Irvine	1966	...
Anne Templeton Lambie★	1968	...
Basil Frank Clarke	1968	...
David Caton Flenley★	1969	1978
David John Crymble Shearman★	1969	1975
Laurance Francis Prescott★	1969	...
Hugh Murdoch MacLeod	1969	...
Edward Housley	1970	...
Niall Diarmid Campbell Finlayson	1973	...
Alexander Thompson Proudfoot	1974	...
Alexander Laird Muir★	1974	...
Hugh Craig Miller	1975	...
Andrew Cairns Douglas★	1975	...
Ronald Foote Robertson, CBE	1975	...
Robert Campbell Heading	1975	...
David Anderson Seaton	1975	...
Alistair Cameron Parker	1978	...
Anthony Douglas Toft★	1978	...

† See Professors of Medicine

	Consultant Physicians	Retired or Resigned, Died
Robin John Winney	1978	...
David Paul de Bono	1979	...
Geoffrey Gower Lloyd	1979	...
Christopher Armstrong Ludlam	1980	...

Professors of Medicine 1929-1982

	Appointed	Retired or Resigned, Died
Edwin Bramwell	1922	1934
Moncrieff Arnot professor of clinical medicine		
David Murray Lyon		
Christison professor of therapeutics	1924	1936
Moncrieff Arnot professor of clinical medicine	1936	1953
William Thomas Ritchie, OBE	1928	1938
professor of medicine		
Edwin Matthew	1934	1936
Moncrieff Arnot professor of clinical medicine		
Sir Derrick Melville Dunlop	1936	1962
Christison professor of therapeutics		
Sir Leybourne Stanley Patrick Davidson	1939	1959
professor of medicine		
Kenneth William Donald, DSC	1959	1977
professor of medicine		
Ronald Haxton Girdwood	1962	1982
Christison professor of therapeutics		
James Scott Robson	1977	...
professor of medicine		
Michael Francis Oliver		
personal chair in cardiology	1978	1979
Duke of Edinburgh professor of cardiology	1979	...

Physicians Consultant

	Appointed	Retired or Resigned, Died
Physician consultant in tuberculosis		
Sir Robert William Philip	1922	1939, died
professor of tuberculosis		
Charles Cameron	1947	1951
professor of tuberculosis		
Physician consultant in psychiatry		
William Malcolm McAlister	1929	1932
Sir David Kennedy Henderson	1932	1954
professor of psychiatry		

	Appointed	Retired or Resigned, Died

Physician consultant in diseases of tropical climates

Lieut.-Colonel Edward David Wilson Greig, CIE	1929	1939
Lieut.-Colonel Edward Humphrey Vere Hodge, CIE	1939	1950

No further appointments were made by the Managers to these posts and the term visiting physician came into usage.

Visiting Physicians

Respiratory disease

Sir John Wenman Crofton★	1952	1977
professor of respiratory diseases		
Andrew Cairns Douglas★	1963	1975[1]
David Caton Flenley★	1978	...
professor of respiratory diseases		

Rheumatic Disease

John George Sclater	1938	1972
John George Macleod	1938	1980
John James Reid Duthie	1947	1977
professor in medicine 1968-1977		
Robert John Giffen Sinclair	1951	1972
George Nuki★	1979	...
professor of rheumatic diseases		

Psychiatry

Thomas Arthur Munro	1954	1966, died
Alexander Kennedy★	1954	1960, died
professor of psychiatry		
Frank James Fish	1956	1963
George Morrison Carstairs★	1961	1973
professor in psychiatry		
Robert Cairns Brown Aitken	1967	1974
John Raymond Smythies	1961	1973
Ian Oswald	1968	...
professor in psychiatry		

Neurology

John Alexander Simpson	1956	1964

Geriatrics

Neil Macmichael	1966	1973
Thomas Grieve Judge	1974	...
James Williamson★	1976	...
professor of geriatric medicine		
Roger Galbraith Smith	1976	...
Norman Arthur Hood	1978	...
Colin Thomas Currie	1979	...

[1] See Medical Department

	Appointed	Retired or Resigned, Died
Medical Genetics		
Alan Eglin Heathcote Emery★	1967	...
professor of medical genetics		
Nutrition		
Arnold Peter Meiklejohn★	1947	1961, died

SURGICAL DEPARTMENT

	Assistant Surgeons	Ordinary Surgeons	Retired or Resigned, Died
George Lyall Chiene	1903	1922	1937
William James Stuart	1907	1923	1938
John William Struthers	1908	1924	1939
Sir Henry Wade, CMG, DSO	1909	1924	1939
Sir David Percival Dalbreck Wilkie, OBE	1912	1924	1938, died
professor of surgery 1924-1938			
Sir John Fraser, Bt, KCVO, MC	1919	1925	1944
Regius professor of clinical surgery 1925-1944			
James Methuen Graham	1919	1928	1946
Alexander Pirie Watson, OBE	1919	1937	1943, died
Francis Evelyn Jardine	1919	1938	1947
Walter Quarry Wood	1923	1939	1954
John James McIntosh Shaw, MC	1924	1939	1940, died WOAS
Sir Walter Mercer	1924	1943	1957
professor of orthopaedic surgery 1948-1957			
William Alexander Cochrane	1924		1944, died
associate surgeon in orthopaedics			
Keith Paterson Brown	1925	1943	1958
Robert Leslie Stewart	1927	1944	1960
Thomas McWalter Miller	1928	1946	1959
Norman McOmish Dott	1930	[1]	1962
associate neurological surgeon			
Donald Stewart Middleton	1931		1942, killed WOAS
Margaret Christine Tod	1933		1937
associate assistant surgeon for radium therapy			
William Alister D'Arcy Adamson	1937	1954	1963
Sir John Bruce, CBE	1938		1947
Regius professor of clinical surgery		1956	1970
James Roderick Johnston Cameron	1938	1958	1966

[1] See Surgical Neurology

	Assistant Surgeon	Ordinary Surgeon	Retired or Resigned, Died
Sir James Rognvald Learmonth, KCVO, CBE		1939	1956
professor of surgery 1939-1956			
Regius professor of clinical surgery 1946-1956			
Robert Ingleton Stirling	1943		1949
Associate assistant surgeon in orthopaedics			
Eric Leslie Farquharson	1945	1959	1971, died
James Sneddon Jeffrey	1945	1954	1969
Andrew Gilchrist Ross Loudon	1945		1953
Thomas Ian Wilson	1945	1966	1973
Hector William Porter	1945		1964, died
James Alexander Ross, MBE	1946	1960	1960
Alexander Burns Wallace	1946		1970
associate plastic surgeon			
David Band	1946		1966
associate urological surgeon			
Andrew Logan	1946	1961	1972
associate thoracic surgeon			
Donald Macleod Douglas	1946		1951
associate assistant surgeon			

		Consultant Surgeons	
Donald McIntosh[e]		1954	1976
Archibald Ian Stewart Macpherson[e]		1954	1978
Sir Michael Francis Addison Woodruff ★[e]		1956	1976
professor of surgical science			
Ian Scott Robertson Sinclair		1958	...
Bernard Nolan		1962	...
Sir James David Fraser, Bt.★		1963	1968
Catherine Carlow Burt		1963	1967
Thomas Jeffray McNair		1963	...
Alan Charles Barclay Dean★		1964	...
James William Wishart Thomson		1964	...
Ian Buchanan Macleod		1969	...
Andrew Patrick McEwan Forrest★		1971	...
Regius professor of clinical surgery			
Thomas Hamilton★		1971	1976
Alexander John Duff		1971	1980
Iain Ferguson MacLaren		1975	...
James Rodway Kirkpatrick		1975	1976
David Craig Carter★		1976	1979
Alasdair Bruce MacGregor		1977	...
Andrew McLaren Jenkins		1977	...
Charles Vaughan Ruckley		1978	...
Thomas Vincent Taylor★		1979	1981

	Consultant Surgeons	Retired or Resigned, Died
Gerald Courteney Davies★	1980	...
Oleg Feoderevich Eremin★	1981	...
David Lee	1982	...

DEPARTMENT OF SURGICAL NEUROLOGY

	Appointed Neurosurgeon	Retired or Resigned, Died
Norman McOmish Dott[1]	1931	1962
professor of neurological surgery 1947-1962		
George Lionel Alexander	1936	1948
Francis John Gillingham	1950	1980
professor of neurological surgery 1962-1980		
Philip Harris	1953	...
John Fraser Shaw	1963	...
Edward Robert Hitchcock★	1966	1978
Alfred James Wanklyn Steers★	1980	...
James Douglas Miller★	1981	...
professor of neurological surgery 1981-		

	Neurologist	
Kate Hermann	1935	1969
Walter Sneddon Watson	1953	1981

	Neurophysiologist	
Ewart Geoffrey Walsh★	1959	1966
Horace Robert Allan Townsend	1966	1980

	Medical psychologist	
James Alexander Lyon Naughton, MC	1976	1982

CARDIOTHORACIC UNIT

The Cardiothoracic Unit was established in 1961 when the thoracic unit of the Eastern General Hospital was transferred to Wards 17/18. Andrew Logan, who had been associate thoracic surgeon since 1946 became surgeon in charge.

	Appointed Consultant	Retired or Resigned, Died
Andrew Logan[c]	1961	1972
John David Wade[c]	1961	1978
Robert John Murray McCormack	1961	1981, died
Philip Raby Walbaum	1961	...
Philip Kennedy Caves★	1973	1975
David John Wheatley★	1976	1979
Evan John William Cameron	1978	...
Kenneth Grant Reid★	1979	...
Christopher Tsoi Mook Sang	1982	...

[1] See surgical department

DEPARTMENT OF UROLOGY

The department was formed in 1967.

	Appointed Consultant	Retired or Resigned, Died
Thomas Ian Wilson[c]	1967[1]	1973
Peter Edmund, CBE, TD[c]	1970	1980
James William Fowler	1973	...
David Anthony Tolley	1980	...

DENTAL DEPARTMENT

	Assistant Surgeon	Surgeon	Retired or Resigned, Died
Douglas Llewellyn George Radford	1921	1924	1946
Robert Charles Scott Dow	1924	1927	1946
Frederick George Gibbs		1927	1957
James Morham		1927	1945
Herbert Moncrieff Sturrock		1927	1941
David Skene Middleton[c]		1927	1966

In 1956 the new Department of Oral Surgery was opened with F. G. Gibbs and D. S. Middleton the initial consultant surgeons.

	Consultant	
John Boyes*[c]	1958	1976
professor of dental surgery 1958-76		
Augustus Edward Duvall	1963	1978
John Ferguson Gould	1967	...
William Donald MacLennon	1966	1982
professor of oral surgery 1978-82		
James Wallace*	1980	...

DEPARTMENT OF ORTHOPAEDIC SURGERY

	Appointed	Retired or Resigned, Died
William Alexander Cochrane[1]	1936	1944, died
Sir Walter Mercer[1c]	1936	1958
professor of orthopaedic surgery 1948-58		
Robert Ingleton Stirling[1]	1943	1949
William Veitch Anderson	1947	1949
Ewan Alistair Jack	1949	1953, died
Iain Alexander George Lawson Dick	1951	1965, died
Douglas Leslie Savill	1951	1973, died
George Patrick Mitchell, MC	1954	1982

[1] See surgical department

	Appointed	Retired or Resigned, Died
John Ivor Pulsford James★e	1958	1979
professor of orthopaedic surgery 1958-79		
James Henry Shielswood Scott	1958	...
Douglas Watson Lamb	1959	...
Robin Sydney Mackwood Ling	1960	1962
John Chalmers	1961	...
William Macdonald McQuillan	1963	...
William Milton Rigal★	1965	1968
William Alexander Souter	1967	...
David Lawrence Hamblin★	1968	1972
Donald Harley Gray★	1972	1975
William John Gillespie	1974	1977
Michael John McMaster	1976	...
James Christie	1979	...
Sean Patrick Francis Hughes★	1979	...
professor of orthopaedic surgery 1979-		
Malcolm Fraser Macnicol	1980	...

VISITING SURGEONS

Post-1948 no further appointments were made as associate surgeons in specialities and the term visiting surgeon came into usage.

Paediatric surgery

Frederick Howard Roberts	1964	1979

Plastic Surgery

Alexander Campbell Buchan	1964	1980
Alastair David Ross Batchelor	1964	...
Anne Bryson Sutherland	1971	...
Antony Charles Harington Watson	1971	...
John Cummack McGregor	1980	...

GYNAECOLOGICAL DEPARTMENT
(DEPARTMENT OF OBSTETRICS AND GYNAECOLOGY)

With the opening of the Simpson Memorial Maternity Pavilion in 1939 assistant gynaecologists and gynaecologists became respectively assistant obstetricians and gynaecologists or obstetricians and gynaecologists. After the advent of the National Health Service appointments were as consultants with initially a hierarchy which disappeared in similar stages.

	Assistant Gynaecologist (O & G)	Gynaecologist (O & G)	Retired or Resigned, Died
Robert William Johnstone, CBE	1922	1926	1946
professor of midwifery 1926-46			
Hugh Stevenson Davidson	1922	1927	1932, died

	Assistant Gynaecologist (O & G)	Gynaecologist (O & G)	Retired or Resigned, Died
James Young	1922	1928	1934
William Francis Theodore Haultain	1926	1932	1947
Douglas Alexander Miller	1927	1934	1957
Ernest Chalmers Fahmy	1928	1947	1957
John Sturrock	1932	1958	1966
Clifford Donald Kennedy	1933	1958	1966

	Consultant (O & G)		Retired or Resigned, Died
James Bruce Dewar	1939		1945
Thomas Nicol MacGregor	1939		1954
William Alexander Liston	1939		1960, died
Robert James Kellar, CBE★ professor of obstetrics and gynaecology 1946-74	1946		1974
George Douglas Matthew	1946		1974
William David Alastair Callum	1947		1976
Donald James MacIntosh Irvine	1954		1967, died
Philip Roger Myerscough	1958		...
Morton Gilmour Pearson	1958		...
John Duncan Ott Loudon	1960		1966
John Gow Robertson	1966		1976
Melville Greig Kerr★	1966		1969
Francis Ronald Clark	1966		1969
Jeremy Rae Braithwaite Livingstone	1968		...
Martin MacArthur Lees	1969		...
David Tennent Baird★ professor of obstetrics and gynaecology 1977-	1970		...
Melville Greig Kerr★ professor of obstetrics and gynaecology 1974-76	1974		1976
Kenneth Boddy	1974		...
George Edward Smart	1976		...
William Alexander Liston	1977		...
Peter William Howie★	1978		1981
Frank William Johnstone★	1978		...
Robert Wayne Shaw★	1981		...

DEPARTMENT OF NEONATAL PAEDIATRICS

	Appointed	Retired or Resigned, Died
Charles McNeil professor of child life and health 1931-1946	1939	1946
Thomas Yule Finlay	1939	1948
Henry Leonard Wallace	1939	1948
John Louis Henderson	1947	1951

	Appointed	*Retired or Resigned, Died*
Richard White Bernard Ellis, OBE★c professor of child life and health 1946-1964	1946	1964
John Thomson★	1939	1965
Douglas Nairn Nicholson	1948	1964
Donald Mackenzie Douglas	1951	1976
John Oldroyd Forfar, MC★c professor of child life and health 1964-1982	1964	1982
James Watson Farquhar★ professor in child life and health 1978-	1955	...
Forrester Cockburn★	1971	1977
David George Dryburgh Barr	1971	...
William Sutcliffe Uttley	1972	...
John Keith Brown	1973	...
Robert Hume★	1980	...

Pre-1948 appointments were as paediatrician (and assistant/associate paediatrician) to the department of obstetrics and gynaecology. Post-1948 as consultant in the department of paediatrics and child health, renamed in 1970 department of neonatal paediatrics.

DERMATOLOGICAL DEPARTMENT[1]

	Assistant Physician	*Physician*	*Retired or Resigned, Died*
Frederick Gardiner	1904	1912	1933, died
Robert Cranston Low	1906	1924	1933
Robert Aitken	1924	1933	1953
George Hector Percival Grant professor of dermatology 1946-1967	1927	1935	1967
George Alexander Grant Peterkin	1932	1953	1971

	Consultant Physician	*Retired or Resigned, Died*
Patrick Wyatville Hannay	1949	1974
George William Beveridge	1965	...
Patrick James Hare Grant professor of dermatology 1968-1980	1968	1980
John Andrew Savin	1971	...
John Alexander Hunter★ Grant professor of dermatology 1981-	1974	...
Ross St Clair Barnetson	1981	...
Paul Kenneth Buxton	1981	...

[1] from 1884-1935 known as the department for diseases of the skin

OPHTHALMIC DEPARTMENT

	Assistant Surgeon	Ordinary Surgeon	Retired or Resigned, Died
Harry Moss Traquair	1913	1927	1941
Ernest Hugh Cameron	1920	1932	1945
Charles William Graham	1927	1942	1953
John Robert Paterson	1931	1946	1962
George Ian Scott, CBE professor of ophthalmology 1954-72	1945	1954	1972
John McAskill	1946	1962	1963, died
Charles Robert Sweeting Jackson	1953	1963	1979

		Consultant Surgeon	
James Hughes		1959	...
Norman Leslie Stokoe		1960	...
James Finbarr Cullen		1962	...
John Nolan★		1964	1967
Geoffrey Thomas Millar		1967	...
Sohan Singh Hayreh★		1968	1972
Hector Bryson Chawla		1970	...
Calvert Inglis Phillips★ professor of ophthalmology 1972-		1972	...
Richard Shayle Bartholomew★		1972	...
Alastair David Adams		1979	...

EAR, NOSE AND THROAT DEPARTMENT

	Assistant Surgeon	Surgeon	Retired or Resigned, Died
George Ewart Martin	1921	1936	1950, died
Ion Simson Hall	1933	1946	1961
John Philip Stewart	1933	1950	1965
Alexander Brownlie Smith	1936	1961	1970
Robert Benny Lumsden	1950	1965	1967
Ian Malcolm Duncan Napier Farquharson	1945	1973	1976

		Consultants	
George Downes McDowall[c]		1949	1978
Kenneth McLay		1963	1982
Ronald Alastair MacNeill		1966	1968
Bryan Archibald Brownhill Dale		1969	...
Arnold George Maran		1976	...
Alastair Ian Grant Kerr		1978	...

VENEREAL DISEASES DEPARTMENT[1]

	Assistant Clinical Medical Officers	Clinical Medical Officers	Retired or Resigned, Died
David Lees DSO,		1919	1934, died
Robert Campbell Lindsay Batchelor Consultant-in-charge (1948-54)	1920	1935	1954
		Consultants	
Marjorie Murrell 'Senior assistant' (1936-48)		1948	1963
Robert Lees[c]		1954	1967
David Hunter Henderson Robertson[c]		1965	…
Mary Taylor Brown		1969	1980
Robert Nicol Traquair Thin		1972	1973
Ivan Ballantyne Tait		1973	1982
Sheila Stewart Robertson Bain		1978	…
Alexander McMillan		1980	…

DEPARTMENT OF ANAESTHETICS

Records for 1930-1948 are incomplete.

	Appointed	Retired or Resigned, Died
Maurice Howard Jones	c. 1920	1944, died
Henry Torrance Thomson	c. 1924	c. 1935
Frederick George Gibbs	c. 1927	1958
David Skene Middleton	c. 1930	1948
John Gillies, CVO, MC (Director 1948-1960)	1932	1960
Lucien Benedict Wevill	1932	1946
Sheina Cooper Helen Watters	1932	1961
George Maxwell Brown	1934	1950
Alexander MacGregor Duff	1934	1939
Mary Lennox Brown	1945	1948
Alexander McCallum Millar	1940	1958
Margot Wilhelmine Goldsmith	1940	1959
Alison Ritchie	1945	1959
Frank Holmes	1948	1977
Harold William Charles Griffiths	1948	1980
Nutting Stuart Fraser	1949	1961
Allan Scrimgeour Brown	1950	…

[1] In 1979 became Department of Genito-urinary Medicine (including Sexually Transmitted Diseases)

	Appointed	*Retired or Resigned, Died*
James Donald Robertson	1955	1982
professor of anaesthetics 1960-1982 (Director[1] 1960-1974)		
Malcolm Campbell Macqueen	1956	1967, died
Alastair Mackenzie McKinlay	1956	1977
Alastair Hugh Bailey Masson	1957	...
Archibald Cousland Milne	1957	...
Donald Bruce Scott	1959	...
Lillie Stewart Dummer	1960	1968
Ainslie Sanderson Crawford	1961	1979
Calvin Fraser Hider	1964	...
William Rennie MacRae	1964	...
Gordon Hill Rae	1965	1975
Dorothy Child	1965	...
Iain Archibald Davidson	1967	...
James Clark McIntyre	1968	...
Lawrence Vaughan Hunter Martin	1968	...
Robert Hood Wright Park	1971	...
James Wilson	1971	...
James Lawrence Jenkinson	1972	...
Alexander Stewart Buchan	1975	...
Evan Llewelyn Lloyd	1975	...
Ann Whitfield	1976	...
Barbara Margaret Leeming	1976	...
Gordon Blair Drummond	1977	...
John Anthony Winston Wildsmith	1977	...
Nigel Andrew Malcolm-Smith	1978	...
David George Littlewood	1979	...
George Laurin Murray Carmichael	1979	...
David Henry Thomson Scott	1980	...
David Taylor Brown	1982	...

RADIOLOGICAL DEPARTMENT

	Appointed (In charge)	*Retired or Resigned, Died*
John Duncan White	1930 (1930)	1934
James Ralston Kennedy Paterson, CBE	1930	1930
John Struthers Fulton	1930	1931
Angus Campbell	1931	1932
Robert Alexander Kemp Harper	1932	1933
Cyril Bellamy	1933	1935
Alfred Ernest Barclay, OBE	1934 (1934)	1935
Robert McWhirter, CBE	1934 (1935)	1970
Francis Miller Gordon	1935	1936

[1] Office of director discontinued 1974

	Appointed (In charge)	Retired or Resigned, Died
James Zuill Walker	1935	1941
Thomas Rankin Harlan	1935	1936
John Paton McGibbon	1936	1952, died
David Wylie Lindsay	1936	1972
Thomas Sprunt	1937	1938
John McWhirter	1937	1938
Bruce Faulds	1938	1939
Joseph Phelan	1938	1947
Robert Morrison	1941	1942
Helen Innes	1942	1943
James Duncan Brown	1943	1947
William Michael Court Brown	1943	1950
Kenneth Arthur Mackenzie	1944	1962
Colm Kelly	1944	1962
Ernest Francis Ridley	1945	1950

Appointments were as radiologist, assistant radiologist or senior assistant radiologist. The senior was known as 'medical officer in charge' (1930-33); 'Radiologist' (1934-45). For Miss M. C. Tod see department of surgery.

In 1946 the Radiological Department was divided into a Department of Radiodiagnosis and a Department of Radiotherapy each initially under a 'Director'—a term which lapsed with changes in the health service. Diagnosis is now undertaken in the 'Department of Radiology' under an 'administrative consultant'. Therapy is carried out under the control of the 'Department of Clinical Oncology—Radiation Oncology Unit'.

DEPARTMENT OF RADIODIAGNOSIS

	Appointed (in charge)	Retired or Resigned, Died
William Stewart Shearer	1945 (1946)	1957, died
Alexander Colin Peter Duguid Thomson, MC	1946	1947
Peter Aitken	1946	1948
David Randolph Maitland	1947	1959
James George Duncan	1953	1968
Thomas Philp	1953 (1979)	...
Andrew Alexander Donaldson	1956	...
Eric Samuel	1958 (1958)	1978
professor of medical radiology 1970-1978		
Michael Derek Sumerling	1959	1980
Graeme Bruce Young	1966	1980
Kenneth Wood	1968	...
Thomas Alexander Seaton Buist	1969	...
William Galloway Miller Ritchie	1973	1975
Alastair Elliot Kirkpatrick	1973	...
Irene Mackenzie Prosser	1975	...
Arthur James Alexander Wightman	1975	...
Doris Nicol Redhead	1978	...

T

	Appointed *(in charge)*	*Retired or* *Resigned, Died*
Jonathan James Kerle Best★ professor of medical radiology 1979-	1979	...
Sylvia Rimmer	1980	1981
Andrew William Duncan	1980	...

DEPARTMENT OF RADIOTHERAPY

	Appointed *(in charge)*	*Retired or* *Resigned, Died*
Robert McWhirter, CBE professor of medical radiology 1947-70	1935 (1946)	1970
Joseph Phelan	1938	1947
William Michael Court Brown	1943	1950
Kenneth Arthur Mackenzie	1944	1962
Ernest Francis Ridley	1945	1950
Mary Ann Jeffrey Torrance Douglas	1952	1979
Walter Disney Rider	1953	1955
John Archibald Orr	1955	1957
reappointed	1963	...
James Gordon Pearson	1955	1970
Joseph Newall	1956	1964
James McLelland	1957	...
Gordon Law Ritchie	1965	...
Allan Ogilvie Langlands	1969	1978
Gaber Aly Newaishy	1970	...
William Duncan★ professor of Radiotherapy 1971-	1971	...
Sidney John Arnott	1974	...
Helen Jean Stewart	1978	1980
Susanne Marion Ludgate	1979	...
Alan Rodger	1981	...

DEPARTMENT OF MEDICAL PHYSICS

	Appointed	*Retired or* *Resigned, Died*
John Raymond Greening professor of medical physics 1966-	1957	...
Peter Tothill	1958	...
James McEwan McIntyre Neilson	1960	...

DEPARTMENT OF CLINICAL CHEMISTRY

	Appointed	*Retired or* *Resigned, Died*
Corbet Page Stewart Reader 1946-62	1923	1962
Samuel Cherrie Frazer	1959	1962
John Andrew Owen	1962	1964

	Appoihted	Retired or Resigned, Died
Lionel Gordon Whitby	1963	…
professor of clinical chemistry 1963-		
Iain Walter Percy-Robb	1968	…
Alastair Fairley Smith	1971	…

The Biochemistry Laboratory (1926) became the Department of Clinical Chemistry in 1946.

BLOOD TRANSFUSION SERVICE FOR THE SOUTH-EAST REGION OF SCOTLAND

	Regional Director	Retired or Resigned, Died
Robert Alexander Cumming, OBE	1947	1974
John David Cash	1974	1978
David Brian Lorimer McLelland	1978	…

PATHOLOGICAL DEPARTMENT

Pathological services have always been provided by members of the University Department of Pathology with the professor variously honorary pathologist (pre-1948), Pathologist-in-chief (1948-1966) and pathologist (post 1966). Staff have been senior pathologists, pathologists and assistant pathologists (pre-1949) with lecturers and senior lecturers (post-1950). Only the dates between which individuals served the hospital are shown. Professors [p], Readers [r], Senior Lecturers [s], are so distinguished.

	First Appointed	Retired or Resigned, Died
James Lorrain Smith[p]	1912	1931, died
Theodore Rettie	1921	1934
Francis Esmond Reynolds[1]	1924	1931
William Gilbert Millar[s]	1925	1939
Alexander Murray Drennan[p]	1931	1953
James Davidson	1922	1934
reappointed	1948	1965
John Henry Biggart[1] (later Kt.)	1934	1937
Agnes Rose MacGregor[r2]	1920	1959
Robertson Fotheringham Ogilvie[s]	1930	1965, died
Alexander Colin Patton Campbell[s1]	1935	1950
William Blackwood[1]	1940	1946
William Forbes[1]	1940	1954
Alastair Mitchell McDonald	1937	1949
Leonard Grant Leitch	1945	1954
Albert Edward Claireaux	1948	1953
Anthony Francis Joseph Maloney[1]	1948	1982, died
Kenneth Rhaney	1948	1954
Edith Kate Dawson	1950	1954
George Lightbody Montgomery, CBE[p]	1954	1971

[1] Neuropathologist   [2] Reader in pathology of diseases of children

The following include only those who attained the grade of senior lecturer. The order is that in which they attained the grade.

	First Appointed	Retired or Resigned, Died
Alun Wynn Williams	1955	1963
Andrew Armitage Shivas	1959	1982
Archibald Douglas Bain	1950	…
Donald Lindsay Gardner	1956	1966
Mary Kynoch MacDonald[r]	1946	…
Stewart Fletcher	1966	…
Brian Edyvean Heard	1966	1972
Angus Erskine Stuart[r]	1956	1978
Alexander Gordon[1]	1969	…
John Dunlop MacGregor	1950	…
Sir Alastair Robert Currie[p]	1972	…
David Thomson	1966	…
Colin Carmichael Bird	1972	1975
David Lamb	1974	…
Thomas Johnstone Anderson	1974	…
Hector MacDonald Cameron, OBE	1974	…
Ian Inglis Smith	1959	…
Andrew Hamilton Wyllie	1972	…
Sybil Monteith Dick McNair	1975	…
Linda Holloway	1978	1979
Margaret Ann MacIntyre	1978	…
Hugh Montgomery Gilmour	1969	…
James Adler Survis	1979	…

BACTERIOLOGICAL DEPARTMENT

Bacteriological services have always been provided by members of the University Department of Bacteriology with the professor as honorary bacteriologist (pre-1948) and bacteriologist-in-chief (post-1948). Otherwise staffing structures were similar to those in the pathological department and where appropriate are similarly distinguished.

	First Appointed	Retired or Resigned, Died
Thomas Jones Mackie[p]	1923	1955, died
William Robertson Logan	1925	1948, died
John Telfer Smeall, MC	1930	1946
Robert James Gerard Rattrie	1946	1948
John Herbertson Bowie[r]	1949	1972
Thomas Bryson Mitchell Durie	1948	…
Ralph William Tonkin	1948	…
James Cameron Gould	1950	1961
Robert Reid Gillies[r]	1952	1976
Adam William Blyth Lawson	1953	1956

[1] Neuropathologist

	First Appointed	Retired or Resigned, Died
Matthew Henderson Robertson	1957	1962
Joan Margaret McWilliam	1957	1966
Robert Cruickshank[p]	1958	1966
Barrie Patrick Marmion[p]	1968	1978
Alastair Milner Macdonald Wilson	1972	1974
Philip Wesley Ross	1973	...
Rex Stafford Miles	1976	...
John Gerald Collee[p]	1978	...

Clinical virologists

Richard Henry Austin Swain[r]	1947	1975
John Forrest Peutherer	1976	...
Elizabeth Edmund	1980	...

SENIOR ADMINISTRATIVE OFFICERS

Board of Managers of The Royal Infirmary of Edinburgh (1929-1948)

Secretaries & Treasurers

Henry Maw	1929-1942
William F. Ferguson	1942-1948

Superintendents

Colonel George David St Clair Thom, CB, AMS	1924-1935
Lt.-Col. Alexander Dron Stewart, CIE, IMS	1935-1948

Lady Superintendents of Nurses

Miss Ellen Frances Bladon	1925-1931
Miss Elizabeth Dunlop Smaill, OBE, ARRC, LLD	1931-1944
Miss Margaret Colville Marshall, OBE, ARRC, LLD	1944-1948

Matron—Simpson Memorial Maternity Pavilion

Miss Jean Page Ferlie, OBE	1939-1948

Board of Management for The Royal Infirmary of Edinburgh and Associated Hospitals (1948-1974)

Secretaries & Treasurers

William F. Ferguson	1948-1957
Tom W. Hurst	1957-1971
George G. Savage	1972-1973

Medical Superintendents

Major General Evelyn Alexander Sutton, CB, CBE, MC, late RAMC	1948-1952
Dr. Sidney Graham McKenzie Francis, TD	1952-1974

Lady Superintendents of Nurses

Miss Margaret Colville Marshall, OBE, ARRC, LLD	1948-1955
Miss Barbara Helen Renton, OBE	1955-1959
Miss Mary Hutcheson Cordiner, OBE	1959-1967
Miss Muriel Florence Cullen	1967-1972

Chief Nursing Officer
Miss Muriel Florence Cullen   1972-1974

Principal Nursing Officer (General Division)
Miss Margaret S. Laing   1972-1974

Matron—Simpson Memorial Maternity Pavilion
Miss Jean Page Ferlie, OBE   1948-1958
Miss Margaret Jane Wilson Taylor   1958-1968
Miss Margaret Gibson Auld   1968-1972

Principal Nursing Officer (Midwifery)
Miss Margaret Gibson Auld   1972-1974

Lothian Health Board—South Lothian District (1974-   )

Divisional Administrator
George D. Robb   1974-1977

Administrators—Royal Infirmary of Edinburgh
John Burton   1975-1978
Ian L. Puckering   1978-

Administrators—Simpson Memorial Maternity Pavilion
William D. Anderson   1974-1975
David C. White   1975-1978
R. Alan Langlands   1978-1981

Community Medicine Specialists—Royal Infirmary of Edinburgh
Dr. Sidney Graham McKenzie Francis, TD   1974-1977
Dr. John Ramsay Wood   1977-1978
Dr. Rosamund Gruer   1978-1979
Dr. Roger Barclay   1979-1982

Community Medicine Specialist—Simpson Memorial Maternity Pavilion
Dr. William Clyne Shepherd   1975-

Divisional Nursing Officer—Royal Infirmary of Edinburgh
Miss Jemima Lunnan Pitillo Robertson   1976-

Divisional Nursing Officer—Simpson Memorial Maternity Pavilion
Miss Bess Jamieson   1974-

Index